T0263565

Non-Alcoholic Steatohepatitis

Guest Editor

STEPHEN A. HARRISON, MD, LTC, MC, FACP

CLINICS IN LIVER DISEASE

www.liver.theclinics.com

Consulting Editor
NORMAN GITLIN, MD

November 2009 • Volume 13 • Number 4

SAUNDERS an imprint of ELSEVIER, Inc.

W.B. SAUNDERS COMPANY

A Division of Elsevier Inc.

1600 John F. Kennedy Boulevard, Suite 1800 • Philadelphia, PA 19103-2899

http://www.theclinics.com

CLINICS IN LIVER DISEASE Volume 13, Number 4
November 2009 ISSN 1089-3261, ISBN-13: 978-1-4377-1237-7, ISBN-10: 1-4377-1237-1

Editor: Kerry Holland
Developmental Editor: Donald Mumford

Clinics in Liver Disease (ISSN 1089-3261) is published quarterly by Elsevier Inc., 360 Park Avenue South, New York, NY 10010-1710. Months of issue are February, May, August, and November. Subscription prices are $218.00 per year (U.S. individuals), $109.00 per year (U.S. student/resident), $333.00 per year (U.S. institutions), $288.00 per year (foreign individuals), $151.00 per year (foreign student/resident), $401.00 per year (foreign instituitions), $251.00 per year (Canadian individuals), $151.00 per year (Canadian student/resident), and $401.00 per year (Canadian institutions). Foreign air speed delivery is included in all *Clinics* subscription prices. All prices are subject to change without notice. **POSTMASTER:** Send address changes to *Clinics in Liver Disease*, Elsevier Health Sciences Division, Subscription Customer Service, 3251 Riverport Lane, Maryland Heights, MO 63043. **Customer Service: Telephone: 1-800-654-2452 (U.S. and Canada); 314-447-8871 (outside U.S. and Canada). Fax: 314-447-8029. E-mail: journalscustomerservice-usa@elsevier.com (for print support); journalsonlinesupport-usa@elsevier.com (for online support).**

Reprints. For copies of 100 or more of articles in this publication, please contact the Commercial Reprints Department, Elsevier Inc., 360 Park Avenue South, New York, NY 10010-1710. Tel.: 212-633-3812; Fax: 212-462-1935; E-mail: reprints@elsevier.com.

Clinics in Liver Disease is covered in *MEDLINE/PubMed (Index Medicus)*.

Printed and bound by CPI Group (UK) Ltd, Croydon, CR0 4YY

Transferred to Digital Print 2011

Contributors

GUEST EDITOR

STEPHEN A. HARRISON, MD, LTC, MC, FACP
Chief of Hepatology, Department of Medicine, Gastroenterology Service, Brooke Army Medical Center, Fort Sam Houston; Clinical Associate Professor of Medicine, University of Texas Health Science Center, San Antonio, Texas

AUTHORS

CURTIS K. ARGO, MD, MS
Assistant Professor, Division of Gastroenterology and Hepatology, University of Virginia Health System, Charlottesville, Virginia

JEFFREY D. BROWNING, MD
Assistant Professor of Internal Medicine and Advanced Imaging Research Center, The University of Texas Southwestern Medical Center, Dallas, Texas

ELIZABETH M. BRUNT, MD
Professor, Department of Pathology and Immunology, Washington University School of Medicine, St. Louis, Missouri

STEPHEN H. CALDWELL, MD
Professor, Division of Gastroenterology and Hepatology, University of Virginia Health System, Charlottesville, Virginia

MICHAEL CHARLTON, MD, FRCP
Department of Gastroenterology and Hepatology, Mayo Clinic and Foundation, Mayo Clinic Transplant Center, Rochester, Minnesota

STEVE S. CHOI, MD
Department of Medicine, Section of Gastroenterology, Durham Veteran Affairs Medical Center, Durham, North Carolina

KENNETH CUSI, MD, FACP, FACE
Professor of Medicine, Diabetes Division, The University of Texas Health Science Center at San Antonio; Audie L. Murphy Veterans Administration Medical Center, San Antonio, Texas

ANNA MAE DIEHL, MD
Chief, Division of Gastroenterology, Duke University School of Medicine; Division of Gastroenterology, Durham Regional Hospital, Durham, North Carolina

STEPHEN A. HARRISON, MD, LTC, MC, FACP
Chief of Hepatology, Department of Medicine, Gastroenterology Service, Brooke Army Medical Center, Fort Sam Houston; Clinical Associate Professor of Medicine, University of Texas Health Science Center, San Antonio, Texas

ASHWANI KAPOOR, MBBS
Fellow, Department of Internal Medicine, Division of Gastroenterology, Hepatology and Nutrition, Virginia Commonwealth University School of Medicine, Richmond, Virginia

EDITH KOEHLER, MD
Department of Gastroenterology and Hepatology, Mayo Clinic and Foundation, Mayo Clinic Transplant Center, Rochester, Minnesota

ARTHUR J. McCULLOUGH, MD
Department of Gastroenterology and Hepatology, Digestive Disease Institute of the Cleveland Clinic; Professor of Medicine, Cleveland Clinic Lerner College of Medicine, Cleveland, Ohio

BRENT A. NEUSCHWANDER-TETRI, MD
Professor, Department of Internal Medicine, Division of Gastroenterology and Hepatology, Saint Louis University School of Medicine, St. Louis, Missouri

MANGESH PAGADALA, MD
Department of Gastroenterology and Hepatology, Digestive Disease Institute of the Cleveland Clinic, Cleveland, Ohio

JOHN M. PAGE, MD
Gastroenterology Fellow, Department of Medicine, Gastroenterology Service, Brooke Army Medical Center, Fort Sam Houston, Texas

ANJANA A. PILLAI, MD
Clinical Instructor, Department of Transplant Surgery, Northwestern University, Feinberg School of Medicine, Chicago, Illinois

VLAD RATZIU, MD, PhD
Université Pierre et Marie Curie, Assistance Publique Hôpitaux de Paris, Hôpital Pitié Salpêtrière, Paris, France

MARY E. RINELLA, MD
Assistant Professor, Division of Hepatology, Northwestern University, Feinberg School of Medicine, Chicago, Illinois

ARUN J. SANYAL, MBBS, MD
Professor of Medicine and Pathology, Department of Internal Medicine, Division of Gastroenterology, Hepatology and Nutrition, Virginia Commonwealth University School of Medicine, Richmond, Virginia

WING-KIN SYN, MBChB, MRCP
Department of Medicine, Division of Gastroenterology, Durham, North Carolina; Centre for Liver Research, Institute of Biomedical Research, University of Birmingham, United Kingdom

KYMBERLY WATT, MD
Department of Gastroenterology and Hepatology, Mayo Clinic and Foundation, Mayo Clinic Transplant Center, Rochester, Minnesota

CLAUDIA O. ZEIN, MD, MSc
Department of Gastroenterology and Hepatology, Digestive Disease Institute of the Cleveland Clinic; Assistant Professor of Medicine, Case Western Reserve University, Cleveland, Ohio

SHIRA ZELBER-SAGI, RD, PhD
Department of Gastroenterology, The Liver Unit, Tel Aviv Sourasky Medical Center, Tel Aviv, Israel; Faculty of Social Welfare and Health Sciences, School of Public Health, Haifa University, Haifa, Israel

Contents

FORTHCOMING ISSUES

February 2010
Liver Disease and Endoscopy
Andres Cardenas, MD, and
Paul J. Thuluvath, MD, *Guest Editors*

May 2010
Healthcare-Associated Viral Hepatitis
Bandar Al Knawy, MD, FRCPC,
Guest Editor

August 2010
Hepatitis B Virus
Naoky Tsai, MD, *Guest Editor*

RECENT ISSUES

August 2009
Novel Therapies in Hepatitis C Virus
Paul J. Pockros, MD, *Guest Editor*

May 2009
Key Consultations in Hepatology
Paul Martin, MD, *Guest Editor*

February 2009
Coagulation and Hemostasis in Liver Disease: Controversies and Advances
Stephen H. Caldwell, MD, and
Arun J. Sanyal, MD, *Guest Editors*

Preface

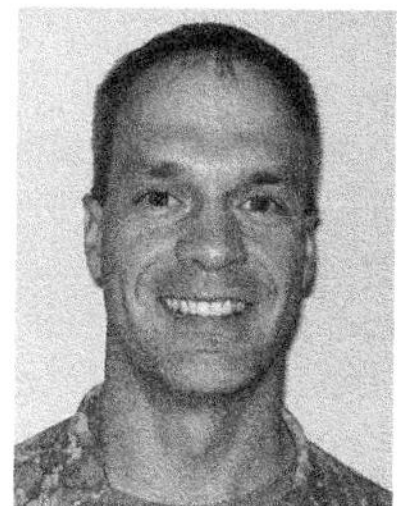

Stephen A. Harrison, MD, LTC, MC, FACP
Guest Editor

Our understanding of nonalcoholic fatty liver disease (NAFLD) has grown exponentially in the past 29 years since Ludwig and colleagues[1] first described the histologic lesions that comprise a subset of NAFLD known as nonalcoholic steatohepatitis (NASH). A recent PubMed search using the term "nonalcoholic fatty liver disease" generated 1475 articles published since 1980, of which 1405 were published since the year 2000. Concern for this liver disease is validated, as NAFLD is becoming, if it has not already become, the number one chronic liver disease in this country and in many others around the world. As the prevalence of obesity and diabetes, both of which are characterized by impairment in insulin signaling, continues to rise, so will the prevalence of NAFLD. We as health care providers are now faced with an epidemic.

How big of a problem is this? Do we just have to worry about liver disease in these patients, or are there extrahepatic problems that deserve attention too? Among patients with NAFLD, are there specific subsets who are likely to progress in their liver disease more quickly? The data in reference to these questions are discussed in the first article of this issue of *Clinics in Liver Disease* by Drs. Argo and Caldwell, who detail the epidemiology and natural history of this disease.

Liver biopsy has long been a mainstay among the hepatologic community in assisting with disease diagnoses. As is pointed out by Dr. Brunt in her article on histopathology of NAFLD, biopsy of hepatic tissue remains the only unequivocal way to make a definitive diagnosis of NASH, identify potential coexisting liver disease such as autoimmune hepatitis, and ensure exclusion of other disease processes. She discusses the salient histopathologic features of both pediatric and adult NASH and the differences that occur among various ethnic groups.

Much has been learned about the pathogenesis of fat accumulation in the liver and its relationship to insulin resistance. Over the past several years, our knowledge of the interaction between insulin resistance and multiorgan lipotoxicity has significantly expanded. For instance, we now know that specific cytokines, induced in part by dysfunctional adipocytes and altered free fatty acid metabolism, trigger the activation and/or alteration of cellular processes that result in the histopathologic lesions seen in patients with NAFLD. Although there is much yet to learn, this edition of *Clinics in Liver*

Clin Liver Dis 13 (2009) xiii–xiv
doi:10.1016/j.cld.2009.08.001

Disease also focuses on mitochondrial dysfunction, endoplasmic reticulum stress, apoptosis, and their relationship to lipotoxicity, as discussed by Drs. Cusi, Wing-Syn, Choi, Diehl, Kapoor, and Sanyal. This exciting data will inevitably guide future therapeutic development in this field.

It is imperative that novel ways to diagnose and triage patients with NAFLD be developed, given the epidemic that exists in our world today. Most patients with NAFLD do not progress in their liver disease, so although performing a liver biopsy is still considered the gold standard for diagnosing NASH, it does not make sense from a global health perspective, and it is not practical to biopsy all patients. Drs. Pagadala, Zein, McCullough, and Browning discuss newer imaging techniques and other noninvasive strategies, currently under development or under clinical investigation, to triage these patients.

Recent data suggest that obese and diabetic patients are at increased risk for hepatocellular carcinoma (HCC). Given the link between these 2 diseases and NAFLD, one would expect that these patients would be at increased risk for HCC. Although prospective, long-term studies are lacking, evidence suggests that this is indeed the case, and the relationship of NAFLD to HCC is discussed by Drs. Page and Harrison. Furthermore, although hepatitis C has traditionally been the number one reason for liver transplantation in this country, more and more transplant centers are seeing patients with underlying NASH cirrhosis or cryptogenic cirrhosis present for liver transplantation. Drs. Koehler, Watt, and Charlton discuss the increasing demand for liver transplantation in this patient population and the subsequent outcomes after surgery.

Although our knowledge of the pathogenesis is expanding rapidly, therapy to reverse or slow this disease process has been challenging. We know that dietary modification and exercise will improve insulin resistance and subsequent NAFLD/NASH. However, many questions still remain. Specifically, what type of diet is preferred? How much weight loss and/or exercise is necessary to effect both biochemical and histopathologic improvement? If patients are unable or unwilling to lose weight or exercise, what other therapies are available that have been proven effective? These issues are discussed by Drs. Neuschwander-Tetri, Ratziu, Zelber-Sagi, and Rinella.

In summary, this collection of up-to-date articles on NAFLD/NASH, put together by leading researchers and clinicians in hepatology and endocrinology, is meant to provide the reader with a front row seat to the current understanding, evaluation, and treatment of this most common liver disease. I would like to personally thank the authors and their families for the time and effort put into their contributions. I would also like to thank Kerry Holland for outstanding editorial support and Dr. Norm Gitlin for allowing me to develop this issue of *Clinics in Liver Disease*.

Stephen A. Harrison, MD, LTC, MC, FACP
Chief of Hepatology, Clinical Associate Professor of Medicine
Department of Medicine, Division of Gastroenterology and Hepatology
Brooke Army Medical Center, University of Texas Health Center San Antonio
3851 Roger Brooke Drive, Fort Sam Houston, Texas 78234, USA

E-mail address:
stephen.harrison@amedd.army.mil (S.A. Harrison)

REFERENCE

1. Ludwig J, Viggiano TR, McGill DB, et al. Nonalcoholic steatohepatitis: Mayo Clinic experiences with a hitherto unnamed disease. Mayo Clin Proc 1980;55:434–8.

Epidemiology and Natural History of Non-Alcoholic Steatohepatitis

Curtis K. Argo, MD, MS*, Stephen H. Caldwell, MD

KEYWORDS

- Fatty liver • Steatohepatitis • Outcomes
- Epidemiology • Obesity

Non-alcoholic fatty liver disease (NAFLD) is the most common chronic liver condition in the United States and in most regions worldwide. The range of conditions defined by this term incorporates hepatic steatosis as a common factor. Although most patients generally have simple hepatic steatosis with no or mild nonspecific inflammation, more active forms that include steatohepatitis can have significant clinical consequences, related to the development of cirrhosis and its complications or comorbid cardiovascular disease. The epidemiology and natural history of NAFLD are important in identifying areas of potential intervention in the disease course and promising therapies, but also in apportioning resources for research and care of patients with this burgeoning disorder.

PREVALENCE OF NAFLD IN ADULTS

NAFLD is one of the most common liver disorders in industrialized countries,[1–7] with type 2 diabetes, obesity, hyperlipidemia, and cardiovascular disease being the most frequently evaluated and cited risk factors for the presence of NAFLD and accelerated disease.[8] The estimated prevalence in the general population ranges between 2.8% and 46% depending on the screening test used (**Fig. 1**).[9] Clearly, no single marker or test has sufficient positive or negative predictive value for NAFLD. Ultrasound and computed tomography (CT) have suboptimal sensitivity; liver enzymes are notably poor predictors of steatosis[10] and significant fibrosis,[11] and the gold standard of liver biopsy is subject to sampling error, differences in histopathologic interpretation, and selection and ascertainment biases.[12] In imaging-based studies, prevalence of steatosis varies between 11.5% in Taiwanese men[13] and 46% in hospitalized, elderly Israeli patients.[14] The only magnetic resonance imaging (MRI)-based and most widely

Division of Gastroenterology and Hepatology, University of Virginia Health System, 1335 Lee Street, MSB 2091, Box 800708, Charlottesville, VA 22908-0708, USA
* Corresponding author.
E-mail address: cka3d@virginia.edu (C.K. Argo).

Clin Liver Dis 13 (2009) 511–531
doi:10.1016/j.cld.2009.07.005

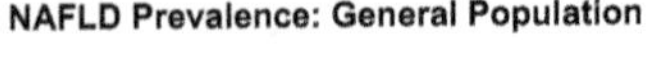

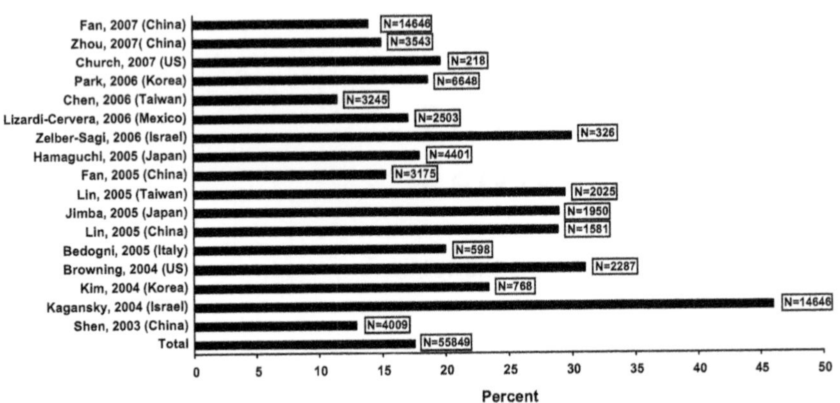

Fig. 1. NAFLD was diagnosed by imaging in all of the studies (ultrasound in 15, computed tomography [CT] in 1, and magnetic resonance [MR] spectroscopy in 1). Prevalence varies by region: Asian countries, N = 45,991, 16.9%; Europe-North America, N = 5606, 23.2%; Middle East, N = 460, 34.7%. (*Adapted from* Lazo M, Clark JM. The epidemiology of non-alcoholic fatty liver disease: a global perspective. Semin Liver Dis 2008;28:341–2; with permission.)

recognized US study demonstrated a NAFLD prevalence of 31% from various ethnicities.[10] When liver enzymes are used as the diagnostic prevalence marker, the rate decreases substantially to between 2.8% and 9.3%, with the highest of this group from a Japanese population.[15] In the United States, a comprehensive, NHANES III dataset-based analysis showed that between 2.8% and 24% of US adults have NAFLD depending on the definition used.[16] From autopsy- and biopsy-based studies, the rates of NAFLD prevalence fall midway between imaging- and enzyme-based studies, with rates between 15.8% in an Indian study[17] and 53% in a well-known Canadian autopsy study.[18] More recent histology-based studies of liver donors estimate the prevalence to be between 17.9% and 38.5%.[9]

CLASSICAL PHENOTYPE OF NAFLD

NAFLD and metabolic syndrome (central obesity, hypertriglyceridemia, hypertension, impaired glucose tolerance, and low high-density lipoprotein [HDL] cholesterol) commonly coexist, with over 90% of NAFLD patients having at least one of these characteristics. NAFLD prevalence increases as the severity and number of metabolic syndrome parameters increases.[19]

The prevalence of NAFLD has accelerated in the last 20 years, paralleling the substantial increase in rates of overweight and obesity in the general population. In the Dionysos study, NAFLD was present in 94% of obese patients (body mass index [BMI] greater than or equal to 30 kg/m^2), 67% of overweight patients (BMI greater than or equal to 25 kg/m^2), and 25% of normal weight patients.[20] The association of more severe obesity portending more severe NAFLD has been established.[21–23] Abdominal obesity also appears to independently predict the presence of NAFLD. Recent studies evaluating waist circumference noted an association between the degree of abdominal obesity and the likelihood of NAFLD.[24] A recent prospective, serum-based study provides more solid support to this concept, as BMI and body fat were predictive of elevated aminotransferases.[15] Bariatric surgery studies provide further corroboration, as up to 95% of morbidly obese patients have NAFLD, and up to 25% have NASH at intraoperative biopsy.[23,25–32]

Insulin resistance (IR), either resulting from or inducing obesity, appears to play a central role in NAFLD pathophysiology. The intersection of NAFLD and type 2 diabetes is important to characterize to best establish the strength and direction of their association. Overall prevalence of NAFLD in type 2 diabetics ranges from 40% to 70%.[33] Several cross-sectional studies have inferred that severe inflammation, hepatocyte ballooning, and fibrosis are associated with type 2 diabetes.[19,22,34] This may result in part because of more severe hepatic fat deposition, as a recent case–control study based on 1H-magnetic resonance spectroscopy assessment found significantly high degrees of steatosis in type 2 diabetics, with up to 200% more liver fat than age-, gender-, and BMI-matched controls.[35] Presence of NAFLD in patients who have type 2 diabetes is a significant clinical distinction, as these patients appear to be at higher risk of cardiovascular morbidity than type 2 diabetics without NAFLD.[36]

NAFLD IN BARIATRIC SURGERY PATIENTS/MORBID OBESITY

Because of the ease of performing intraoperative liver biopsy in bariatric surgery patients (BMI greater than or equal to 40 kg/m^2 or BMI greater than or equal to 35 kg/m^2 with medical comorbidities), the high prevalence of NAFLD in this population is well-established. In pooled analysis, the rate of steatosis from studies of this population is 61%, with a rate of NASH of 36%. Fibrosis is present in 16% of patients, and cirrhosis is present in approximately 2%.[9] These studies have demonstrated convincingly that steatosis, NASH, and fibrosis are at least partially reversible after weight loss occurs postoperatively,[27] although there appears to be a small proportion of patients who develop accelerated NASH after significant and rapid weight loss after gastroplasty.[37]

NONCLASSICAL PHENOTYPE OF NAFLD: NORMAL WEIGHT PATIENTS

Although NAFLD and NASH are more common among obese patients, it is recognized widely that a fraction of NAFLD patients do not meet weight criteria of obesity. Not surprisingly, this is more common among Asian patients (even with adjusted criteria), although it is recognized increasingly in Western countries.[5] In China, it has been reported that up to 40% of patients with NASH do not meet ethnicity-adjusted BMI for overweight or obesity.[13,38,39] Most lower BMI NAFLD/NASH patients, however, have central obesity and can be described as metabolically obese, which includes findings of insulin resistance in spite of normal BMI.[40,41] Whether a separate group of lower BMI patients with primary lipoprotein abnormalities but without insulin resistance exists can be conjectured but remains unproven.

FAMILIAL ASSOCIATIONS, GENETICS, AND ETHNICITY IN NAFLD

There have been three studies reporting clustering of NASH and cryptogenic cirrhosis in one or more first-degree relatives of index cases of NASH.[42–44] In the two earlier studies, an association with obesity, diabetes, and features of metabolic syndrome were evident as a common thread.[45] From this group of studies, a case-control aggregation analysis revealed a possible maternal linkage supporting a genetic predisposition. Although it previously was estimated that about 20% of index cases of NASH have a positive family history, more recent studies suggest that this might be a substantial underestimation. Whether a positive family history influences severity remains uncertain but warrants consideration when evaluating patients for liver biopsy or more aggressive pharmacologic therapy.

Familial clustering could represent inherited genetic predisposition, but it should be recalled that common environmental exposures such as dietary habits or typical activity levels also could play a significant role. The finding of insulin resistance and impaired skeletal muscle mitochondrial metabolism in the offspring of patients with type 2 diabetes suggests a more prominent genetic risk related to intracellular fat metabolism, however.[46] More convincingly, Schwimmer and colleagues[47] recently performed a prospective investigation of the prevalence of fatty liver (greater than 5% triglyceride) by H^1 MR (proton magnetic resonance) spectroscopy among siblings and parents of overweight probands with and without fatty liver. They detected fatty liver in 17% of siblings and 37% of parents of the overweight group without fatty liver compared with a striking prevalence of 59% and 78% respectively among siblings and parents of the overweight group with fatty liver. A correlation between liver fat and BMI was evident in both groups, but it was much stronger in the group of relatives from probands with NAFLD, suggesting a very strong genetic component in the tendency to deposit fat in the liver.

Similar to familial clustering, ethnic variation in the prevalence of NAFLD/NASH has been described in a growing number of studies that consistently have shown that fatty liver is less common among African Americans and most common in the United States among people of Hispanic descent.[48,49] These associations are paralleled by previously described ethnic differences in body fat distribution.[49–54] In the most definitive of these studies, Browning and colleagues[10] prospectively assessed liver steatosis in 2287 subjects using H^1 MR spectroscopy. The percent of subjects with steatosis was significantly lower among African Americans (24%) compared with non-Hispanic whites (33%) and Hispanics (45%) in this cross-sectional study. Although steatosis correlated with obesity and insulin resistance among Hispanics, this relationship was weaker in the African American group.

A similar pattern has been observed among adult diabetic patients in the general medicine setting undergoing liver ultrasound, where steatosis was significantly more evident among non-African Americans with diabetes.[55] From Westin's prevalence study in California, the prevalence in US citizens of primarily Asian descent is about the same as whites, although at a relatively lower BMI and with a more pronounced gender difference.[49] NAFLD clearly is emerging in Asian populations, especially in regions with significant industrialization. In the study from Fan and Farrell, it was noted that the prevalence in China (15% overall) has doubled in the past decade.[38]

Ethnic variation also has revealed a paradoxic degree of dissociation between fatty liver and insulin resistance with which NAFLD has been linked so closely. This issue has been explored extensively in a recent prospective study from the Dallas Heart Study Group.[56] Despite similar levels of insulin resistance compared with Hispanic Americans, the African American patients had lower intraperitoneal fat, liver fat, and blood triglycerides although liver fat correlated to intraperitoneal fat in all groups. Interestingly, a somewhat similar paradox has been observed in the experimental setting. Variation in hepatic lipogenic gene expression was observed in the B6 ob/ob mouse strain where, paradoxically, greater hepatic steatosis was associated with relatively less insulin resistance.[57]

From the foregoing discussion, it seems clear that substantial genetic risk exists in the development of steatosis and perhaps in the development of cell injury and subsequent disease severity. These associations are consistent with the previously described genetic variation in obesity and diabetes and ethnic variation in lipoprotein metabolism.[58–62] Moreover, from the perspective of the thrifty genome evolutionary concept, this situation suggests the evolution of two types of metabolic syndromes, which might explain the existence of such marked ethnic variation in NAFLD epidemiology.[63] Several candidate genetic polymorphisms have been described related either to lipogenic genes or genes altering the response to oxidative stress.[64–79] A leading candidate, however, has emerged recently that may fundamentally underlie ethnic variation. PNPLA3 (patatin-like phospholipase domain-containing protein 3) is a liver-expressed transmembrane phospholipase also known as adiponutrin that is up-regulated during adipocyte differentiation. Romeo and colleagues[80] recently reported that homozygotes for a particular PNPLA3 polymorphism were more likely to have steatosis and evidence of cell injury.[81] Moreover, the allele was more common among Hispanic Americans compared with African Americans, indicating that this allele may be a major determinant of ethnic variation. Although its role relative to other genetic variables remains to be established, genetic variation in PNPLA3 may prove to be a significant predictor of severe steatosis under conditions of calorie excess.

MITOCHONDRIOPATHIES AND LIPODYSTROPHIES ASSOCIATED WITH NAFLD

The evident histologic abnormalities involving mitochondria in NAFLD have fueled speculation that manifestations usually associated with primary mitochondriopathies may occur in NAFLD patients.[82,83] Several isolated elements of systemic mitochondrial disease have been observed in NASH patients, including opthalmoplegia, deafness, depression, gut dysmotility, lipomatosis, and neurodegenerative diseases.[84] Concerted investigation of these phenomena has not occurred, but Al-Osaimi and colleagues[85] reported presence of disconjugate gaze palsy in NASH patients. Components of the metabolic syndrome, specifically insulin resistance and dyslipidemia, are found in patients affected by maternally inherited diabetes and deafness (MIDD) syndrome, Madelung disease, and symmetric lipomatosis, all three of which are associated with mitochondrial DNA mutations.[86–88] Interestingly, hepatic mitochondrial DNA mutations have been identified in some patients with NASH and cryptogenic cirrhosis.[89,90] Dedicated investigation of histologic and molecular abnormalities in NAFLD and NASH may uncover significant clues to vital pathophysiological mechanisms of these disorders.

Similar to the primary mitochondriopathies, the exact relationships between NAFLD and the group of disorders known as the lipodystrophies remain to be fully examined. These disorders, whether acquired or inherited, are characterized by fatty liver, diabetes, hypertriglyceridemia, panniculitis, and focal or diffuse loss of subcutaneous fat, and they are thought to result from failure of differentiation of preadipocytes, possibly because of leptin deficiency.[91–93] Similar experimental models have also been described.[94,95] Among females with the acquired variety, cirrhosis also has been observed.[95,96] The diagnosis hinges on recognition of body phenotypes, demonstration of atrophy of various fat depots, and associated low leptin levels.

Recognition of the rare generalized forms of lipodystrophy is especially important, as leptin therapy has been reported to improve this disorder.[97,98] How frequently partial forms of these disorders are overlooked in patients with NAFLD or NASH is unknown, as the diagnosis can be difficult, and the diagnostic tools are not commonly available. Reports of generalized lipodystrophy in patients with typical features of metabolic syndrome and reports of focal forms of lipodystrophy associated with NAFLD suggest that this association is probably not as rare as believed, and it could underlie variation in drug response in NASH therapy.[99,100] Lipodystrophy also can be seen with antihuman immunodeficiency virus (HIV) therapy, which is perhaps the most common acquired form of this disorder. Drug-induced mitochondrial dysfunction has been implicated, although efforts at manipulating various agents in anti-HIV therapy have met with variable success in reversing or slowing this condition.[101]

NAFLD IN PEDIATRIC PATIENTS

Just as the worldwide epidemic of obesity in adults has been mirrored in children, determining the prevalence of NAFLD in the pediatric population has been difficult because of the lack of reliable disease markers, the invasiveness of liver biopsy, and a relative lack population-based studies. As a result, secondary surrogates such as aminotransferases and ultrasound imaging have been the basis for diagnosis in most studies estimating prevalence to date.

Some population-based prevalence studies using surrogate markers of NAFLD have shown a range of 2.6% to 17.3% depending on the age range of the subjects. Larger, population-based studies in adolescents in the United States and Korea showed rates of abnormal alanine aminotransferase (ALT) to be 3% and 3.2%, respectively, in similarly aged cohorts.[102,103] A Japanese ultrasound-based study of 810 patients showed that 2.6% of preadolescents had steatosis.[104] When restricting the focus to obese adolescents, multiple studies demonstrated NAFLD rates ranging from 10% to 77%.[102,104–106] The single autopsy study in 742 US children demonstrated a higher rate of NAFLD of 9.6%, with rates of NAFLD increasing with age within the cohort. NAFLD appears to be more common in boys than girls in an almost 2:1 ratio.[107] Similar to adults, ethnicity appears to be a significant predictor of NAFLD in children, with Hispanics having the highest risk, and African Americans having the lowest risk to develop NAFLD.[108]

CRYPTOGENIC CIRRHOSIS

Based on a number of epidemiologic studies of cryptogenic cirrhosis patients after transplant and more recent serial histologic studies, it is estimated that antecedent NASH underlies two thirds to three fourths of cryptogenic cirrhosis cases. The epidemiologic association was compiled recently in a review of six prior studies.[109] Compared with cirrhotic control groups, the prevalence of obesity was increased among cryptogenic cirrhosis in all six series examined, and diabetes was increased in five of the six series.[110–114] This relationship also is observed in other regions of the world including Asia and Central America.[112,115–117] Indeed, ethnic variation that mirrors that reported in epidemiologic studies of NASH also has been described in cryptogenic cirrhosis.[42,118] Further discussion of this topic is available in the Natural History portion of this article.

LIVER TRANSPLANTATION AND DE NOVO AND RECURRENT NAFLD

The proportion of orthotopic liver transplants occurring secondary to NASH cirrhosis is increasing rapidly. In data from United Network for Organ Sharing, 3.5% of transplants occurred in patients with confirmed NASH cirrhosis in 2005 compared with only 0.1% of transplants in 1996.[119] Over the same period, transplants for cryptogenic cirrhosis decreased from 9.6% in 1996 to 6.6% in 2005, which most likely represents greater acceptance of the diagnosis of NASH-related late-stage cirrhosis. NAFLD and NASH patients, however, also are perceived to be under-represented on transplant waiting lists because of exclusive comorbidities such as obesity, cardiovascular disease, and diabetes mellitus. As recognition of NAFLD and NASH continues to improve, the obesity epidemic continues to worsen, the hepatitis C indication for transplantation decreases, and the ability to manage pre-transplantation metabolic syndrome complications improves, substantially more patients will present for transplantation because of NASH cirrhosis in the coming decade.

NAFLD and NASH undoubtedly recur after transplantation in patients who undergo liver transplant for NASH or cryptogenic cirrhosis. Approximately 25% of patients develop steatosis within the first year, and nearly 50% develop it by 4 years after transplantation, with about 30% to 50% of those patients exhibiting histologic evidence of NASH.[120–125] Risk factors for recurrence include pre- and post-transplantation obesity and diabetes mellitus and post-transplantation weight gain and hypertriglyceridemia.[119] In one series, post-transplantation survival was impacted negatively in those patients with recurrent NASH.[124]

Several small case series have described instances of de novo NAFLD occurring in patients who have undergone liver transplantation for other indications. Patients who underwent transplantation for PBC, alpha-1 antitrypsin deficiency, alcohol, and hepatitis C infection have been documented to develop new-onset NAFLD after transplantation. Onset occurred more frequently in patients with preservation injury on 1-week post-transplantation protocol biopsy.[126,127]

Risk factors for recurrent or de novo NAFLD identified in cross-sectional, post-transplantation studies include obesity, diabetes mellitus/insulin resistance, decreased HDL-cholesterol, elevated total cholesterol, and hypertension. These risk factors are present more frequently in post-transplant patients than in the general population, at least in part because of the use of corticosteroids and calcineurin inhibitor-based immunosuppression.[120]

DRUG- AND TOXIN-ASSOCIATED NASH

Environmental exposures have been associated with NASH, although the relative prevalence and relationship to underlying genetic or other risks remain uncertain. Petrochemical workers have been the best characterized such group.[128] Typical features of common NASH including insulin resistance are less apparent in these patients, although progressive disease has been observed.[129] More recently, NASH has been observed in nonobese chemical workers with high-level exposure to vinyl chloride.[130] Interestingly, sinusoidal dilation appeared to be a somewhat unique and characteristic finding in this group. Among medicines implicated in causing histologic NASH, tamoxifen has perhaps the most compelling evidence, although several other agents often are mentioned.[131] The relationship between these exposures and underlying and sometimes unrecognized risk for obesity-related NASH remains to be established, however, and some skepticism is warranted.

NATURAL HISTORY OF NAFLD

Much work is ongoing to elucidate the mechanisms for progression of NAFLD to cirrhosis, but the overall body of literature suffers from lack of controlled, longitudinal studies, use of nonstandard definitions of the condition, variable collection of clinical parameters, and referral and publication bias. Although many potential predictors have been investigated, histology at initial presentation appears to have the best predictive value. Benign fatty liver appears to have very little likelihood of developing into advanced fibrosis over a typical lifetime, but the probability of the development of cirrhosis in patients with steatosis and fibrosis alone and steatosis with nonspecific, low-grade inflammation is less clear. Inflammation, whether satisfying the current histopathological criteria for NASH, appears to have predictive power for progression to advanced fibrosis. Patients without inflammation, even in those with fibrosis at presentation, however, appear to have less likelihood of developing advanced fibrosis, suggesting that pre-existing fibrosis in those patients with steatosis but without inflammation may be caused by a coexistent disorder (**Fig. 2**).[132]

HISTOLOGIC SPECTRUM AND PROGRESSION OF NAFLD

Cross-sectional and longitudinal biopsy studies constitute the best available evidence for establishing the probability of developing progressive fibrosis caused by NAFLD. Cross-sectional studies are naturally substantially limited by lack of follow-up. Longitudinal studies with paired biopsies carry the obvious benefit of providing firm follow-up data on which to establish long-term predictors, but they are limited by referral, selection, and ascertainment biases and tend to portray patients with more severe disease and thus poorer outcomes. Other potential problems such as variable time intervals between biopsies and inconsistent collection of clinical data can be controlled reasonably well with statistical methods. Sampling variability is problematic in all histologic studies, and defining the extent of its effect is critical to understanding the limitations of liver biopsy. Variability is a problem of all data collection methods, however, and liver biopsy continues to represent the diagnostic gold standard in NAFLD and NASH studies.

Cross-sectional studies have contributed significantly to the understanding of the importance of the severity of NAFLD at the time of presentation. These studies aid in decision making regarding undertaking a liver biopsy during the diagnostic phase of evaluation and provide guidance to providers from other disciplines in identifying

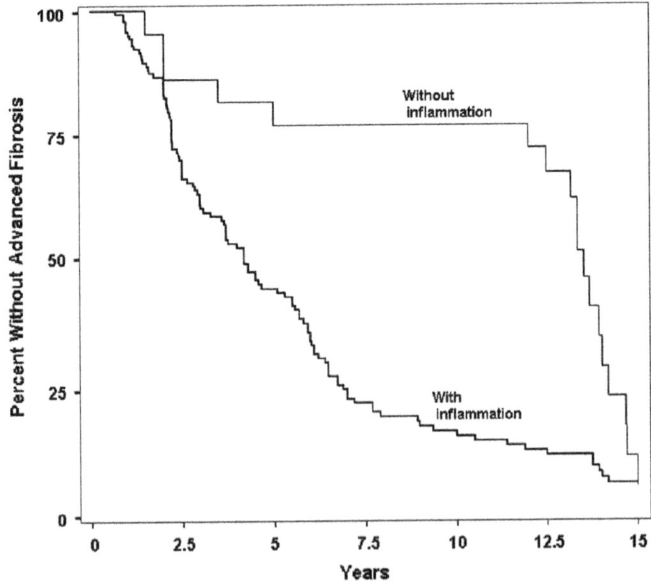

Fig. 2. This Kaplan-Meier survival curve demonstrates the difference in progression to advanced fibrosis (stage 3 or 4 fibrosis) stratified by the presence of any inflammation on the initial index biopsy in patients included in paired biopsy, natural history studies of NASH. Patients with advanced fibrosis on their initial biopsy were not included in this analysis secondary to lack of possibility of progression to the defined endpoint. (*From* Argo CK, Northup PG, Al-Osaimi AM, et al. Systematic review of risk factors for fibrosis progression in non-alcoholic steatohepatitis. J Hepatol. 2009;51:371–9; with permission.)

patients with high risk for advanced liver disease secondary to NAFLD who may benefit from hepatology consultation. Several risk factors consistently arise from these studies as predictors for presence of fibrosis. These include age (especially over 50 years), BMI over 28 to 32 kg/m^2, insulin resistance/diabetes mellitus, and abnormal aminotransferases.[8,19,23,133–137] Most of these risk factors were examined in univariate fashion, but age, BMI, hypertension (HTN), ALT, insulin resistance, and necroinflammation on initial biopsy were shown in multivariate analyses to independently predict the presence of fibrosis.[19,23,135,137]

Longitudinal, paired biopsy studies provide a more rigorous evaluation of these risk factors for developing advanced fibrosis in NAFLD without therapy. Several cohorts from various geographic locations with longer follow-up intervals have been characterized recently, and the results regarding fibrosis development are consistent.[110,137–145] If the scope of these studies is restricted to those patients with NASH defined as steatosis with lobular inflammation or steatosis with fibrosis alone,[3] these cohorts reflect a population that is predominantly female (61%), obese (63%), insulin-resistant (38% frankly diabetic), and in the fifth decade of life (mean age, 47 years). Approximately one third of patients had advanced fibrosis (stage 3 or 4 fibrosis) by the end of the follow-up period (mean, 5.3 years). Progression of fibrosis occurred more frequently than improvement (38% versus 21%), although most patients did not have a change in fibrosis. Progression to advanced fibrosis, however, was associated with age and the presence of inflammation on the initial, presenting biopsy. These findings draw renewed attention to the significance of nonspecific inflammation in the setting of steatosis and suggest that expansion of the histologic criteria of NASH to include steatosis with nonspecific inflammation may be beneficial. Previously it had been held widely that this patient group (NAFLD stage 2) had a low likelihood of developing complications of advanced fibrosis. The results of this study, however, suggest that patients with any inflammation in the setting of steatosis, when controlled for initial fibrosis, had 2.5 times the likelihood of developing advanced fibrosis.[132]

SURVIVAL AND LONG-TERM OUTCOMES IN NAFLD

The long-term clinical outcome in patients with NAFLD has been controversial, although it long has been recognized that the prognosis varies with the presence or absence of histologic injury (ie, NASH versus simple steatosis) and that the outcomes are tied closely into other conditions associated with metabolic syndrome. For example, variable clinical outcomes were evident in one of the early publications classifying NAFLD into histologic types wherein the risk of liver disease-related death was most evident in the group with NASH as opposed to simple steatosis.[3]

These findings since have been supported strongly by four papers that describe the long-term clinical course of patients with NAFLD (**Table 1**). In the first of these, Adams and colleagues[135] reported on 420 NAFLD patients identified between 1980 and 2000 with a mean follow-up of 7.6 years (range 0.1 to 23.5 years). During follow-up, seven patients died from liver-related causes, making it the third leading cause of death compared with the 13th leading cause in the comparison population. Thirteen patients (3.1%) developed liver-related complications including two patients with hepatocellular cancer. Ekstedt and colleagues[144] published a cohort control study of 129 NAFLD patients in 2006 followed over a mean of 13.7 years. Diminished survival was evident but only in the group with histologic NASH as opposed to simple steatosis. Seven (5.4%) patients in the NASH group developed end-stage liver disease, including two with hepatocellular cancer. Compared with the general population,

Table 1
A clearer picture of the natural history of NAFLD is emerging from longitudinal outcome studies that combined show the expected course of 1512 patients, most of whom first were diagnosed in the 1980s with non-alcoholic fatty liver. With the burgeoning epidemic of obesity in the interval since the inception of these cohorts, it remains to be seen whether these patterns remain stable. The accelerated rate of liver-related complications evident in the Ekstedt study is especially concerning.

	Adams 2005	Ekstedt 2006			Ong 2008		Rafiq 2009	
	NAFLD[a]	NASH	Risk	NNFL[b]	NAFLD	AHR[c]	NASH	NNFL
N	435	71	—	58	817	—	57	74
Age at diagnosis	49 ± 15	55 ± 12	—	47 ± 12	—	—	54 ± 12	53 ± 25
Males/Females	213/222	—	—	—	—	—	24/48	45/29
Era at diagnosis	1980–2000	1988–1993	—	1988–1993	1988–1994	—	1979–1987	1979–1987
Follow-up (y)	7.6 ± 4	13.7 ± 1.3	—	13.7 ± 1.3	8.4	—	14.98 (median)	19.5 (median)
Advanced cirrhosis[d]	13 (3.1%)	7 (9.8%)	—	0	—	—	—	—
HCC	2 (0.5%)	2 (2.8%)	—	0	—	—	—	—
Deaths (due to):	53 (12.6%)	19 (26.7%)	—	7 (12%)	80 (9.7%)	—	—	—
Coroonary artery disease	13 (2.9%)	11 (15.5%)	2 ×[e]	5 (8.6%)	20 (2.4%)	—	7 (12.3)	15 (20.3)
Cancer[f]	15 (3.4%)	4 (5.6%)	—	1 (1.7%)	19 (2.3%)	—	5 (8.8)	9 (12.2)
Liver[g]	7 (1.6%)	2 (2.8%)	10 ×[h]	0	5 (0.6%)	9.2	10 (17.5%)	2 (2.7%)[i]

[a] The Adams study included patients with both biopsy-defined and noninvasively defined fatty liver.
[b] The authors have used the term NNFL to indicate non-NASH fatty liver disease in patients with low or no ethanol exposure.
[c] AHR in Ong's study indicates adjusted hazard ratio for dying from liver-related complications compared with a control reference population.
[d] Advanced cirrhosis indicates development of ascites, variceal bleeding, jaundice, or encephalopathy.
[e] 2× indicates a two fold risk of dying from coronary disease comparing NASH with NNFL.
[f] Cancer indicates nonprimary liver malignancy.
[g] Liver indicates death caused by a liver-related problem.
[h] 10 × indicates a tenfold increased risk of liver-related death in NASH versus NNFL.
[i] The difference shown in Rafiq's report in liver-related deaths between NASH and NNFL was significantly different between NASH and NNFL.

the authors showed a tenfold increase in the risk of liver-related death and a twofold increase in the risk of cardiovascular disease death.

In another study, Rafiq and colleagues[146] reviewed the subsequent course of patients included in the original Matteoni cohort. With a median follow-up of 18.5 years, 10 of 57 (17.5%) patients with baseline NASH died from progressive liver disease compared with 2 of 74 (2.7%) patients with simple steatosis. Finally, in a population study based on the NHANES 3 data set with a median follow-up of 8.7 years, Ong and colleagues[147] demonstrated increased overall mortality and increased liver-related mortality (hazard ratios = 1.038 and 9.32, respectively) in 817 subjects with presumed NAFLD compared with 10,468 nonliver disease controls. More recently, a potentially severe course has been documented in pediatric patients also.[148]

Emerging from these studies are several common threads. Overall mortality in people with NASH is increased, and the risk of dying from liver disease complications is increased markedly in NASH compared with people with non-NASH fatty liver (NNFL). Among patients diagnosed with NASH, the 10-year risk of developing advanced complications of portal hypertension appears to be on the order of 5%. Among those who develop advanced disease, the risk of hepatocellular cancer (HCC) is estimated to be about 5% to 7%. If the patient is diagnosed initially with NASH-related cirrhosis, however, Hui and colleagues[149] demonstrated that the risk of developing a major complication of portal hypertension is 17%, 23%, and 52% at 1, 3, and 10 years respectively. Whether the risk of HCC is similar to that of hepatitis C-related cirrhosis or significantly less remains controversial.[149,150] A risk for HCC has been recognized in noncirrhotic fatty liver, however, making this condition potentially one of substantially greater impact on overall health concerns in the coming years.[151–153]

Another common thread is that, despite the increased rate of liver-related death and morbidity in patients with NASH, the number one and number two causes of death in this population remain cardiovascular disease and nonhepatic malignancy. Whether these relationships are stable over time or presently are changing with increasing obesity in younger patients is uncertain. Moreover, to what extent the coexistence of occult liver disease in patients with vascular disease or cancer impacts management and response to treatment remains to be explored.

CRYPTOGENIC CIRRHOSIS IN THE PATIENT WITH METABOLIC SYNDROME

For many years, the overall impact of NASH was obscured further by its relationship to cryptogenic cirrhosis.[45] Although originally used to describe the occurrence of unexplained steatohepatitis, Ludwig's 1980 description of NASH is equally applicable to many cases of cryptogenic cirrhosis

> *"...we have encountered patients who did not drink, who had not been subject to bypass surgery, and who had not taken drugs that may produce steatohepatitis, yet had in their liver biopsy specimens changes that were thought to be characteristic of alcoholic liver disease. In these instances, the biopsy evidence sometimes caused clinicians to persevere unduly in their attempts to wrench from the patient an admission of excessive alcohol or to obtain a confirmation of such habits from relatives of the patients. Thus, the misinterpretation of the biopsy in this poorly understood and hitherto unnamed condition caused embarrassment to the patient and physician."*[1]

The first observation that NASH can progress to a form of cirrhosis with loss of characteristic histologic findings is because of the salient observations of Powell and colleagues in a landmark paper documenting the natural history of NASH.[110,154] Although 5% to 10% of patients with suspected NASH eventually may be shown to actually have ethanol-related liver disease,[144,155] most such patients across an increasingly large number of studies have major risks for metabolic syndrome, especially obesity and type 2 diabetes mellitus.[45] Most such patients are female, about 60 years old, with minimal liver enzyme abnormalities, a history of obesity, and diabetes.[45] Given the risks of coronary disease in NASH patients generally and in males in particular, it is possible that this discrepancy in the prevalence of NASH is attributable to drop-out among male patients caused by coronary disease, although this remains at present only conjecture.

Most studies linking cryptogenic cirrhosis to NASH have focused on clinical and epidemiologic associations as previously discussed. Although the finding of late-stage NASH frequently includes loss of characteristic steatosis on conventional light microscopy, paired biopsies among patients who come to medical attention at both early and late stages of the disease occur infrequently for several reasons. For example, patients with a history of biopsy-proven NASH who present with a late-stage complication of portal hypertension may not undergo a second biopsy. On the other hand, patients presenting with an initial complication of portal hypertension may have had no prior evaluation. Moreover, among those with a remote prior biopsy, such specimens are commonly unavailable because of limitations on tissue repositories.

Although such histologic pairs are uncommon, two studies recently have emerged in comparing paired biopsies among cryptogenic cirrhosis patients either postmortem,[156] or undergoing a second biopsy or liver transplantation with available explant tissue.[157] Initial results from these abstracts confirm loss of steatosis with progressive fibrosis in cryptogenic cirrhosis. The mechanism of this process remains to be elucidated. It may involve diminished insulin exposure caused by portosystemic shunting, changes associated with cirrhotic malnutrition, or potentially re-population of the liver with physiologically unique progenitor cells as native cells drop out. Because NASH is a relatively long-term disease often extending over 10 to 20 years, the discarding of specimens after 10 years remains an impediment to better understanding of this disease.

OCCULT MORBIDITY AND CHANGING EPIDEMIOLOGY OF NAFLD

Existing natural history studies draw from populations encountered in the 1980s and 1990s and cannot account for the changing epidemiology that has occurred in the interval because of the increasing prevalence of obesity in the general population, in pediatric patients, and in groups not traditionally thought of as having significant obesity such as the Asian population. These changing patterns raise the probability that what has been seen in the past 10 to 15 years is a harbinger of problems to come.

Existing data indicate that the mortality rate in NASH is approximately 15% from cardiovascular disease and 7% from liver disease-related complications roughly 15 years from the diagnosis of NASH. The risk of cirrhosis-related death among patients with NASH compared with control populations is increased about tenfold, however, while the risk of death from heart disease is increased about twofold. Considering that the epidemiology of obesity has changed drastically over the past 15 years with increasing prevalence among younger patients, it is not clear how these relative risks of mortality related to NAFLD will change over the coming decades.

Moreover, the prospect of increasing numbers of patients with coexisting severe coronary and progressive liver disease raises numerous management questions, especially regarding issues of anticoagulation (for example in patients with coronary stents and coexisting cirrhosis) and the use of statin agents. Another recent population-based study supports the close relationship between NAFLD and cardiovascular disease.[158] The development of cirrhosis in an obese, diabetic patient raises further issues relevant to the primary care physician. For example, edema or ascites in such patients may be caused by portal hypertension and common use of nonsteroidal anti-inflammatory drugs. Portal hypertensive fluid retention may be ameliorated by withdrawal of such agents because of the renal effects. Depression may be the unrecognized result of hepatic encephalopathy and responsive to cathartics, and dyspnea may be due to unrecognized hepatopulmonary syndrome. Most of these emerging issues await further clinical research.

SUMMARY

NAFLD will present increasingly greater challenges over the next decade. The prevalence of this disorder shows no signs of slowing in any region of the world, and many predict it eventually may overtake all other forms of liver disease as the most common reason for liver transplantation and liver disease-related death in some regions. NAFLD undoubtedly is aligned closely with obesity, insulin resistance, and the metabolic syndrome, but differences according to age, ethnicity, and medical comorbidities exist. Histologic subtype at initial diagnosis appears prognostic, although new questions have been raised about the fibrosis progression in those patients with steatosis with nonspecific inflammation. Prognosis related to cirrhotic complications and HCC appear to be similar to other etiologies. Further research to better understand the pathophysiologic mechanisms of genetic and metabolic differences as they relate to fibrosis progression and development of complications of cirrhosis related to NAFLD will be critical to predicting the worldwide public health impact of this omnipresent disorder.

REFERENCES

1. Ludwig J, Viggiano TR, McGill DB, et al. Nonalcoholic steatohepatitis: an expanded clinical entity. Mayo Clin Proc 1980;55:434–8.
2. Schaffner F, Thaler H. Nonalcoholic fatty liver disease. Prog Liver Dis 1986;8: 283–98.
3. Matteoni CA, Younossi ZM, Gramlich T, et al. Nonalcoholic fatty liver disease: a spectrum of clinical and pathological severity. Gastroenterology 1999;116: 1413–9.
4. Sheth SG, Gordon FH, Chopra S. Nonalcoholic steatohepatitis. Ann Intern Med 1997;126:137–45.
5. Itoh S, Youngel T, Kawagoe K. Comparison between nonalcoholic steatohepatitis and alcoholic hepatitis. Am J Gastroenterol 1987;82:650–4.
6. Diehl AM, Goodman Z, Ishak KG. Alcohol-like liver disease in nonalcoholics. Gastroenterology 1988;95:1056–62.
7. Neushwander-Tetri BA, Caldwell SH. Nonalcoholic steatohepatitis: summary of an AASLD single-topic conference. Hepatology 2003;37:1202–19.
8. Angulo P, Keach JC, Batts KP, et al. Independent predictors of liver fibrosis in patients with nonalcoholic steatohepatitis. Hepatology 1999;30:1356–62.
9. Lazo M, Clark JM. The epidemiology of nonalcoholic fatty liver disease: a global perspective. Semin Liver Dis 2008;28:339–50.
10. Browning JD, Szczepaniak LS, Dobbins R, et al. Prevalence of hepatic steatosis in an urban population in the United States: impact of ethnicity. Hepatology 2004;40:1387–95.

11. Mofrad P, Contos MJ, Haque M, et al. Clinical and histologic spectrum of nonalcoholic fatty liver disease associated with normal ALT values. Hepatology 2003;37:1286–92.
12. Ratziu V, Charlotte F, Heurtier A, et al. Sampling variability of liver biopsy in nonalcoholic fatty liver disease. Gastroenterology 2005;125:1898–906.
13. Chen CH, Huang MH, Yang JC, et al. Prevalence and risk factors of nonalcoholic fatty liver disease in an adult population of Taiwan: metabolic significance of nonalcoholic fatty liver disease in nonobese adults. J Clin Gastroenterol 2006; 40:745–52.
14. Kagansky N, Levy S, Keter D, et al. Nonalcoholic fatty liver disease: a common and benign finding in octogenarian patients. Liver Int 2004;24:588–94.
15. Suzuki A, Angulo P, Lymp J, et al. Chronological development of elevated aminotransferases in a nonalcoholic population. Hepatology 2005;41:64–71.
16. Clark JM. The epidemiology of nonalcoholic fatty liver disease in adults. J Clin Gastroenterol 2006;40(Suppl 1):S5–10.
17. Amarapurkar A, Ghansar T. Fatty liver: experience from western India. Ann Hepatol 2007;6:37–40.
18. Wanless IR, Lentz JS. Fatty liver hepatitis (steatohepatitis) and obesity: an autopsy study with analysis of risk factors. Hepatology 1990;12:1106–10.
19. Marchesini G, Bugianesi E, Forlani G, et al. Nonalcoholic fatty liver, steatohepatitis, and the metabolic syndrome. Hepatology 2003;37:917–23.
20. Bellentani S, Bedogni G, Miglioli L, et al. The epidemiology of fatty liver. Eur J Gastroenterol Hepatol 2004;16:1087–93.
21. Clark JM, Brancati FL, Diehl AM. Nonalcoholic fatty liver disease. Gastroenterology 2002;122(6):1649–57.
22. Ong JP, Elariny H, Collantes R, et al. Predictors of nonalcoholic steatohepatitis and advanced fibrosis in morbidly obese patients. Obes Surg 2005;15:310–5.
23. Dixon JB, Bhathal PS, O'Brien PE. Nonalcoholic fatty liver disease: predictors of nonalcoholic steatohepatitis and liver fibrosis in the severely obese. Gastroenterology 2001;121(1):91–100.
24. Jakobsen MU, Berentzen T, Sorensen TI, et al. Abdominal obesity and fatty liver. Epidemiol Rev 2007;29:77–87.
25. Kral JG, Thung SN, Biron S, et al. Effects of surgical treatment of the metabolic syndrome on liver fibrosis and cirrhosis. Surgery 2004;135:48–58.
26. Lima ML, Mourao SC, Diniz MT, et al. Hepatic histopathology of patients with morbid obesity submitted to gastric bypass. Obes Surg 2005;15:661–9.
27. Dixon JB, Bhathal PS, Hughes NR, et al. Nonalcoholic fatty liver disease: improvement in liver histological analysis with weight loss. Hepatology 2004; 39:1647–54.
28. Moretto M, Kupski C, Mottin CC, et al. Hepatic steatosis in patients undergoing bariatric surgery and its relationship to body mass index and comorbidities. Obes Surg 2003;13:622–4.
29. Boza C, Riquelme A, Ibanez L, et al. Predictors of nonalcoholic steatohepatitis (NASH) in obese patients undergoing gastric bypass. Obes Surg 2005;15: 1148–53.
30. Shalhub S, Parsee A, Gallagher SF, et al. The importance of routine liver biopsy in diagnosing nonalcoholic steatohepatitis in bariatric patients. Obes Surg 2004; 14:54–9.
31. Beymer C, Kowdley KV, Larson A, et al. Prevalence and predictors of asymptomatic liver disease in patients undergoing gastric bypass surgery. Arch Surg 2003;138:1240–4.

32. Harnois F, Msika S, Sabate JM, et al. Prevalence and predictive factors of nonalcoholic steatohepatitis (NASH) in morbidly obese patients undergoing bariatric surgery. Obes Surg 2006;16:183–8.
33. Tolman KG, Fonseca V, Tan MH, et al. Narrative review: hepatobiliary disease in type 2 diabetes mellitus. Ann Intern Med 2004;141:946–56.
34. Marchesini G, Brizi M, Morselli-Labate AM, et al. Association of nonalcoholic fatty liver disease with insulin resistance. Am J Med 1999;107:450–5.
35. Kotronen A, Juurinen L, Hakkarainen A, et al. Liver fat is increased in type 2 diabetic patients and underestimated by serum alanine aminotransferase compared with equally obese nondiabetic subjects. Diabetes Care 2008;31:165–9.
36. Targher G, Bertolini L, Poli F, et al. Nonalcoholic fatty liver disease and risk of future cardiovascular events among type 2 diabetic patients. Diabetes 2005;54:3541–6.
37. Luyckx FH, Desaive C, Thiry A, et al. Liver abnormalities in severely obese subjects: effect of drastic weight loss after gastroplasty. Int J Obes Relat Metab Disord 1998;22:222–6.
38. Fan JG, Li F, Cai XB, et al. The importance of metabolic factors for the increasing prevalence of fatty liver in Shanghai factory workers. J Gastroenterol Hepatol 2007;22:663–8.
39. Fan J-G, Farrell GC. Epidemiology of nonalcoholic fatty liver disease in China. J Hepatol 2009;50:204–10.
40. Nguyen-Day T-B, Nichaman MZ, Church TS, et al. Visceral and liver fat are independent predictors of metabolic risk factors in men. AM J Physiol Endocrinol Metab 2003;284:E1065–71.
41. Banerji MA, Faridi N, Atluri R, et al. Body composition, visceral fat, leptin, and insulin resistance in Asian Indian men. J Clin Endocrinol Metab 1999;84:137–44.
42. Struben VM, Hespenheide EE, Caldwell SH. Nonalcoholic steatohepatitis and cryptogenic cirrhosis within kindreds. Am J Med 2000;108:9–13.
43. Willner IR, Waters B, Patil SR, et al. Ninety patients with nonalcoholic steatohepatitis: insulin resistance, familial tendency, and severity of disease. Am J Gastroenterol 2001;96:2957–61.
44. Abdelmalek MF, Liu C, Shuster J, et al. Familial aggregation of insulin resistance in first-degree relatives of patients with nonalcoholic fatty liver disease. Clin Gastroenterol Hepatol 2006;4:1162–9.
45. Caldwell SH, Oelsner DH, Iezzoni JC, et al. Cryptogenic cirrhosis: clinical characterization and risk factors for underlying disease. Hepatology 1999;29:664–9.
46. Petersen KF, Dufour S, Befroy D, et al. Impaired mitochondrial activity in the insulin-resistant offspring of patients with type 2 diabetes. N Engl J Med 2004;350:664–71.
47. Schwimmer JB, Celedon MA, Lavine JE, et al. Heritability of nonalcoholic fatty liver disease. Gastroenterology 2009;136:1585–92.
48. Caldwell SH, Harris DM, Hespenheide EE. Is NASH underdiagnosed among African Americans? Am J Gastroenterol 2002;97:1496–500.
49. Weston SR, Leyden W, Murphy R, et al. Racial and ethnic distribution of nonalcoholic fatty liver in persons with newly diagnosed chronic liver disease. Hepatology 2005;41:372–9.
50. Perry AC, Applegate EB, Jackson ML, et al. Racial differences in visceral adipose tissue but not anthropometric markers of health-related variables. J Appl Physiol 2000;89:636–43.

51. Yanoyski JA, Yanovski SZ, Filmer KM, et al. Differences in body composition of black and white girls. Am J Clin Nutr 1996;64:833–9.
52. Dowling HJ, Pi-Sunyer FX. Race-dependent health risks of upper body obesity. Diabetes 1993;42:537–43.
53. Mahmood S, Taketa K, Imai K, et al. Association of fatty liver with increased ratio of visceral to subcutaneous adipose tissue in obese men. Acta Med Okayama 1998;52:225–31.
54. Perseghin G, Scifo P, Pagliato E, et al. Gender factors affect fatty acid-induced insulin resistance in nonobese humans: effects of oral steroidal contraception. J Clin Endocrinol Metab 2001;86:3188–96.
55. Al-Osaimi, Sundaram V, Nadkarni M, et al. Risk factors of non-alcoholic fatty liver disease in a large cohort of noninsulindependent diabetic patients. Hepatology 1995;42:1095 [abstract].
56. Guerrero R, Vega GL, Grundy SM, et al. Ethnic differences in hepatic steatosis: an insulin resistance paradox? Hepatology 2009;49:791–801.
57. Lan H, Rabaglia ME, Stoehr JP, et al. Gene expression profiles of nondiabetic and diabetic obese mice suggest a role of hepatic lipogenic capacity in diabetes susceptibility. Diabetes 2003;52:688–700.
58. Samaras K, Spector TD, Nguyen TV, et al. Independent genetic factors determine the amount and distribution of fat in women after the menopause. J Clin Endocrinol Metab 1997;82:781–5.
59. Carey DP, Nguyen TV, Campbell LV, et al. Genetic influences on central abdominal fat: a twin study. Int J Obes Relat Metab Disord 1996;20:722–6.
60. Laws A, Stefanick ML, Reaven GM. Insulin resistance and hypertriglyceridemia in nondiabetic relatives of patients with noninsulin-dependent diabetes mellitus. J Clin Endocrinol Metab 1989;69:343–7.
61. Lillioja S, Mott DM, Zawadzki JA, et al. In vivo insulin action is familial characteristic in nondiabetic Pima Indians. Diabetes 1987;36:1329–35.
62. Sumner AE, Finley KB, Genovese DJ, et al. Fasting triglyceride and the triglyceride-HDL cholesterol ratio are not markers of insulin resistance in African Americans. Arch Intern Med 2005;165:1395–400.
63. Caldwell SH, Ikura Y, Iezzoni JC, et al. Has natural selection in human populations produced two types of metabolic syndrome (with and without fatty liver)? J Gastro Hepatol 2007;22(Suppl 1):S11–9.
64. Sreekumar R, Rosado B, Rasmussen D, et al. Hepatic gene expression in histologically progressive nonalcoholic steatohepatitis. Hepatology 2003;38:244–51.
65. Trujillo KD, Vizcarra SN, Lopez RO, et al. Nonalcoholic steatohepatitis related to morbid obesity: genetic and clinical risk factors [abstract]. Gastroenterology 2005;128:A542.
66. Merriman RB, Aouizerat BE, Yankovich M, et al. Variants of adipocyte genes affecting free fatty acid flux in patients with nonalcoholic fatty liver disease [abstract]. Hepatology 2003;34:A508.
67. Huang H, Merriman RB, Chokkalingam AP. Novel genetic markers associated with risk of nonalcoholic fatty liver disease. Gastroenterology 2005;128:A684.
68. Aitman TJ. CD36, insulin resistance, and coronary heart disease. Lancet 2001;357:651–2.
69. Miyaoka K, Kuwasako T, Hirano K. CD36 deficiency associated with insulin resistance. Lancet 2001;357:686–8.
70. Mendler M-H, Turlin B, Moirand R, et al. Insulin resistance-associated hepatic iron overload. Gastroenterology 1999;117:1155–63.

71. Hegele RA, Anderson CM, Wang J, et al. Association between nuclear lamin A/C R482Q mutation and partial lipodystrophy with hyperinsulinemia, dyslipidemia, hypertension, and diabetes. Genome Res 2000;10:652–8.
72. Capel ID, Dorrell HM. Abnormal antioxidant defense in some tissues of congenitally obese mice. Biochem J 1984;219:41–9.
73. Watson AM, Poloyac SM, Howard G, et al. Effect of leptin on cytochrome p-450, conjugation, and anti-oxidant enzymes in the ob/ob mouse. Drug Metab Dispos 1999;27:695–700.
74. Sastre J, Pallardo FV, Liopos J, et al. Glutathione depletion by hyperphagia-induced obesity. Life Sci 1989;45:183–7.
75. Strauss RS. Comparison of serum concentrations of α-tocopherol and β-carotene in a cross-sectional sample of obese and nonobese children (NHANES III). J Pediatr 1999;134:160–5.
76. Lee M, Hyun D, Halliwell B, et al. Effect of the over expression of wild-type or mutant alpha-synuclein on cell susceptibility to insult. J Neurochem 2001;76: 998–1009.
77. Lee M, Hyun D, Jenner P, et al. Effect of overexpression of wild-type and mutant Cu/Zn-superoxide dismutases on oxidative damage and antioxidant defenses: relevance to Down's syndrome and familial amyotrophic lateral sclerosis. J Neurochem 2001;76:957–65.
78. Powell EE, Edwards-Smith CJ, Hay JL, et al. Host genetic factors influence disease progression in chronic hepatitis C. Hepatology 2000;31:828–33.
79. Dixon JB, Bhathal PS, Jonsson JR. Profibrotic polymorphisms predictive of advanced liver fibrosis in the severely obese. J Hepatol 2003;39:967–71.
80. Romeo S, Kozlitina J, Xing C, et al. Genetic variation in PNPLA# confers susceptibility to nonalcoholic fatty liver disease. Nat Genet 2008;40:1461–5.
81. Weiskirchen R, Wasmuth HE. The genes that underlie fatty liver: the harvest has begun. Hepatology 2009;49:692–4.
82. Caldwell SH, Swerdlow RH, Khan EM. Mitochondrial abnormalities in nonalcoholic steatohepatitis. J Hepatol 1999;31:430–4.
83. Schon EA, Bonilla E, DiMauro S. Mitochondrial DNA mutations and pathogenesis. J Bioenerg Biomembr 1997;29:131–49.
84. Sozo A, Arrese M, Glasinovic JC. Evidence of intestinal bacterial overgrowth in patients with NASH. Gastroenterology 2001;120:A118 [abstract].
85. Al-Osaimi AM, Berg CL, Caldwell SH. Intermittent disconjugate gaze: a novel finding in nonalcoholic steatohepatitis and cryptogenic cirrhosis. Hepatology 2005;41:943.
86. Feliciani C, Amerio P. Madelung's disease: inherited from an ancient Mediterranean population? [letter]. N Engl J Med 1999;340:1481.
87. Vila MR, Gamez J, Solano A, et al. Uncoupling protein-1 mRNA expression in lipomas from patients bearing pathogenic mitochondrial DNA mutations. Biochem Biophys Res Commun 2000;278:800–2.
88. Guillausseau P-J, Massin P, Dubois-LaForgue D, et al. Maternally inherited diabetes and deafness: a multicenter study. Ann Intern Med 2001;134:721–8.
89. Bohan A, Droogan O, Nolan N, et al. Mitochondrial DNA abnormalities without significant deficiency of intramitochondrial fatty acid beta-oxidation enzymes in a well-defined subgroup of patients with nonalcoholic steatohepatitis (NASH). Hepatology 2000;32:A387 [abstract].
90. Carrozzo R, Hirano M, Fromenty B. Multiple mtDNA deletions features in autosomal-dominant and -recessive diseases suggest distinct pathogeneses. Neurology 1998;50:99–106.

91. Phan J, Reue K. Lipin, a lipodystrophy and obesity gene. Cell Metab 2005;1: 73–83.
92. Garg A. Lipodystrophies. Am J Med 2000;108:143–52.
93. Garg A. Acquired and inherited lipodystrophies. N Engl J Med 2004;350: 1220–34.
94. Cortés VA, Curtis DE, Sukumaran S, et al. Molecular mechanisms of hepatic steatosis and insulin resistance in the AGPAT2-deficient mouse model of congenital generalized lipodystrophy. Cell Metab 2009;9:165–76.
95. Case records of the Massachusetts General Hospital. N Engl J Med 1975;292: 35–41.
96. Chandalia M, Garg A, Vuitch F, et al. Postmortem findings in generalized lipodystrophy. J Clin Endocrinol Metab 1995;80:3077–81.
97. Ebihara K, Kusakabe T, Hirata M, et al. Efficacy and safety of leptin-replacement therapy and possible mechanisms of leptin actions in patients with generalized lipodystrophy. J Clin Endocrinol Metab 2007;92:532–41.
98. Park JY, Javor ED, Cochran EK, et al. Long-term efficacy of leptin replacement in patients with Dunnigan-type familial partial lipodystrophy. Metabolism 2007;56: 508–16.
99. Powell EE, Searle J, Mortimer R. Steatohepatitis associated with limb lipodystrophy. Gastroenterology 1989;97:1022–4.
100. Collet-Gaudillat C, Billon-Bancel A, Beressi JP. Long-term improvement of metabolic control with pioglitazone in a woman with diabetes mellitus related to Dunnigan syndrome: a case report. Diabetes Metab 2009;35:151–4.
101. Herranz P, Lucas R, Perez-Espana L, et al. Lipodystrophy syndromes. Dermatol Clin 2008;26:569–78.
102. Strauss RS, Barlow SE, Dietz WH. Prevalence of abnormal serum aminotransferase values in overweight and obese adolescents. J Pediatr 2000;136:727–33.
103. Park HS, Han JH, Choi KM, et al. Relation between elevated serum alanine aminotransferase and metabolic syndrome in Korean adolescents. Am J Clin Nutr 2005;82:1046–51.
104. Franzese A, Vajro P, Argenziano A, et al. Liver involvement in obese children. Ultrasonography and liver enzyme levels at diagnosis and during follow-up in an Italian population. Dig Dis Sci 1997;42:1428–32.
105. Tazawa Y, Noguchi H, Nishinomiya F, et al. Serum alanine aminotransferase activity in obese children. Acta Paediatr 1997;86:238–41.
106. Barshop NJ, Sirlin CB, Schwimmer JB, et al. Review article: epidemiology, pathogenesis, and potential treatments of paediatric nonalcoholic fatty liver disease. Aliment Pharmacol Ther 2008;28:13–24.
107. Schwimmer JB, McGreal N, Deutsch R, et al. Influence of gender, race, and ethnicity on suspected fatty liver in obese adolescents. Pediatrics 2005;115: e561–5.
108. Schwimmer JB, Deutsch R, Kahen T, et al. Prevalence of fatty liver in children and adolescents. Pediatrics 2006;118:1388–93.
109. Maheshwari A, Thuluvath PJ. Cryptogenic cirrhosis and NAFLD: are they related? Am J Gastroenterol 2006;101:664–8.
110. Powell EE, Cooksley WG, Hanson R, et al. The natural history of nonalcoholic steatohepatitis: a follow-up study of forty-two patients for up to 21 years. Hepatology 1990;11:74–80.
111. Poonawala A, Nair SP, Thuluvath PJ. Prevalence of obesity and diabetes in patients with cryptogenic cirrhosis: a case–control study. Hepatology 2000;32: 689–92.

112. Sakugawa H, Nakasone H, Nakayoshi T, et al. Clinical characteristics of patients with cryptogenic liver cirrhosis in Okinawa, Japan. Hepatogastroenterology 2003;50:2005–8.
113. Nair S, Verma S, Thuluvath PJ. Obesity and the effect on survival in patients undergoing orthotopic liver transplantation in the United States. Hepatology 2002;35:105–9.
114. Heneghan MA, Zolfino T, Muiesan P, et al. An evaluation of long-term outcomes after transplantation for cryptogenic cirrhosis. Liver Transplant 2003;9:921–8.
115. Duseja A, Nanda M, Das A, et al. Prevalence of obesity, diabetes mellitus, and hyperlipidemia in patients with cryptogenic cirrhosis. Trop Gastroenterol 2004; 25:15–7.
116. Kojima H, Sakuri S, Matsumura M, et al. Cryptogenic cirrhosis in the region where obesity is not prevalent. World J Gastroenterol 2006;12:2080–5.
117. Tellez-Avila F, Sanchez-Avila F, Garcia–Saenz-de-Sicilia M, et al. Prevalence of metabolic syndrome, obesity, and diabetes type 2 in cryptogenic cirrhosis. World J Gastroenterol 2008;14:4771–5.
118. Browning JD, Kumar KS, Saboorian MH, et al. Ethnic differences in the prevalence of cryptogenic cirrhosis. Am J Gastroenterol 2004;99:292–8.
119. Angulo P. Nonalcoholic fatty liver disease and liver transplantation. Liver Transpl 2006;12:523–34.
120. Contos MJ, Cales W, Sterling RK, et al. Development of nonalcoholic fatty liver disease after orthotopic liver transplantation for cryptogenic cirrhosis. Liver Transpl 2001;7:363–73.
121. Sutedja DS, Gow PJ, Hubscher SG, et al. Revealing the cause of cryptogenic cirrhosis by post-transplant liver biopsy. Transplant Proc 2004;36:2334–7.
122. Ong J, Younossi ZM, Reddy V, et al. Cryptogenic cirrhosis and post-transplantation nonalcoholic fatty liver disease. Liver Transpl 2001;7:797–801.
123. Molloy RM, Komorowski R, Varma RV. Recurrent nonalcoholic steatohepatitis and cirrhosis after liver transplantation. Liver Transpl Surg 1997;3:177–8.
124. Charlton MR, Kondo M, Roberts SK. Liver transplantation for cryptogenic cirrhosis. Liver Transpl Surg 1997;3:359–64.
125. Lim LG, Cheng CL, Wee A, et al. Prevalence and clinical associations of post-transplant fatty liver disease. Liver Int 2007;27:76–80.
126. Morales E, Garcia R, Saksena S, et al. Recurrent and de novo nonalcoholic steatohepatitis (NASH) following orthotopic liver transplantation (OLT). J Hepatol 2000;32:57 [abstract].
127. Poordad F, Gish R, Wakil A, et al. De novo nonalcoholic fatty liver disease following orthotopic liver transplantation. Am J Transplant 2003;3:1413–7.
128. Cotrim HP, De Freitas LA, Freitas C, et al. Clinical and histopathological features of NASH in workers exposed to chemicals with or without associated metabolic conditions. Liver Int 2004;24:131–5.
129. Cotrim HP, Carvalho F, Siqueira AC, et al. Nonalcoholic fatty liver and insulin resistance among petrochemical workers. JAMA 2005;294:1618–20.
130. Cave MC, Falkner KC, Joshi-Barve S, et al. Industrial toxin associated steatohepatitis (TASH) develops in the absence of obesity and is associated with many of the traditional biomarkers and mechanisms of NASH. Hepatology 2008;48: 1118 [abstract].
131. Osman KA, Osman MM, Ahmed MH. Tamoxifen-induced nonalcoholic steatohepatitis: where are we now, and where are we going? Expert Opin Drug Saf 2007; 6:1–4.

132. Argo CK, Northup PG, Al-Osaimi AM, et al. Systematic review of risk factors for fibrosis progression in nonalcoholic steatohepatitis. J Hepatol 2009;51:371–9.
133. Garcia-Monzon C, Martin-Perez E, Iacono OL, et al. Characterization of pathogenic and prognostic factors of nonalcoholic steatohepatitis associated with obesity. J Hepatol 2000;33:716–24.
134. Park KS, Lee YS, Park HW, et al. Factors associated or related to with pathological severity of nonalcoholic fatty liver disease. Korean J Intern Med 2004;19:19–26.
135. Adams LA, Lymp JF, St Sauver J, et al. The natural history of nonalcoholic fatty liver disease: a population-based cohort study. Gastroenterology 2005;129: 113–21.
136. Gramlich T, Kleiner DE, McCullough AJ, et al. Pathologic features associated with fibrosis in nonalcoholic fatty liver disease. Hum Pathol 2004;35:196–9.
137. Ratziu V, Giral P, Charlotte F, et al. Liver fibrosis in overweight patients. Gastroenterology 2000;118:1117–23.
138. Harrison SA, Torgerson S, Hayashi PH. The natural history of nonalcoholic fatty liver disease: a clinical histopathological study. Am J Gastroenterol 2003;98: 2042–7.
139. Evans CD, Oien KA, MacSween RN, et al. Nonalcoholic steatohepatitis: a common cause of progressive chronic liver injury? J Clin Pathol 2002;55:689–92.
140. Adams LA, Sanderson S, Lindor KD, et al. The histological course of nonalcoholic fatty liver disease: a longitudinal study of 103 patients with sequential liver biopsies. J Hepatol 2005;42:132–8.
141. Hui AY, Wong VW, Chan HL, et al. Histological progression of nonalcoholic fatty liver disease in Chinese patients. Aliment Pharmacol Ther 2005;21:407–13.
142. Lee RG. Nonalcoholic steatohepatitis: a study of 49 patients. Hum Pathol 1989; 20:594–8.
143. Bacon BR, Farahvish MJ, Janney CG, et al. Nonalcoholic fatty liver disease: an expanded clinical entity. Gastroenterology 1994;107:1103–9.
144. Ekstedt M, Franzen LE, Mathiesen UL, et al. Long-term follow-up of patients with NAFLD and elevated liver enzymes. Hepatology 2006;44:865–73.
145. Fassio E, Alvarez E, Dominguez N, et al. Natural history of nonalcoholic steatohepatitis: a longitudinal study of repeat liver biopsies. Hepatology 2004;40:820–6.
146. Rafiq N, Bai C, Fang Y, et al. Long-term follow-up of patients with nonalcoholic fatty liver. Clin Gastroenterol Hepatol 2009;7:234–8.
147. Ong JP, Pitts A, Younossi ZM. Increased overall mortality and liver-related mortality in nonalcoholic fatty liver disease. J Hepatol 2008;49:608–12.
148. Feldstein AE, Charatcharoenwitthaya P, Treeprasertsuk S, et al. The natural history of nonalcoholic fatty liver disease in children: a follow-up study for up to 20 years. Gut July 21, 2009 [epub ahead of print].
149. Hui JM, Kench JG, Chitturi S, et al. Long-term outcomes of cirrhosis in nonalcoholic steatohepatitis compared with hepatitis C. Hepatology 2003;38:420–7.
150. Ratziu V, Bonyhay L, Di Martino V, et al. Survival, liver failure, and hepatocellular carcinoma in obesity-related cryptogenic cirrhosis. Hepatology 2002;35: 1485–93.
151. Bullock RE, Zaitoun AM, Aithal GP, et al. Association of nonalcoholic steatohepatitis without significant fibrosis with hepatocellular carcinoma. J Hepatol 2004;41:685–6.
152. Maeda T, Hashimoto K, Kihara Y, et al. Surgically resected hepatocellular carcinomas in patients with nonalcoholic steatohepatitis. Hepatogastroenterology 2008;55:1404–6.

153. Zen Y, Katayanagi K, Tsuneyama K, et al. Hepatocellular carcinoma arising in nonalcoholic steatohepatitis. Pathol Int 2001;51:127–31.
154. Caldwell SH, Crespo DM. The spectrum expanded: cryptogenic cirrhosis and the natural history of nonalcoholic fatty liver disease. J Hepatol 2004;40:578–84.
155. Hayashi PH, Harrison SA, Torgerson S, et al. Cognitive lifetime drinking history in nonalcoholic fatty liver disease: some cases may be alcohol-related. Am J Gastroenterol 2004;99:76–81.
156. Yatsuji S, Hashimoto E, Noto H, et al. Clinicopathological features in nonalcoholic steatohepatitis autopsy cases. Gastroenterology 2008;134:S1917 [abstract].
157. Lee VD, Kleiner DE, Al-Osaimi AM, et al. Histological characteristics of patients with cryptogenic cirrhosis and prior biopsy showing NASH. Hepatology 2007; 46:1138 [abstract].
158. Dunn W, Xu R, Wingard DL, et al. Suspected nonalcoholic fatty liver disease and mortality risk in a population-based cohort study. Am J Gastroenterol 2008;103: 2263–71.

Histopathology of Non-Alcoholic Fatty Liver Disease

Elizabeth M. Brunt, MD

KEYWORDS

• NASH • Steatosis • Histologic lesions

As noted in other articles in this issue, evaluation of liver biopsy, or resection/explant, remains the only unequivocal manner for diagnosis of non-alcoholic fatty liver disease (NAFLD) or non-alcoholic steatohepatitis (NASH), semiquantitative assessment of the particular lesions (scoring), diagnosis of concurrent disease processes, and exclusion of other pathologic processes as the cause of clinical liver disease. Serologic evaluation can exclude many possible concurrent processes. Laboratory testing is best for excluding viral hepatitides (hepatitis B and C), alpha 1-antitrypsin deficiency, and C282Y homozygous, which is the most common form of hereditary hemochromatosis. However, it is now recognized that serology alone can be a source of confusion in other potential liver diseases, such as autoimmune hepatitis and possibly primary biliary cirrhosis (PBC), because antinuclear antibody (ANA), and less commonly anti-smooth muscle antibody (ASMA) and anti-mitochondrial antibody (AMA), may occur in 2% to 40% of patients who have NAFLD.[1] On the other hand, biopsy may be necessary to definitively exclude the presence of autoimmune liver disease in the presence of ANA greater than or equal to 1:160 or ASMA greater than or equal to 1:40.[2] Alternatively, NAFLD and NASH may be coexistent with any other form of chronic liver disease[3] and careful liver biopsy evaluation is the best method of discerning this. Finally, Wilson disease may, or may not, share many histopathologic features of NASH (eg, macrovesicular steatosis, Mallory-Denk bodies[MDB], lipofuscin, iron deposition); thus, if there is any clinical suspicion of this possibility, analysis of the tissue from the paraffin block for quantitative copper analysis is the recommended assay.

Current imaging methodologies can detect steatosis with increasing accuracy,[4,5] but cannot detect inflammation or precirrhotic fibrosis or remodeling of the liver parenchyma.[6] Imaging also cannot assess types or localization of hepatic steatosis. With the increased use of rodents to study NAFLD/NASH, careful analysis or reading highlights the fact that liver tissue evaluations reported in many of the popular animal models of NAFLD/NASH often do not imitate many of the significant aspects of the

Department of Pathology and Immunology, Washington University School of Medicine, 660 S. Euclid Ave, Box 8118, St. Louis, MO 63110, USA
E-mail address: ebrunt@wustl.edu

Clin Liver Dis 13 (2009) 533–544
doi:10.1016/j.cld.2009.07.008
1089-3261/09/$ – see front matter

human disease, despite similar terminology applied by investigators.[7] This review will focus on the findings in human disease.

As briefly mentioned, liver biopsy is useful not only for diagnosis and grading but also for exclusion of NAFLD/NASH. There is an under-recognized but repeatedly reported finding in human studies worth noting: not all obese, or obese and diabetic, individuals have fatty liver or fatty liver disease. This is true in the bariatric series[8] and other series of evaluations for elevated liver tests[9] or studies of lipid and glucose metabolism in obesity.[10–12] In addition, not all individuals with NAFLD or NASH have otherwise unexplained elevated ALT; thus, while considered a useful screening tool when positive, ALT may not be considered either diagnostic or exclusive of the presence of NAFLD/NASH. This finding is noted in children and adults. Even in the setting of normal ALT, individuals with features of metabolic syndrome have features of NAFLD and the entire spectrum of histologic lesions of NASH, including fibrosis and cirrhosis; the former has been noted by imaging,[10] and the latter by histopathologic evaluations in adults[13,14] and children.[15]

Finally, liver biopsy evaluation has served as the gold standard against which a variety of clinical tests have been developed to predict NASH or fibrosis.[16] Many of these clinical test algorithms are discussed elsewhere in this issue.

Liver biopsy is not without its own difficulties, the most significant of which is sampling concerns. Several studies with different designs have shown differences in histologic findings based on: (1) the lobes from which the biopsy is taken,[17,18] (2) lengths of needles employed,[18–20] (3) numbers of passes for the biopsy,[20,21](4) surgical versus nonsurgical attainment of the biopsy tissue,[1] and (5) pathologists' abilities to reproducibly evaluate the different features of the disease.[22] While these are very real concerns that can potentially impact results of comparative studies,[20,23] each of these concerns can be sufficiently addressed so that the role of an adequate liver biopsy can be accepted in patient evaluation, management, and study designs. Ultimately, the use of a sufficiently large needle for biopsy procurement,[18,20] more than a single core of tissue[20] and the overall expertise of the liver pathologist,[24] will assure the best assessment. Despite significant interobserver variations in interpretation of lesions of NAFLD and NASH between pathologists, all studies to date have shown high intraobserver kappa agreement.[20,22]

There are two remaining concerns that are not completely addressed. One relates to the differences in capsule/parenchyma ratio. The right hepatic lobe is typically larger than the left, and thus has a smaller ratio. Needle biopsies from the left lobe may, therefore, include more of the immediate subcapsular parenchyma, and thus, include greater amounts of the connective tissue elements associated with the capsule and potentially larger portal tracts. The latter may even lead to confusion for size evaluation of portal tracts. One animal model of NASH has shown there are differences in the amounts and types of steatotic droplets in the subcapsular versus deep parenchyma based on whole sections of the livers.[25] Furthermore, comparisons of pre- and post-biopsies from bariatric patients will, almost by definition, have biopsies from the left lobe for the prebiopsy and from the right lobe for the postbiopsy. Whether this is truly an appropriate comparison for the lesions of NAFLD and NASH has not been critically assessed.

The second concern relates to the attainment of liver biopsies during a surgical procedure. The aggregation of polymorphonuclear leukocytes (PMN) during surgery is a well-recognized process by pathologists and is referred to as "surgical hepatitis." Whether this results from anesthetic-related cytokine release or to organ manipulation is not clear. In most areas of surgical pathologic evaluation of the liver tissue, this finding is irrelevant as one is evaluating resection specimens for tumor, or even biopsies for grading and staging of a known disease, such as hepatitis C in which the infiltrates are not PMN. However, in NAFLD/NASH, lobular inflammatory infiltrates are included in the systematic evaluation for diagnosis and necroinflammatory grade, and in contrast to other chronic necroinflammatory diseases of the liver, such as hepatitis C, PMN infiltrates may be a component of the lobular inflammation of NASH. Thus, whether the infiltrates of PMN is surgical hepatitis or inflammation secondary to steatohepatitis cannot be discerned, and the pathologist cannot accurately assess this significant lesion. If biopsies are performed very early in the procedure, and before organ manipulation, there is a better chance that surgical hepatitis may not occur.

Other potential confounders in liver biopsy interpretation include the under-studied differences in liver tissue from individuals who are overweight, obese, and morbidly obese. Just as clinical studies likely include otherwise obviously uncharacterized subjects with "not (yet) otherwise diagnosed liver disease" as NAFLD/NASH, thus rendering the diagnostic category as "trash,"[26] histologic studies are not uniform in specific lesions considered necessary for patient accrual or in methods of evaluation. This lack of uniformity may largely explain why some of the early studies had such discrepant results. Two studies in bariatric patients reported the incidence of steatosis and steatohepatitis of 22% and 70% in one study,[27] compared with 72% and 25%, respectively, in another with strict histologic criteria.[28] There is also an assumption that the liver biopsies of adult clinic patients and patients who are bariatric surgery patients should have similar histologic findings, but careful review of the studies from bariatric surgery indicates this may not always be the case. The most significant lesion reported to date in this category is the finding of isolated portal fibrosis[29]; whether this finding results from weight-cycling, weight reduction before surgery, larger portal tracts of the left lobe subcapsular biopsies, or is a true finding in this population has not been clarified. In addition, distribution of steatosis may differ in the bariatric population; the predominant zone 3 steatosis of patients who are nonbariatric has not been consistently reported. Clearly, careful histopathologic review is needed in the liver tissues obtained in bariatric studies.

Finally, cirrhosis can lead to challenges in imaging and liver biopsy interpretation in NASH. Although the reasons are not understood, the fact that cirrhotic livers in NASH may or may not retain features of steatosis, with or without inflammatory activity and foci of residual perisinusoidal fibrosis, can lead to problems in assignment of a diagnosis beyond cryptogenic.

HISTOPATHOLOGIC FINDINGS OF ADULT AND PEDIATRIC NON-ALCOHOLIC FATTY LIVER DISEASE/NON-ALCOHOLIC STEATOHEPATITIS

Each of the several reports in the 1960s (in Europe), 1970s, and 1980s highlighted the concept that a liver disease with histology similar to that of alcoholic liver disease, specifically alcoholic steatohepatitis, existed in overweight individuals who were commonly women, and commonly diabetic, but who did not consume alcohol.[1] From these reports grew a common misperception that the two are indistinguishable in their histopathologic manifestations. This concept, in reality, is only partly true; while features such as steatosis and mild steatohepatitis may occur in either group, there are lesions of more advanced alcoholic hepatitis that are not reported in NAFLD/NASH. These include canalicular cholestasis, extensive deposition of dense perisinusoidal collagen, and cholangiolitis. In cirrhosis caused by alcohol, copper deposition may occur. Large, dense MDB (Mallory's hyaline) are also more common in alcoholic hepatitis than in NASH. Finally, noncirrhotic alcoholic hepatitis may actually exist without steatosis; this is not true in noncirrhotic NAFLD/NASH.[30,31]

As may be anticipated, adults and children (2–19 years) may, or may not, have differing patterns of the lesions associated with NAFLD/NASH: steatosis, lobular and portal inflammation, hepatocyte ballooning, and fibrosis. The first study to codify these differences labeled the adult pattern as Type 1, and the pediatric pattern as Type 2.[32] The former consists of zone 3 predominant macrovesicular steatosis, ballooning, and when present, perisinusoidal fibrosis. Lobular inflammation is not necessarily concentrated in zone 3, but may be. Type 2 NASH is not as uniform. There may be panacinar steatosis, or steatosis concentrated in the periportal (zone 1) hepatocytes. In either case, ballooning, as identified in adults, is unusual or even absent, and lobular inflammation is commonly very mild, if present. However, portal tract expansion by chronic inflammation or fibrosis is commonly observed. Groups that have attempted to apply these criteria to pediatric biopsies have noted that while some fulfill these criteria for types 1 or 2, many, if not most, have some combinations of the lesions.[33–35] When present, a very reliable finding of pediatric NAFLD is zone 1 steatosis[34]; which has been termed the "indefinite for NASH, zone 1 pattern" by the National Institute of Diabetes and Digestive and Kidney Disease sponsored Non-alcoholic Steatohepatitis Clinical Research Network (NASH CRN) Pathology Committee, and is noted more often in pediatric biopsies than adult biopsies.

Just as there are recognized differences in prevalence and severity of NAFLD among various ethnic groups, histologic differences are also being reported.[36–38] Giday and colleagues[36] found only 2% NAFLD in a retrospective review of 320 liver biopsies, the majority of which (94%) were from African American subjects. None of the biopsies had evidence of steatohepatitis although the subjects with NAFLD had dyslipidemia and a body mass index greater than or equal to 30. In a bariatric population of 238 subjects, African Americans had significantly lower rates of steatosis, steatohepatitis, and fibrosis than either Caucasians or Hispanics.[38] Additionally, in a mixed urban population in which 238 liver biopsies had evidence of NAFLD, 15% were African American, 13% Hispanic and 7% Asian, and the remainder were Caucasian. Mohanty and colleagues[37] noted this ethnic distribution was significantly different from clinic and hospital patients (44% African American, 68% African American, respectively); thus, African Americans were significantly under-represented in the NAFLD group, despite similar metabolic features. Comparing the NAFLD biopsies, there was less significant steatosis (grade 3) in the African Americans and Asians compared with Caucasians, higher percentage of biopsies with ballooning in Asians, and greater percentage of biopsies with MDB in Hispanics. The majority of all groups had fibrosis scores greater than or equal to 2, although the highest percent with cirrhosis (9.4%) was in the Hispanic biopsies. To date, different specific findings between ethnic groups in large pediatric series have not been detected,[39,40] but the small numbers of African Americans, despite similar rates of obesity and diabetes, parallels that of adults.[34] A recent study confirmed the greater susceptibility of Hispanic adults, and lesser susceptibility of African American adults for hepatic steatosis based on the presence of an allele of *PNPLA3*[41]; thus, once studies such as this are extended to the pediatric population, it is possible that similar findings will be reported.

Histologic differences are also noted based on gender. In pediatric series, boys are more commonly affected with the severe features, whereas in adults, women predominate. The clinical features associated with severity in biopsy findings (ie, greater insulin resistance/diabetes and obesity) have correlated with the histologic findings, but the exact reasons for the gender effect have not been identified.[1]

Criteria for differentiating NAFLD from the necroinflammatory process referred to as NASH are developed in adults, but not as well in pediatrics.[1] In the former, these include the presence of a combination of lesions: zone 3 steatosis (commonly macrovesicular), lobular inflammation of some degree, and hepatocellular ballooning of some degree. Portal chronic inflammation is commonly present, as is zone 3 perisinusoidal fibrosis, however neither are considered required lesions for diagnosis.[42] It is apparent that the diagnosis rests not only on the presence of specific lesions but also on a pattern of injury; thus, a definite diagnosis will fit the description above, whereas, as used by the Pathology Committee of the NASH CRN, other possible diagnostic choices may include not steatohepatitis, indefinite, zone 3 pattern, and indefinite zone 1 pattern.[34] The presence of steatosis alone, or in combination with lobular or portal inflammation, therefore can be referred to as NAFLD, but does not fulfill criteria of steatohepatitis.

Many clinical investigators have used the term "simple steatosis" for which pathologists have no equivalent tissue lesions. While this is likely referring to liver with at least the minimal amount of steatosis to be considered NAFLD (5% or 3%, depending on the reference),[12,43] whether or not mild inflammation is also present is not inferred from this moniker. From unpublished personal experience, it is quite uncommon to find steatosis without any type of inflammation in liver biopsies. Likewise, as is recognized in pathophysiologic evaluations of NAFLD,[44] there is truly nothing simple about the presence of steatosis in hepatocytes, and the term "isolated steatosis" may be more appropriate. Steatosis is considered the first hit in the popular two-hit theory of NASH.[45] It is also now recognized that the steatosis not only results from aberrations in lipid metabolism, and is the background upon which the pathways of inflammation, mitochondrial dysfunction, endoplasmic reticulum stress, hepatocyte death, and fibrosis occur, but is also a marker of systemic processes including insulin resistance[46] and aberrant glucose disposal by skeletal muscle, and a risk of cardiovascular dysfunction.[12,47–49]

STEATOSIS IN NON-ALCOHOLIC FATTY LIVER DISEASE/NON-ALCOHOLIC STEATOHEPATITIS

In noncirrhotic livers, steatosis is necessary and sufficient for a histologic diagnosis of NAFLD, but is necessary and not sufficient for a diagnosis of NASH. In cirrhosis, all the lesions of steatosis and steatohepatitis may be absent.

The most common form of steatosis in NAFLD/NASH in adults and children is the large droplet steatosis, referred to as macrovesicular. This may be comprised of a single droplet that displaces the cytoplasm and nucleus peripherally, or may be comprised of a mixture of small and large droplets with similar cytoplasmic and nuclear displacement. At times, the smaller droplets appear in a ring-formation around the larger one. The significance of this is unknown, but current investigations into lipid droplet formation may eventually shed light.[50,51]

True microvesicular steatosis is comprised of nearly unappreciable or uncountable droplets that cause the cytoplasm to appear foamy and the centrally retained nucleus is commonly indented. This type of steatosis characterizes acute fatty liver of pregnancy, and other processes of beta-oxidation defects. This type of steatosis is most likely not what is referred to in surgical literature relating to liver transplant as "microvesicular"[52]; in that context, "microvesicular steatosis," or "small droplets of steatosis" (small open spaces in frozen section tissue) has not been shown to be harmful to graft outcome, in contrast with macrovesicular steatosis, and may even be questioned as true steatosis[53] True microvesicular steatosis may or may not be present in NAFLD/NASH, is never the predominant form, and when present, is usually in a nonzonal distribution in patches of contiguous hepatocytes.[54] These hepatocytes often contain megamitochondria. To date, clinical correlations with the presence of true microvesicular steatosis have not been done in NAFLD/NASH.

Studies have shown high correlations among pathologists in assessment of amounts of steatosis in formalin-fixed, paraffin embedded liver biopsies.[22] Likewise, clinical correlations are shown with the pathologist's assessment of steatosis, and lipid content as assessed by either biochemical results, or by MR imaging.[55] The assessment for steatosis is much more challenging in frozen sections of liver tissue, although the exact reasons why liver tissue has artifacts similar to steatotic spaces have not been elucidated.

The localization of steatosis may aid in determination of underlying pathogenesis. Processes more commonly considered with zone 3 predominance include adult NAFLD, alcoholic steatosis or steatohepatitis, many drugs, and metabolic abnormalities (such as lipodystrophy) that result in NAFLD. Zone 1 predominance is most commonly related to pediatric NAFLD, hepatitis C, cachexia or protein-calorie malnutrition, AIDS, total parenteral nutrition, cystic fibrosis, phosphorous poisoning, corticosteroids and amiodarone.[1]

As noted above, pediatric NAFLD/NASH, and occasionally adult NAFLD/NASH, may also have panacinar (diffuse) steatosis, or may have scattered droplets that are graded as azonal. Localization may be aided by consideration of zonal sparing; use of the trichrome stain may aid in this assignment. Panacinar steatosis may or may not occupy the entire surface of the biopsy, but the steatotic hepatocytes are uniformly present across the acini. Azonal steatosis, on the other hand, is characterized by nonuniformity of the fat droplets.

INFLAMMATION IN NON-ALCOHOLIC FATTY LIVER DISEASE/NON-ALCOHOLIC STEATOHEPATITIS

Inflammation in NAFLD/NASH is either lobular and portal, or one of these. The lobular infiltrates in NAFLD/NASH may be mixed acute (polymorphonuclear leukocytes) and chronic (mononuclear cells, including lymphocytes, monocytes and plasma cells and eosinophils) cell types, or only the latter. Portal inflammation is mononuclear with or without lipogranulomas. It is highly unusual for acute inflammation to predominate in portal tracts; in fact, if this is the finding, the differential considerations of alcoholic liver disease with cholangiolitis or biliary obstruction are warranted. Portal chronic inflammation may range from absent to moderate/marked in otherwise uncomplicated NASH.[56] When disproportionate to the lobular findings, consideration of another, concomitant process should be considered; concurrence rates are approximately 5% for NASH and other forms of chronic hepatitis.[3,57] Portal chronic inflammation is most notable in three settings of NASH: pediatric liver biopsies, resolution of NASH following treatment,[58] and in cases of severe steatohepatitis of adults or children.[59] The last was shown with a correlative study of clinical and histologic features from 728 adults and 205 children from the NASH CRN. In neither adults nor children did portal chronic inflammation correlate with serum ALT levels, presence or absence of ANA or ASMA, or with grades of lobular inflammation.[59] The potential causes of increased portal inflammation with resolution of other features of steatohepatitis are not known at the current time.

Frequently overlooked in NASH are the increase in Kupffer cell aggregates and the loss of the usual zone 1 predominance of this cell type.[60] In fact, in NASH, Kupffer cells aggregate in zone 3. Likewise, often overlooked is the fact that centrizonal inflammation may be so intense as to cause confusion with a portal area. Part of the confusion may stem from the more commonly recognized artery branch in zone 3 in severe NASH as has been reported in alcoholic liver disease[61] and in abstract form in NASH.[62] The absence of a bile duct, however, clarifies the fact that this location is zone 3 and not portal.

Lipogranulomas may occur in NAFLD/NASH in three areas: perivenular, lobular, and portal. The first and last are fibro-inflammatory lesions, whereas in the lobules, a lipogranuloma can be as small as a single droplet of macrovesicular steatosis surrounded by a pigmented Kupffer cell. Eosinophils may be present in any form of lipogranuloma. In contrast with alcoholic liver disease in which lipogranulomas may represent regression of injury,[30] significance has not been attributed to these structures in NAFLD/NASH. The pathologist needs to distinguish the fibrosis associated with them from true collagen deposition in the perivenular area or in the portal tracts.

CELLULAR INJURY/DEATH IN NON-ALCOHOLIC FATTY LIVER DISEASE/NON-ALCOHOLIC STEATOHEPATITIS

Three histologic features are recognized as representing hepatocellular injury/death: ballooning, acidophil bodies, and spotty necrosis. Another poorly recognized feature in NASH is the presence of zone 3 lipofuscin pigment; whether this may be related to oxidative stress in these hepatocytes has not been studied. Hepatocellular ballooning can be challenging to recognize. In the fully developed form, the affected cells are quite enlarged and the cytoplasm is flocculent. These cells may or may not also contain lipid droplets[63] or MDB[64] (Mallory's hyaline). It is not uncommon to note perisinusoidal fibrosis in association with ballooned hepatocytes. These cells are most often noted in zone 3. Recently, the use of immunostains for K8/18, the two cytoskeletal keratin filaments of hepatocytes, has shown loss of the normally abundant hepatocellular positivity and relative clearing of K8/18 from the cytoplasm; this stain will also highlight the MDB.[65] In addition to steatosis and lobular inflammation, ballooning is considered a required feature by liver pathologists for the distinction between steatohepatitis (with ballooning) and steatosis (without ballooning).[42]

The other two forms of cell death, spotty necrosis and apoptosis, are not limited to zone 3. The former results from lytic necrosis of hepatocytes with resultant reticulin collapse, Kupffer cell phagocytosis, and occasional mononuclear cell aggregates. Apoptosis is the well-characterized ATP-dependent result of intrinsic and extrinsic pathways that result in caspase activation. Severity of activity and numbers of acidophil (apoptotic bodies) are correlated.[66–68] Immunohistochemical stains for M30, a K18 fragment that results from apoptosis, have shown graduated presence in normal, steatotic livers and livers with steatohepatitis.[69]

FIBROSIS IN NON-ALCOHOLIC FATTY LIVER DISEASE/NON-ALCOHOLIC STEATOHEPATITIS

At the current time, there is general agreement on the patterns and progression of fibrosis in NASH; this was first formalized in a proposal for staging NASH in 1999,[56] and has been modified to include observations from treatment trials[70] and pediatric NAFLD.[32] The earliest stage in adults is zone 3, perisinusoidal (chicken wire) fibrosis; this type of fibrosis resembles a piece of mesh and the collagen fibers in it may be delicate (1a in the NASH CRN system) or dense (1b in the NASH CRN system). Because this is a lesion not predictably seen in children, the earliest stage for pediatric biopsies is portal expansion (1c in the NASH CRN system). Additional fibrosis may occur in the portal and periportal regions (stage 2); with progression, bridging between central areas, between central and portal areas, or between portal areas may occur (stage 3). Cirrhosis is the final stage (stage 4). In adult biopsies, perisinusoidal fibrosis continues to be present in stage 2 and may or may not persist in stages 3 (bridging) and 4 (cirrhosis). The presence of elastic fibers suggests maturity of collagen deposition; a recent study has taken advantage of this and shown elastic fibers to be present in stages 3 and 4 but not in the lower stages.[71] The investigators suggest this may be useful in deriving stage when it is in question. As with any liver biopsy, subcapsular parenchyma should be excluded from staging.

SEMIQUANTITATIVE SCORING SYSTEMS FOR HISTOPATHOLOGIC LESIONS IN NON-ALCOHOLIC FATTY LIVER DISEASE/NON-ALCOHOLIC STEATOHEPATITIS

Recent reviews of NAFLD/NASH have focused on the different methods extant for evaluation of lesions.[72,73] It is worthwhile to realize what the methods were created to do. The originally proposed scoring system[56] was developed for semiquantitative assessment of necroinflammatory activity (grade) and fibrosis (stage) for steatohepatitis in a fashion similar to those for other forms of chronic liver disease, specifically chronic hepatitis.[74] The method proposed for grading included collective assessments of steatosis amount, lobular and portal inflammation, and ballooning. The latter features (ballooning and inflammation) were the driving features for progression of grade, not steatosis. The NIDDK NASH CRN system[54] was developed to assign scores for evaluating pre- and post liver biopsies in studies; as such, the entire spectrum of NAFLD, including the then-recognized different pattern for children, was included. This method was derived by a group after multiple blinded readings of the study set, and has been validated as such. This is a feature-based system in which equal weighting is given to three features for grade: steatosis amount, lobular inflammation, and ballooning. From addition of these features, the NAS (NAFLD Activity Score) is derived. Fibrosis scores (stage) is as described above.

FUTURE DEVELOPMENTS IN PATHOLOGY

As has been noted throughout this review, there remain several areas that need further fundamental histologic study. Furthermore, sound histologic evaluation will likely remain the cornerstone of clinical trials, animal studies into pathophysiology, and development of noninvasive assays. Whether or not noninvasive markers will be as informative as a carefully evaluated liver biopsy will remain an open question.

REFERENCES

1. Brunt EM, Tiniakos DG. Alcoholic and nonalcoholic fatty liver disease. In: Odze RD, Goldblum JR, editors. Surgical pathology of the GI tract, Liver, biliary tract and pancreas. 2nd edition. Philadelphia: Elsevier; 2009. p. 1007–14.
2. Vuppalanchi R, Chalasani N. Nonalcoholic fatty liver disease and nonalcoholic steatohepatitis: selected practical issues in their evaluation and management. Hepatology 2009;49:306–17.
3. Brunt EM, Ramrakhiani S, Cordes BG, et al. Concurrence of histologic features of steatohepatitis with other forms of chronic liver disease. Mod Pathol 2003;16:49–56.
4. Sharma P, Martin DR, Pineda N, et al. Quantitation analysis of T2 correction in single voxel magnetic resonance spectroscopy of hepatic lipid fraction. J Magn Reson Imaging 2009;29:629–35.
5. Cassidy FH, Yokoo T, Aganovic L, et al. Fatty liver disease: MR imaging techniques for the detection and quantification of liver steatosis. Radiographics 2009;29:231–60.
6. Joy D, Thava VR, Scott BB. Diagnosis of fatty liver disease: is biopsy necessary? Eur J Gastroenterol Hepatol 2003;15:539–43.
7. Brunt EM. Do you see what i see? The role of quality histopathology in scientific study. Hepatology 2008;47:771–4.

8. Machado M, Marques-Vidal P, Cortez-Pinto H. Hepatic histology in obese patients undergoing bariatric surgery. J Hepatol 2006;45:600–6.
9. Neuschwander-Tetri BA. Nonalcoholic steatohepatitis: an evolving diagnosis. Can J Gastroenterol 2000;14(4):321–6.
10. Browning JD, Szczepaniak LS, Dobbins R, et al. Prevalence of hepatic steatosis in an urban population in the United States: impact of ethnicity. Hepatology 2004; 40:1387–95.
11. Fabbrini E, deHaseth D, Deivanayagam S, et al. Alterations in fatty acid kinetics in obese adolescents with increased intrahepatic triglyceride content. Obesity (Silver Spring) 2009;17:25–9.
12. Fabbrini E, Mohammed BS, Magkos F, et al. Alterations in adipose tissue and hepatic lipid kinetics in obese men and women with nonalcoholic fatty liver disease. Gastroenterol 2008;134:424–31.
13. Mofrad P, Contos MJ, Haque M, et al. Clinical and histologic spectrum of nonalcoholic fatty liver disease associated with normal ALT values. Hepatology 2003; 37:1286–92.
14. Fracanzani AL, Valenti L, Bugianesi E, et al. Risk of severe liver disease in nonalcoholic fatty liver disease with normal aminotransferase levels: a role for insulin resistance and diabetes. Hepatology 2008;48:792–8.
15. Manco M, Alisi A, Nobili V. Risk of severe liver disease in NAFLD with normal ALT levels: a pediatric report [Letter to the Editor]. Hepatology 2008;48:2087–8.
16. Wieckowska A, Feldstein AE. Diagnosis of nonalcoholic fatty liver disease: invasive versus noninvasive. Semin Liver Dis 2008;28:386–95.
17. Merriman RB, Ferrell LD, Patti MG, et al. Correlation of paired liver biopsies in morbidly obese patients with suspected nonalcoholic fatty liver disease. Hepatology 2006;44(4):874–80.
18. Larson SP, Bowers SP, Palekar NA, et al. Histopathologic variability between the right and left lobes of the liver in morbidly obese patients undergoing roux-en-Y bypass. Clin Gastroenterol Hepatol 2007;5:1329–32.
19. Bedossa P, Dargere D, Paradis V. Sampling variability of liver fibrosis in chronic hepatitis C. Hepatology 2003;38:1449–57.
20. Vuppalanchi R, Unalp A, Van Natta ML, et al. Effects of liver biopsy sample length and number of readings on histologic yield for nonalcoholic fatty liver disease. Clin Gastroenterol Hepatol 2009;7:481–6.
21. Ratziu V, Charlotte F, Heurtier A, et al. Sampling variability of liver biopsy in nonalcoholic fatty liver disease. Gastroenterol 2005;128:1898–906.
22. Brunt EM. Pathology of fatty liver disease. Mod Pathol 2007;20:S40–8.
23. Neuschwander-Tetri BA. Fatty liver and the metabolic syndrome. Curr Opin Gastroenterol 2007;23:193–8.
24. Rousselet M-C, Michalak S, Dupre F, et al. Sources of variability in histological scoring of chronic viral hepatitis. Hepatology 2005;41:257–64.
25. Tetri LH, Basaranoglu M, Brunt EM, et al. Severe NAFLD with hepatic necroinflammatory changes in mice fed trans fats and a high-fructose corn syrup equivalent. Am J Physiol Gastrointest Liver Physiol 2008;295:G987–95.
26. Cassiman D, Jaeken J. Nash may be trash. Gut 2008;57:141–4.
27. Garcia-Monzon C, Martin-Perez E, Iacono OL, et al. Characterization of pathogenic and prognostic factors of nonalcoholic steatohepatitis associated with obesity. J Hepatol 2000;33(5):716–24.
28. Dixon JB, Bhatal PS, O'Brien PE. Nonalcoholic fatty liver disease: predictors of nonalcoholic steatohepatitis and liver fibrosis in the severely obese. Gastroenterol 2001;121:91–100.

29. Abrams GA, Kunde SS, Lazenby AJ, et al. Portal fibrosis and hepatic steatosis in morbidly obese subjects: a spectrum of nonalcoholic fatty liver disease. Hepatology 2004;40:475–83.
30. Yip WW, Burt AD. Alcoholic liver disease. Semin Diagn Pathol 2007;23:149–60.
31. Lefkowitch JH. Morphology of alcoholic liver disease. Clin Liver Dis 2005;9(1): 37–53.
32. Schwimmer JB, Behling C, Newbury R, et al. Histopathology of pediatric nonalcoholic fatty liver disease. Hepatology 2005;42:641–9.
33. Nobili V, Marcellini M, Devito R, et al. NAFLD in children: a prospective clinical-pathological study and effect of lifestyle advice. Hepatology 2006;44:458–65.
34. Patton HM, Lavine JE, Van Natta ML, et al. Clinical correlates of histopathology in pediatric nonalcoholic steatohepatitis. Gastroenterol 2008;135:1961–71.
35. Carter-Kent CA, Yerian LM, Brunt EM, et al. Nonalcoholic steatohepatitis in children: a multicenter clinicopathological study [abstract]. Hepatology 2008;48:804.
36. Giday SA, Shiny Z, Naab T, et al. Frequency of nonalcoholic fatty liver disease and degree of hepatic steatosis in African-American patients. J Natl Med Assoc 2006;98:1613–5.
37. Mohanty SR, Troy TN, Huo D, et al. Influence of ethnicity on histological differences in nonalcoholic fatty liver disease. J Hepatol 2009;50:797–804.
38. Kallwitz ER, Guzman G, TenCate V, et al. The histologic spectrum of liver disease in African-American, non-Hispanic white and Hispanic obesity surgery patients. Am J Gastroenterol 2009;104:64–9.
39. Wieckowska A, Feldstein AE. Nonalcoholic fatty liver disease in the pediatric population: a review. Curr Opin Pediatr 2005;17:636–41.
40. Patton HM, Sirlin CB, Behling C, et al. Pediatric nonalcoholic fatty liver disease: a critical appraisal of current data and implications for future research. J Pediatr Gastroenterol Nutr 2006;43:413–27.
41. Romeo S, Kozlitina J, Xing C, et al. Genetic variation in *PLPLA3* confers susceptibility to nonalcoholic fatty liver disease. Nat Genet 2008;40:1461–5.
42. Brunt EM. Nonalcoholic steatohepatitis. Semin Liver Dis 2004;24:3–20.
43. Leevy CM. Fatty liver: a study of 270 patients with biopsy proven fatty liver and a review of the literature. Medicine 1962;41:249–76.
44. Tiniakos DG, Vos M, Brunt EM. Nonalcoholic steatohepatitis: Pathology and Pathophysiology. Ann Rev Pathol, in press.
45. Day CP, James OF. Steatohepatitis: a tale of two "hits"? Gastroenterol 1998; 114(4):842–5.
46. Wasada T, Kasahara T, Wada J, et al. Hepatic steatosis rather than visceral adiposity is more closely associated with insulin resistance in the early stage of obesity. Metab Clin Exp 2008;57:980–5.
47. Rubinstein R, Lavine JE, Schwimmer JB. Hepatic, cardiovascular, and endocrine outcomes of the histologic subphenotypes of nonalcoholic fatty liver disease. Semin Liver Dis 2008;28:380–5.
48. Korenblat KM, Fabbrini E, Mohammed BS, et al. Liver, muscle, and adipose tissue insulin action is directly related to intrahepatic triglyceride content in obese subjects. Gastroenterol 2008;134:1369–75.
49. Misra VL, Khashab M, Chalasani N. Nonalcoholic fatty liver disease and cardiovascular risk. Curr Gastroenterol Rep 2009;11:50–5.
50. Straub BK, Stoeffel P, Heid H, et al. Differential pattern of lipid droplet-associated proteins and de novo perilipin expression in hepatocyte steatogenesis. Hepatology 2008;47:1936–46.

51. Bell M, Wang H, Chen H, et al. Consequences of lipid droplet coat protein down-regulation in liver cells: abnormal lipid droplet metabolism and induction of insulin resistance. Diabetes 2008;57:2037–45.
52. McCormick L, Petrowsky H, Jochum W, et al. Use of severely steatotic grafts in liver transplantation. Ann Surg 2007;246:940–8.
53. Feng S. Steatotic livers for liver transplantation - life saving but at a cost. Nat Clin Pract Gastroenterol Hepatol 2008;5:360–1.
54. Kleiner DE, Brunt EM, Van Natta M, et al. Design and validation of a histological scoring system for nonalcoholic fatty liver disease. Hepatology 2005;41(6): 1313–21.
55. Vuppalanchi R, Cummings OW, Saxena R, et al. Relationship among histologic, radiologic, and biochemical assessments of hepatic steatosis. J Clin Gastroenterol 2007;41:206–10.
56. Brunt EM, Janney CG, Di Bisceglie AM, et al. Nonalcoholic steatohepatitis: a proposal for grading and staging the histological lesions. Am J Gastroenterol 1999;94(9):2467–74.
57. Brunt EM, Clouston AD. Histologic features of fatty liver disease. In: Bataller R, editor. International hepatology updates. Barcelona: Permanyer Press; 2007. p. 95–110.
58. Brunt EM, Tiniakos DG. Pathological features of NASH. Front Biosci 2005;10: 1475–84.
59. Brunt EM, Kleiner DE, Wilson LA, et al. Portal chronic inflammation in nonalcoholic fatty liver disease (NAFLD): a histologic marker of advanced NAFLD-Clinicopathologic correlations from the nonalcoholic steatohepatitis clinical research network. Hepatology 2009;46:809–20.
60. Lefkowitch JH, Haythe J, Regent N. Kupffer cell aggregation and perivenular distribution in steatohepatitis. Mod Pathol 2002;15:699–704.
61. Yabes A, Ferrell LD. Arterialization of central zones in alcoholic cirrhosis [abstract]. Mod Pathol 2006;18:289.
62. Ferrell L, Belt P, Bass N. Arterialization of central zones in nonalcoholic steatohepatitis [abstract]. Hepatology 2007;46:732.
63. Caldwell SH, Redick JA, Chang CY, et al. Enlarged hepatocytes in NAFLD examined with osmium fixation: does microsteatosis underlie cellular ballooning in NASH? Am J Gastroenterol 2006;101:1677–8.
64. Zatloukal K, French SW, Denk H, et al. From Mallory to Mallory-Denk inclusion bodies: what, how and why? Exp Cell Res 2007;313:2033–49.
65. Lackner C, Gogg-Kammerer M, Zatloukal K, et al. Ballooned hepatocytes in steatohepatitis: The value of keratin immunohistochemistry for diagnosis. J Hepatol 2008;48:821–8.
66. Yeh M, Belt P, Brunt EM, et al. Acidophil body index may help diagnosing nonalcoholic steatohepatitis. Mod Pathol 2009;22:326A.
67. Feldstein AE, Canbay A, Angulo P, et al. Hepatocyte apoptosis and fas expression are prominent features of human nonalcoholic steatohepatitis. Gastroenterol 2003;125:437–43.
68. Ribeiro PS, Cortez-Pinto H, Sola S, et al. Hepatocyte apoptosis, expression of death receptors, and activation of NF-kappaB in the liver of nonalcoholic and alcoholic steatohepatitis patients. Am J Gastroenterol 2004;99(9): 1708–17.
69. Wieckowska A, Zein NN, Yerian LM, et al. *In vivo* assessment of liver cell apoptosis as a novel biomarker of disease severity in nonalcoholic fatty liver disease. Hepatology 2006;44:27–33.

70. Neuschwander-Tetri BA, Brunt EM, Wehmeier KR, et al. Improvement in nonalcoholic steatohepatitis following 48 weeks of treatment with the PPAR-g ligand rosiglitazone. Hepatology 2003;38:1008–17.
71. Nakayama H, Itoh H, Kunita S, et al. Presence of perivenular elastic fibers in nonalcoholic steatohepatitis fibrosis stage III. Histol Histopathol 2008;23:407–9.
72. Bondini S, Kleiner DE, Goodman ZD, et al. Pathologic assessment of nonalcoholic fatty liver disease. Clin Liver Dis 2007;11:17–23.
73. Brunt EM. Nonalcoholic fatty liver disease. In: Burt AD, Portmann BG, Ferrell LD, editors. MacSween's pathology of the liver. 5th edition. Edinburgh: Churchill Livingstone; 2007. p. 367–98.
74. Brunt EM. Grading and staging the histopathological lesions of chronic hepatitis: the Knodell histology activity index and beyond. Hepatology 2000;31:241–6.

Role of Insulin Resistance and Lipotoxicity in Non-Alcoholic Steatohepatitis

Kenneth Cusi, MD, FACP, FACE[a,b,*]

KEYWORDS

- Insulin resistance • Lipotoxicity • NAFLD
- NASH • Type 2 diabetes mellitus

At first glance, obesity, the metabolic syndrome (MetS), type 2 diabetes mellitus (T2DM), cardiovascular disease (CVD), and non-alcoholic fatty liver disease (NAFLD) and non-alcoholic steatohepatitis (NASH) appear to be very different and separate entities. However, they are closely linked by a common underlying metabolic abnormality: adipose tissue insulin resistance leading to multiorgan "lipotoxicity." Although the degree of compromise of each end-organ varies from patient to patient and the causes remain poorly understood, dysfunctional fat accounts today for a large portion of the medical complications that clinicians, and in particular hepatologists, see regularly in their practice. However, it should be noted that NAFLD/NASH typically develops within a broader range of FFA-induced metabolic abnormalities that affect not only the liver, but also other tissues such as skeletal muscle, pancreatic beta-cells, and the vascular bed. This is because most organs are poorly suited to store large amounts of excess free fatty acids (FFA), as typically seen in obesity and type 2 diabetes mellitus (T2DM). However, it has become evident that progression from simple steatosis to NASH is not just a consequence of FFA-derived triglyceride (TG) accumulation but rather an inadequate hepatocyte adaptation to toxic lipid-derived metabolites (ie, unsaturated fatty acids, lipid peroxidation products and others) with activation of multiple inflammatory pathways, mitochondrial dysfunction, and endoplasmic reticulum (ER) stress, leading in the end to cellular apoptosis. The aim of this review is to examine mechanisms by which lipotoxicity causes widespread

[a] Diabetes Division, The University of Texas Health Science Center at San Antonio, Room 3.380S, 7703 Floyd Curl Drive, San Antonio, TX 78284-3900, USA
[b] Audie L. Murphy Veterans Administration Medical Center, San Antonio, TX 78284-3900, USA
* Diabetes Division, The University of Texas Health Science Center at San Antonio, Room 3.380S, 7703 Floyd Curl Drive, San Antonio, TX 78284-3900, USA.
E-mail address: cusi@uthscsa.edu

Clin Liver Dis 13 (2009) 545–563
doi:10.1016/j.cld.2009.07.009
liver.theclinics.com
1089-3261/09/$ – see front matter

metabolic havoc and how clinicians may improve patient care by understanding the close relationship between the FFA-induced metabolic abnormalities and the development of NAFLD/NASH.

INSULIN RESISTANCE: GENETIC VERSUS ACQUIRED FACTORS

Although obesity plays a major role in the development of insulin resistance in human disease and is becoming a major public health problem, it should be noted that the presence of insulin resistance is the result of a complex combination of genetic and many different acquired factors, such as sedentary lifestyle, medications, chronic illnesses, aging, and many other environmental factors (**Fig. 1**).[1] However, it should not be forgotten that there is an intrinsic genetic component to insulin resistance that is frequently overlooked as obesity is becoming more and more prevalent. For example, nonobese healthy subjects with a strong family history of T2DM (ie, having both parents with T2DM or one parent and multiple siblings) are extremely insulin

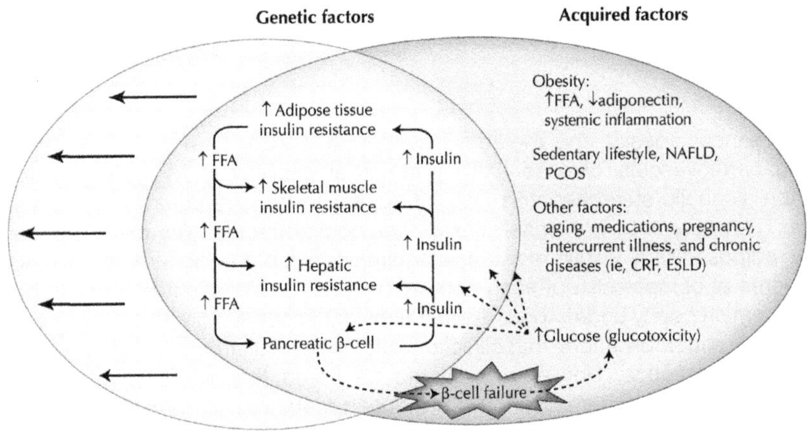

Current Diabetes Reports DR 09-3-1-02 fig. 1
324 pts. W/234 pts. D (27 x 19p6)
Author: Cusi Editor: Mardi Artist: Heather

Fig. 1. Interaction between genetic and acquired factors in the development of insulin resistance (IR) and β-cell dysfunction in humans. In modern society, acquired factors, in particular obesity and lipotoxicity, are playing an increasing role (indicated by *arrows* overlapping on the genetic background) in accelerating the development of type 2 diabetes mellitus (T2DM) in genetically predisposed subjects. Genes may determine adipose tissue, liver, and muscle IR. Increased rates of lipolysis and elevated plasma free fatty acid (FFA) from insulin-resistant adipose tissue may further exacerbate the genetically determined liver and muscle IR by promoting the accumulation of ectopic fat in both tissues. Both insulin resistance and elevated plasma FFA promote pancreatic β-cell hypersecretion, at least initially. Chronic hyperinsulinemia downregulatea muscle/liver insulin signaling and promotes hepatic steatosis. Once β-cell failure develops, hyperglycemia (glucotoxicity) becomes an additional insult (on top of lipotoxicity and hyperinsulinemia) to target tissues. Development of obesity, sedentary lifestyle, aging, and many other environmental factors would accelerate the onset of the described events in subjects genetically predisposed to T2DM. CRF, chronic renal failure; ESLD, end-stage liver disease; JAFLD, non-alcoholic fatty liver disease; PCOS, polycystic ovary syndrome. (*Reproduced from* Cusi K. Lessons learned from studying families genetically predisposed to type 2 diabetes mellitus. Curr Diab Rep 2009;9:200–7; with permission.)[1]

resistant even though they are lean and have no clinical feature of the metabolic syndrome (ie, absence of impaired fasting glucose [>100 mg/dL], hypertension, high TG/low HDL-C or central obesity). The presence of insulin resistance in these subjects strongly speaks to the hereditability of insulin resistance and why lean nondiabetic individuals may still develop NASH and other metabolic conditions. When these lean nondiabetic individuals with a strong family history of T2DM are carefully studied, they reveal severe hepatic, muscle, and adipose tissue insulin resistance and subtle defects in β-cell function. It is likely that many of these individuals have NAFLD despite having normal liver transaminases, as suggested from some small studies.[1,2] In most nonobese subjects, metabolic adaptation allows freedom from the development of metabolic complications such as NAFLD/NASH or T2DM for decades. However, the widespread development of obesity is drastically changing this, accelerating sometimes by decades the presence of disease.

This review will focus on the acquired component of obesity as it relates to insulin resistance and lipotoxicity in human disease. **Fig. 1** illustrates how in Westernized societies, more than ever before, obesity is playing an increasing role to negatively impact the individual's genetic background and accelerate the onset of metabolic diseases. Insulin-resistant adipose tissue, as observed in individuals with increased adiposity, likely worsens genetically determined insulin resistance in liver and muscle. Moreover, compensatory pancreatic β-cell hypersecretion can down-regulate muscle and liver insulin signaling while further promoting hepatic steatosis, because insulin-induced hepatic lipogenesis appears intact in insulin-resistant subjects.[1,2] The onset of FFA-induced β-cell failure with subsequent hyperglycemia and diabetes adds another stimulus for hepatic steatogenesis (see **Fig. 1**). Finally, it should also be noted that an individual who is perfectly insulin sensitive may become insulin resistant with just a 24- to 72-hour increase in plasma FFA to levels observed in obesity (reviewed in Cusi[1]). Thus, any chronic elevation of plasma FFA appears particularly deleterious to normal metabolism in humans.

THE IMPACT OF OBESITY IN THE TWENTY-FIRST CENTURY

When talking about the role of obesity, it appears of paramount importance to start with a clear definition of this condition. The most accepted direct measures of body fat include underwater weighing, bioimpedance, and dual energy x-ray absorptiometry. However, these tests are not widely available and not suitable for routine clinical practice, thus the reason why the body mass index (BMI) is the preferred alternative. A normal BMI is between 18.5 and 25 kg/m^2. Overweight is defined as having a BMI between 25 and 29.9 kg/m^2 and obese if greater than 30 kg/m^2. BMI is a simple and inexpensive way to quantify body fat and cardiovascular risk, but many factors modify considerably the health risks associated with obesity, including ethnicity, age, gender, cardiorespiratory fitness, and body fat distribution. For example, females and older adults have a higher proportion of adiposity for any given BMI compared with younger subjects, in particular males.[3] Meta-analysis examining the impact of ethnicity have concluded that estimates of body fat using BMI overestimate in African Americans the percentage of body fat relative to that of Caucasians.[4] Central fat distribution appears to be particularly harmful as visceral fat accumulation is associated more frequently with NAFLD[5] and NASH,[6] as well as with T2DM, more severe insulin resistance, dyslipidemia (elevated TG and low HDL-C levels), systemic inflammation, and an overall higher risk of CVD.

Between 1960 and 2002, the average height has increased by 1.0 to 1.5 inches in the general population, while weight has increased by approximately 25 lbs in both genders in the same period (or 14.8% in men and 17.2% in women).[7] Both reduced levels of physical activity[8] and increased caloric intake[9] appear to account for this. We live in the paradox of a world in which more people are overweight and obese than those undernourished (about 1 billion compared with 850 million, respectively).[10] Health care expenditures increase exponentially when the BMI is 30 kg/m^2 or higher.[11,12] In the United States, almost 1 of 3 children ages 2 to 19 (31.9%) and two of three adults are overweight or obese (64.5%)[12] resulting in medical care expenses for obesity-associated conditions of about $117 billion or nearly 10% of the total health care costs. Obesity is increasing at alarming rates among Hispanic and African American women, particularly those who are more socially disadvantaged.[11,12] In this regard, the social network appears to play a key role in the development of obesity. In a recent report from the Framingham Heart Study with follow-up between 1971 and 2003 the chances of a person becoming obese increased up to 57% if he or she had a spouse, sibling, or friend who became obese.[13] Obesity early in life predicts the future development of MetS, T2DM, and coronary heart disease (CHD) and significantly shortens life expectancy.[11]

INSULIN RESISTANCE AND LIPOTOXICITY: THE LINK BETWEEN THE EPIDEMICS OF OBESITY AND NON-ALCOHOLIC FATTY LIVER DISEASE?

Excess energy intake in obesity leads to an increase in adipocyte size (fat storage) with failure of fat cells to fully adapt in terms of proliferation and differentiation.[14] Hypertrophic fat cells are under considerable metabolic stress. Under normal conditions, the ER adapts to meet the demand related to protein and TG synthesis. However, when nutrients are in pathologic excess, this overwhelms the ER activating the unfolded protein response (UPR) and triggering the development of insulin resistance through a host of mechanisms, including c-jun N-terminal kinase (JNK) activation, inflammation, and oxidative stress (more on this elsewhere in this publication).[14] Once adipose tissue is dysfunctional (as in obesity, T2DM, and NAFLD) it impairs glucose and lipid homeostasis by two major mechanisms: (1) by acting as an "endocrine organ," releasing a myriad of fat-derived cytokines; and (2) by FFA-induced ectopic fat deposition and "lipotoxicity." Both pathways promote systemic inflammation and insulin resistance with activation of intracellular inflammatory pathways and eventual cellular collapse and apoptosis, resulting in devastating effects on glucose and lipid homeostasis.

Adipose Tissue as an "Endocrine Organ"

We refer the reader to a number of recent in-depth reviews,[14] although a few aspects merit attention. It is now well established that adipocytes are actively involved in the secretion of many inflammatory cytokines previously believed to be secreted only by macrophages or simply unknown (ie, tumor necrosis factor-α [TNF-α] interleukin-6 [IL-6], resistin, monocyte chemoattractant protein-1 [MCP-1], plasminogen activator inhibitor-1 [PAI-1], visfatin, angiotensinogen, retinol-binding protein-4 [RBP-4], and so forth). Adipocytokines mediate insulin resistance either through promoting serine phosphorylation (inhibition) of key insulin signaling steps (ie, insulin receptor substrate (IRS)-1 mediated by TNF-α or IL-6-induced I-Kappa-B kinase-beta (an inhibitor of NF kappa B kinase) and JNK pathways) in liver and muscle, or indirectly by activating macrophages with release of a host of cytokines near adipose tissue cells that promote adipose tissue insulin resistance, increased plasma FFA, and ultimately lipotoxicity. Adipose tissue is infiltrated with macrophages, and the content of toxic ceramides in adipocytes has been recently reported to be increased in subjects with NAFLD.[15] Dysfunctional adipocyte function is also characterized by reduced plasma adiponectin levels as reported in NAFLD and in NASH, as well as in obesity and T2DM.[6,16–18] The important role of adiponectin is illustrated in the ob/ob mice overexpressing adiponectin: they are completely rescued from the diabetic phenotype at the expense of morbid obesity, offering an interesting paradox of how fat cells can adapt and store pathologic amounts of fat while remaining insulin sensitive.[19]

Lipotoxicity: Adipose Tissue as the Source of Excessive Free Fatty Acids and Ectopic Fat Deposition

The term "lipotoxicity" describes the deleterious effects of excess FFA and ectopic fat accumulation to cause organ dysfunction and/or cellular death. In obesity, excessive food intake combined with high FFA output from insulin-resistant adipose tissue surpasses the storage and oxidative capacity of tissues such as skeletal muscle, liver, or pancreatic β-cells. FFAs are redirected into harmful pathways of nonoxidative metabolism with intracellular accumulation of toxic metabolites. As discussed later in this article, it is important to emphasize that it is not TG accumulation per se that is uniquely harmful, but rather the lipid-derived metabolites that trigger the formation of reactive oxygen species (ROS) and activation of inflammatory pathways.

TYPE 2 DIABETES MELLITUS AND NON-ALCOHOLIC STEATOHEPATITIS: A COMMON METABOLIC SOIL?

T2DM develops secondary to a progressive decline in pancreatic β-cell function over time (defined as when the fasting plasma glucose [FPG] is >125 mg/dL or a 2-hour OGTT is >199 mg/dL). T2DM is a direct consequence of lipotoxicity promoting insulin resistance and accelerating pancreatic β-cell failure. Elevated plasma FFAs are associated with the progression from "prediabetes" to T2DM (reviewed in Cusi[1]). People with "pre-diabetes" have either impaired fasting glucose (IFG) defined as an FPG between 100 and 125 mg/dL, impaired glucose tolerance (IGT) when the FPG is between 140 to 199 mg/dL after a 2-hour oral glucose tolerance test (OGTT), or both. Based on these definitions, more than one-third of adults aged 60 years or older had "prediabetes" (~57 million), whereas diabetes mellitus affected approximately 25 million Americans. Just in 2007, there were 1.6 million new cases of diabetes diagnosed in people aged 20 years and older with $174 billion spent in direct and indirect medical costs. By 2030 it is estimated that between approximately 30 and 38 million people will have diabetes in the United States and between 333 and 360 million worldwide.[20]

It is well established that obesity is fueling this "epidemic" of T2DM and that both conditions are key contributors to the development of increasing numbers of patients with NAFLD. Diabetes is much more commonly seen in hepatology clinics than in recent years. Elevated plasma FFA concentration, a hallmark of obesity-related adipose tissue insulin resistance, is strongly linked to the development of T2DM.[21–23] Both "prediabetes" and undiagnosed T2DM are common in patients with NAFLD and NASH. Although no large study has systematically screened with an oral glucose tolerance test (OGTT) patients with NAFLD or NASH, in our hands we have found that more than 70% of patients with NASH have disordered glucose metabolism (either IFG, IGT, or T2DM). We have diagnosed IGT or T2DM in a large number of patients referred to us with NAFLD/NASH by means of systematically screening them with a 75-g OGTT. Whether patients with NAFLD/NASH may be a population that in whom it is specially warranted to consider screening for T2DM deserves further evaluation, but an early diagnosis of T2DM may allow early intervention and prevention of diabetes complications. That disorders in glucose metabolism are so common is not totally unexpected, as most patients with NASH are obese and have hepatic and muscle insulin resistance. However, it does have significant clinical implications, as NASH appears to follow a more aggressive course in the presence of hyperglycemia,[24] placing a growing number of diabetic patients at risk of progressive liver disease.

ROLE OF EXCESS FREE FATTY ACIDS ON SKELETAL MUSCLE INSULIN RESISTANCE

The ability of FFA to inhibit glucose metabolism has been known for decades. Initially, Randle and colleagues[25] demonstrated that incubation of rat muscle with FFA diminished insulin-stimulated glucose uptake and proposed a "glucose fatty-acid cycle" (better known later as the Randle cycle) that revolved around the notion that cardiac and skeletal (diaphragm) muscle could shift readily back and forth between carbohydrate and fat as sources of energy for oxidation, depending on substrate availability. More recently, with the observation that obesity and T2DM are characterized by an impairment in insulin signaling,[26] it is well established that FFA and intramyocellular lipid accumulation (IMCL) disrupt early steps of insulin signaling in vitro and in animal studies.[27–29] In our laboratory we have recently demonstrated that FFA-induced muscle insulin resistance can be easily elicited with very small increases in plasma FFA and is dose-dependent (**Fig. 2**A).[29] In this study, plasma FFA were increased from normal (~300 μmol/L) to levels typically seen in obesity and T2DM (~700 μmol/L) into the pharmacologic range (~1,700 μmol/L) in lean healthy subjects. As observed in **Fig. 2**B, a 4-hour lipid infusion was sufficient to translate into a broad inhibition of muscle insulin signaling. These data help to understand why even a mild expansion in adipose tissue mass (as seen in overweight subjects) may cause insulin resistance and that lipotoxicity is fully established in frankly obese individuals.

Insulin resistance in muscle is associated with an increase in IMCL and of a variety of lipid-derived toxic metabolites, including fatty acyl CoAs, ceramides, and diacylglycerol (DAG). These lipid-derived metabolites activate pathways including both protein kinase C activation of βII and δ isoforms and Iκβ/NFκβ pathways.[30] T2DM is characterized by mitochondrial defects (decreased function and/or number) with decreased muscle oxidation.[1,31] Fatty acids cause mitochondrial DNA fragmentation, caspase-3 cleavage, production of reactive oxygen species, and apoptosis.[32] Within our group, Richardson and colleagues[33] have reported that a chronic (2-day) lipid infusion significantly reduces proliferators-activated receptor-α cofactor-1 (PGC-1) gene expression and other nuclear-encoded mitochondrial genes in healthy subjects, along with an increase in the expression of collagen/extracellular matrix genes. This is in striking similarity to defects observed in NASH[34] and suggests that excess FFA flux and lipotoxicity may be the link between functional and structural abnormalities in different tissues. As proof-of-concept, a decrease in plasma FFA concentration by acipimox, a nicotinic acid analog and inhibitor of adipose tissue lipolysis, improves muscle insulin sensitivity in nondiabetic subjects with a strong family history of T2DM,[35] as well as in obese and T2DM subjects.[36]

ROLE OF EXCESS FREE FATTY ACIDS IN INDUCING PANCREATIC β-CELL LIPOTOXICITY AND DIABETES

In NAFLD/NASH, obesity, MetS, polycystic ovary disease, and other insulin-resistant states there is a compensatory rise in insulin secretion in an attempt by the pancreatic beta cell to keep the day-long plasma glucose levels within the normal range. As the fasting plasma glucose rises from normal to approximately 120 mg/dL, there is a gradual loss of insulin secretion, which is rather severe by the time insulin-resistant subjects develop IGT.[1] This is generally followed by a more accelerated loss once fasting hyperglycemia develops.[37]

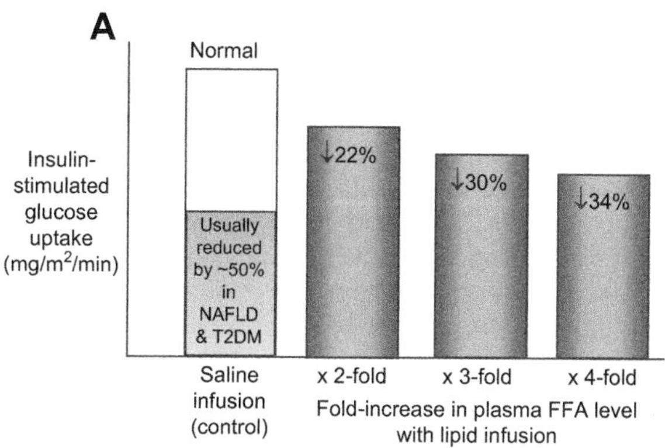

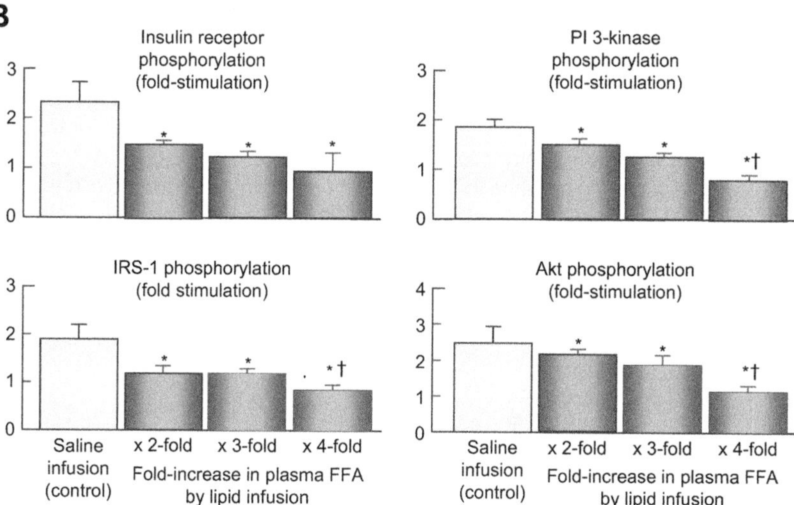

Fig. 2. Dose-dependent effect of an acute elevation in plasma FFA on insulin sensitivity (*A*) and insulin signaling (*2B*) in healthy nondiabetic subjects in skeletal muscle obtained by vastus lateralis muscle biopsies of lean healthy subjects. Reproduced is the effect of saline (open columns) versus lipid (20% triglyceride emulsion, filled columns) infusion at 30, 60, and 90 ml per hour on the percent reduction in insulin receptor (*A*), and IRS-1 tyrosine phosphorylation, PI 3-kinase activity associated with IRS-1, and serine phosphorylation of Akt. **P* < .01–.05, lipid versus saline; †*P* < .05, 90- versus 30-ml per hour lipid infusion rates. (*Data from* Belfort R, Mandarino L, Kashyap S, et al. Dose-response effect of elevated plasma free fatty acid on insulin signaling. Diabetes 2005;54:1640–8.)

The concept of β-cell lipotoxicity was championed initially by Unger[38] in a series of studies in leptin-unresponsive Zucker diabetic fatty (ZDF) rats, where an excess in saturated fatty acids would enter the ceramide pathway and lead to the activation of the NF-Kβ pathway with formation of reactive oxygen species (ROS) and lipoapoptosis. If ceramide production was prevented, β-cell lipotoxicity could be averted. More recently, it has been proposed that there is increased glucose-responsive palmitate esterification and lipolysis in rodent islets in the presence of a lipotoxic environment[39] and/or that beta-cell dysfunction may be attributable to a marked depletion of insulin stores without necessarily a reduction in beta-cell mass or TG accumulation.[40] In any case, the potential for FFA to cause β-cell lipotoxicity and apoptosis in vitro and in vivo varies upon the cell line or animal model, but has been an attractive hypothesis to explain the development of T2DM in humans.

In humans, it is important to understand the role of FFA for normal insulin secretion and compensation during insulin-resistant states in humans (reviewed in Cusi and DeFronzo[1] and McGarry[31]). This is best illustrated by reviewing the glucose–fatty acid cross-talk that controls insulin secretion. In the fasting state, plasma FFA (not glucose) is the primary energy substrate for sustaining insulin secretion. Following a meal, pancreatic β-cells switch from using fatty acids to using glucose as the preferred energy source, so that plasma FFAs go from being the preferred fuel (fasting) to being stored within the β-cell (fed state) for future needs. However, a chronic increase of plasma FFA concentration may paradoxically be deleterious to β-cell function in subjects genetically predisposed to develop T2DM as outlined in the following paragraphs.

Studies in humans have shown that an acute fatty acid increase can stimulate insulin secretion,[31] but chronic exposure to increased levels of fatty acids (~24–48 h) may impair β-cell function in vitro[41] and in vivo.[42] In lean healthy subjects, a prolonged lipid infusion (ie, 48 hours) stimulates insulin secretion.[43] In subjects genetically prone to T2DM, such as nondiabetic individuals with both parents having T2DM, we observed that a modest but sustained increase in plasma FFA concentration for 3 days to levels seen in obesity clearly impair insulin secretion (**Fig. 3**).[44] This was the first documentation in humans that lipotoxicity may play a central role in the development of T2DM in genetically predisposed subjects. We have recently shown that it is specifically FFA-induced lipotoxicity, not glucotoxicity, that impairs insulin secretion in these diabetes-prone subjects[45] and that β-cell lipotoxicity can be rapidly induced

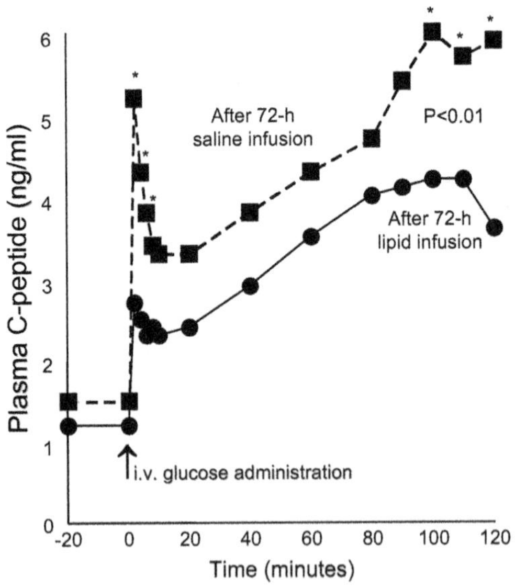

Fig. 3. Effect of a chronic physiologic elevation of plasma FFA by means of a low-dose lipid infusion on glucose-stimulated insulin secretion in subjects genetically predisposed to T2DM (ie, both parents with T2DM). A sustained elevation in plasma had significantly impaired insulin secretion in these subjects, but not in individuals without a family history of T2DM (not shown). (*Data from* Kashyap S, Belfort R, Gastalddelli A, et al. A sustained increase in plasma free fatty acids impairs insulin secretion in nondiabetic subjects genetically predisposed to develop type 2 diabetes. Diabetes 2003;52:2461–74.)[44]

by just an acute (1-hour) pharmacologic increase in plasma FFA in these subjects prone to T2DM.[46]

Taken together, although β-cell failure in T2DM is multifactorial, one may speculate that FFA-induced β-cell lipotoxicity links the epidemiologic observation of chronically elevated plasma FFA with T2DM.[21–23] This view also helps explain why IGT and T2DM are so prevalent in patients with NAFLD/NASH, as these patients are often obese and have elevated plasma FFA. Moreover, NAFLD/NASH patients are characterized by severe hepatic insulin resistance, which poses an extraordinary demand on insulin secretion to maintain normal glucose homeostasis at the expense of accelerating beta-cell failure in subjects genetically predisposed to T2DM.[1]

FREE FATTY ACIDS, HEPATIC INSULIN RESISTANCE, AND NON-ALCOHOLIC STEATOHEPATITIS

Free Fatty Acids and Hepatic Insulin Resistance

Although plasma FFAs play a key role in sustaining hepatic energy needs for gluconeogenesis and insulin tightly regulates gluconeogenesis, glycogenolysis, and the rate of endogenous (~90% hepatic) glucose production (EGP), excess FFA supply and insulin resistance as observed in obesity, NAFLD/NASH or T2DM alter this delicate metabolic balance in many ways. FFAs fuel gluconeogenesis and inhibit insulin suppression of EGP.[1] Moreover, elevated FFA has recently been shown to blunt the ability of hyperglycemia to inhibit glycogenolysis,[47] possibly contributing to the excessive rate of EGP observed in patients with T2DM. Although insulin inhibits hepatic very low density lipoprotein (VLDL) secretion under normal physiologic conditions, in insulin-resistant individuals hyperinsulinemia accounts for the typical dyslipidemia of patients with NAFLD/NASH as it promotes hepatic VLDL secretion and lowers plasma HDL-C levels.[48] Moreover, in insulin-resistant patients with NAFLD, adipose tissue hormone-sensitive lipase (HSL) is resistant to the action of insulin leading to enhanced increased rates of lipolysis and FFA availability for hepatic lipogenesis. In rodents, the combination of high plasma insulin and FFA levels are the most steatogenic and induce a greater reduction in gene expression of mitochondrial oxidation genes than either alone or in the presence of hyperglycemia.[49] At the molecular level, hepatic lipogenesis is driven by chronic hyperinsulinemia that stimulates hepatic sterol regulatory element binding protein1c (SREBP-1c) activity, and to a lesser extent by hyperglycemia, that stimulates hepatic carbohydrate response element binding protein (ChREBP).[50,51] Elevated plasma FFA are also known to inhibit insulin signaling and cause insulin resistance by activating the NF-Kβ pathway.[52,53] In rat liver, FFA-induced insulin resistance and hepatocyte inflammation can be prevented by salicylate administration.[54] Based on a large body of evidence in vitro, in vivo, and pilot human studies on the role of inflammation on insulin resistance and diabetes,[55] an ongoing randomized controlled clinical trial is fully exploring the anti-inflammatory role of salicylates in patients with T2DM.[56] However, chronic fat overload leads to mitochondrial dysfunction, accumulation of DAG, release of ROS, and activation of multiple inflammatory pathways (ie, JNK, NF-Kβ).[52,54,57–59]

In lean healthy subjects, induction of hepatic insulin resistance is fairly rapid following lipid infusion (within 2–4 h)[1,31] and worsens in a dose-dependent manner as plasma FFAs are experimentally increased.[29] Both metabolic pathways of glucose metabolism are affected, with FFA causing a stimulation of hepatic gluconeogenesis[60] and glycogenolysis.[61] Hepatic insulin resistance may develop with minimal (or even without) hepatic steatosis as measured by magnetic resonance spectroscopy (MRS).[45] Adaptation to FFA-induced hepatic insulin resistance in lean[44,45] and obese[62] healthy subjects involves a reduction of insulin clearance and the development of chronic hyperinsulinemia, which explains why insulin levels may be markedly increased in patients with NAFLD or NASH. A reduction of plasma FFA concentration by acipimox (a nicotinic acid derivative that inhibits HSL and the release of FFA from adipose tissue) partially restores hepatic insulin sensitivity.[35,36] Taken together, these studies highlight the close relationship between increased FFA supply and hepatic insulin sensitivity.

Free Fatty Acids and Hepatic Steatosis: Sources of Liver Fat and Role of Diet

The numerous molecular defects that lead to hepatic steatosis and NASH exceed the scope of this article, so we refer the reader to recent in-depth reviews.[34,50,51,58,63–65] However, a few aspects deserve comment in the context of lipotoxicity in NASH. It is now well established that in insulin-resistant states, adipose tissue is the primary source of FFA for hepatic TG synthesis,[1,31,48] accounting for approximately 70% of the FFA used for hepatic fat synthesis,[66,67] while de novo lipogenesis (DNL) is responsible for approximately 5% of hepatic TG, although in NASH it is as high as 26% of hepatic TG content.[66] Export of synthesized TG through VLDL secretion may alleviate lipid accumulation, although inhibition of VLDL secretion in a mouse model of hepatic steatosis lacking microsomal TG transfer protein (*Mttp*$^{\Delta/\Delta}$) promoted marked steatosis but did not cause hepatic necroinflammation, activation of the NF-Kβ pathway, or insulin resistance.[68]

Activation of Hepatocyte Inflammatory Pathways by Excess Free Fatty Acid Supply

It has been suggested that there is an altered composition of the fat that accumulates in NASH. For example, there is considerable debate about the relative role of saturated versus unsaturated fatty acids in the development of NASH. For instance, in the rodent model of NASH induced by a methionine-choline-deficient (MCD) diet (which cause steatosis, necroinflammation, and fibrosis), increasing the amount of polyunsaturated fatty acids (PUFA) causes a similar steatosis compared with an MCD diet with more saturated fat, but only the PUFA-rich MCD diet led to severe hepatic lipid peroxidation and histologic inflammation.[69] Although intriguing, whether this applies to NASH in humans is uncertain as these findings are in contrast to the depletion of hepatic long-chain PUFA reported in subjects with fatty liver disease.[70,71] Another important observation is that the activity of stearoyl-CoA desaturase 1 (SCD1), the rate-limiting enzyme in monounsaturated fatty acid synthesis for the assembly VLDL particles, is low in obese subjects with NAFLD.[72] Again, its role in NASH remains to be fully explored.

Another observation in subjects with NASH is that there is an increase in triacylglycerol (TAG) and DAG and in the TAG/DAG ratio.[73] This may be consistent with the toxic role of saturated FFA extensively studied in vitro. Human hepatocytes incubated with unsaturated FFA accumulate large amounts of TG without harm, but saturated fatty acids such as palmitate (that is poorly incorporated into TG) readily causes apoptosis. This has led to the hypothesis that unsaturated fatty acids rescue palmitate-induced apoptosis by channeling palmitate away from apoptotic pathways and into less harmful TG pools.[74] Recently, interest has developed in hepatic phosphatase and tensin homolog deleted on chromosome 10 (PTEN), a tumor suppressor that when deleted increases hepatic insulin sensitivity but causes steatosis.[75,76] In livers of rats with steatosis and subjects with the metabolic syndrome, PTEN expression is clearly down-regulated. Inhibition of PTEN function can be induced in hepatocytes in vitro by incubation with unsaturated fatty acids,[76] something that deserves further understanding in terms of its role in the development of NAFLD in humans.

Excessive accumulation of saturated FFA in hepatocytes causes significant ER stress and apoptosis.[51] Saturated FFAs also induce mitochondrial dysfunction and oxidative stress by mechanisms dependent on lysosomal disruption and activation of cathepsin B.[65] As proof-of-concept, FFA-induced hepatocyte apoptosis may be prevented by glycyrrhizin, the major bioactive component of licorice root extract, as it stabilizes lysosomal membranes, inhibits cathepsin B expression/enzyme activity, and avoids FFA-induced mitochondrial oxidative stress.[77] Further evidence that it is not TG per se but their channeling into lipid-derived toxic pathways that causes lipotoxicity comes from obese, diabetic db/db mice fed an MCD diet, in which inhibition of acyl-coenzyme A:diacylglycerol acyltransferase (DGAT) 2 (the enzyme that catalizes the final step in TG synthesis) by means of an antisense oligonucleotide (ASO) results in improvement in hepatic steatosis but exacerbates oxidative stress, liver injury, and fibrosis.[50]

IS NON-ALCOHOLIC STEATOHEPATITIS A FAILURE TO ADAPT TO A LIPOTOXIC ENVIRONMENT?

From the above evidence, one may speculate that several steps take place over time in the development of NASH in humans (**Fig. 4**). The "first step" for the development of NASH appears to be a rich source of fatty acids for hepatic TG synthesis. In our experience, performing metabolic studies in patients with NAFLD or NASH, whether patients are lean or obese, there is almost universally *adipose tissue insulin resistance*

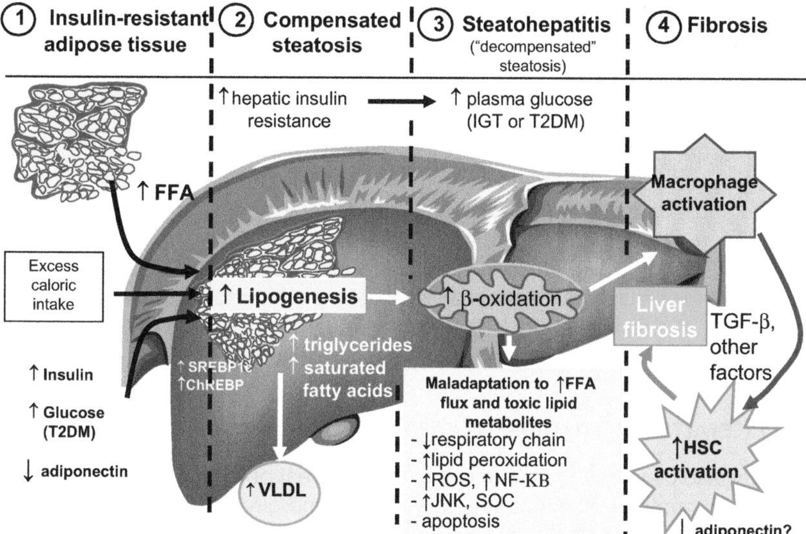

Fig. 4. Possible role of adipose tissue insulin resistance and lipotoxicity in the progression from NAFLD and NASH. (1) In the setting of obesity or T2DM, increased rates of lipolysis and plasma FFA, combined with hyperinsulinemia and hyperglycemia, stimulate excessive hepatic TG synthesis. (2) Steatosis in turn may (i) exacerbate hepatic insulin resistance, (ii) stimulate VLDL secretion, and (iii) increase mitochondrial beta-oxidation. If a new steady-state is achieved, only benign steatosis takes place. (3) If mitochondrial function cannot adapt to the increased FFA flux and respiratory oxidation collapses, lipid-derived toxic metabolites activate inflammatory pathways and hepatocyte lipotoxicity leading to necroinflammation. Endoplasmic reticulum stress and the unfolded protein response also participate in the pathogenesis of NASH. (4) The cross-talk between hepatocytes, macrophages, and hepatic stellate cells (HSC) determines the degree of the fibrogenic response and potential progression to cirrhosis. (*From* Cusi K. Non-alcoholic fatty liver disease in type 2 diabetes mellitus. Curr Opin Endocrinol Diabetes Obes 2009;16:141–9; with permission.)[83]

that creates the conditions for a "lipotoxic environment." This insulin resistance may be genetically determined,[78] or more commonly, a combination of genetic and acquired factors (see **Fig. 1**). Adipose tissue also plays an important role as a powerhouse of inflammatory cytokines in insulin-resistant states[55] and in the secretion of adiponectin.[79] This hormone has many molecular (ie, regulation of hepatocyte AMP-activated protein kinase [AMPK] activity, hepatic stellate cell [HSC] fibrogenesis, and so forth) and systemic anti-inflammatory effects[79] and plasma adiponectin levels are low in patients with NAFLD or NASH.[6,80,81] Moreover, we have recently reported that the increase in plasma adiponectin levels during pioglitazone treatment plays an important role in the reversal of insulin resistance and histologic improvement in patients with NASH.[6] The development of FFA-induced *hepatic steatosis* and the presence of a TG pool from where lipid-derived toxic metabolites may potentially activate inflammatory pathways becomes a likely "second step" toward NASH. Hepatic fat accumulation would vary based on the magnitude of the insult, such as the rate of FFA flux to the liver from exogenous (food overload) and endogenous sources, the presence of hyperinsulinemia and/or hyperglycemia (ie, T2DM), as well as genetic factors that determine the metabolic "flexibility" of the liver to this environment, as has been reported in humans at the level of skeletal muscle.[82] In this regard, it is likely that inherent genetic variations in the expression of mitochondrial-related energy regulators such as AMPK, PGC-1α, Peroxisome proliferator-activated receptor (PPAR)-β, PPAR-α, and others play a decisive role in progressing from "bland steatosis" to severe NASH.[34,78] The "third step" would involve FFA-induced lipotoxicity with mitochondrial collapse, ER stress, ROS formation, and activation of inflammatory pathways (extensively reviewed elsewhere in this publication and in references[34,50,51,58,63–65,83]). Finally, perhaps the least understood step is why only a small fraction of patients with NASH progress to fibrosis and cirrhosis. Of note, a recent preliminary report noted that middle-aged nonobese T2DM subjects had a significant defect in hepatic energy homeostasis, possibly in mitochondrial function, as measured by a reduced generation of γATP and hepatic phosphorus metabolites as assessed by 31P/1H MRS despite similar levels of hepatic fat.[84] So what started as adipose tissue insulin resistance may lead decades later to cirrhosis, a final "forth" step (see **Fig. 4**) dependent upon the incompletely understood cross-talk between hepatocytes, Kupffer cells, and activated hepatic stellate cells.[50,58,78]

ROLE OF FREE FATTY ACIDS TO PROMOTE CARDIOVASCULAR DISEASE

Lipotoxicity also plays an active role in the development of CV disease and endothelial dysfunction in humans. For instance, there is an emerging literature suggesting that NAFLD may be associated with increased CV disease[85] and that CV events are more common in patients with NAFLD when matched with subjects without fatty liver disease.[86] Many reasons may account for this: patients with NAFLD/NASH may be more insulin resistant, have worse subclinical inflammation (eg, hsCRP, IL-6, TNF-alpha), more severe dyslipidemia, and/or be directly affected by myocardial lipotoxicity (see later in this article).

Either way, a chronic increase in FFA availability is detrimental to the heart and vascular bed and promotes cardiovascular disease. For instance, increasing plasma FFA concentration for just a few hours causes endothelial dysfunction in vitro, in animal models and in humans.[87] We have observed that just a mild elevation in plasma FFA to levels observed in T2DM for 48 to 72 hours by means of a lipid infusion increases blood pressure[88] and induces the production of markers of systemic inflammation (ie, soluble intercellular adhesion molecule [ICAM] and vascular adhesion molecule [VCAM], endothelin [ET]-1) in lean healthy subjects.[89] Moreover, we have recently expanded these observations by showing that a 48-hour increase in plasma FFA concentration also increases soluble E-Selectin (sE-Selectin), myeloperoxidase (MPO), and total plasminogen activator inhibitor-1 (tPAI-1), indicators of a procoagulant state and associated with abnormal vascular reactivity.[90] Of interest, FFA impairs nitric oxide production by endothelial cells through the activation of an IKKβ-mediated response,[91] the same inflammatory pathways activated by FFA in muscle and liver, once again providing a unifying framework for lipotoxicity-induced damage across different tissues.

It has been long postulated that myocardial TG accumulation may predispose to cardiac dysfunction.[92] However, MRS has just recently been validated to measure TG accumulation in the human myocardium.[93] With the use of this technique, several investigators have demonstrated an elevation in myocardial fat content and/or an association between hepatic and cardiac lipid accumulation combined with

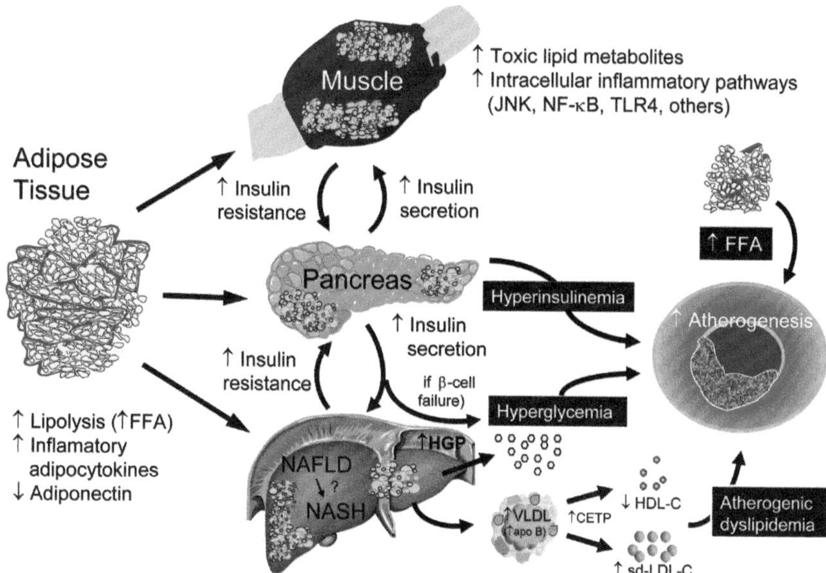

Fig. 5. Schematic representation integrating the role of adipose tissue insulin resistance, ectopic fat, and lipotoxicity in the development of NASH, T2DM, and CVD in humans. Dysfunctional fat releases excessive amounts of FFA and a host of inflammatory cytokines. This leads to ectopic fat deposition in tissues poorly adapted to this lipid overload. In muscle and liver this causes TG accumulation and the channeling of fat into harmful metabolic pathways with formation of toxic lipid metabolites, which results in alterations in glucose metabolism (insulin resistance) and activation of intracellular inflammatory pathways. This elicits a compensatory increase in insulin secretion, but in subjects genetically predisposed to T2DM it leads to beta-cell failure and/or lipotoxicity. Hepatic insulin resistance causes an increase in HGP and TG secretion with the typical dyslipidemia of the metabolic syndrome. FFA can directly cause endothelial dysfunction and activate inflammatory pathways as well. In the end, the combination of these factors (elevated plasma FFA, insulin, glucose, and dyslipidemia) aggregate to cause CVD. HGP, hepatic glucose production; FFA, free fatty acids; JNK, c-jun N-terminal kinase; NF-kB, nuclear receptor kappa beta; TLR4, toll-like receptor 4; NAFLD, non-alcoholic fatty liver disease; NASH, non-alcoholic steatohepatitis; VLDL, very low density lipoprotein; HDL-C, high density lipoprotein cholesterol; sd-LDL, small, dense low density lipoprotein.

abnormalities in cardiac metabolism. For instance, subjects with either glucose intolerance or T2DM have a significant increase in myocardial TG content.[94] The same group showed that short-term treatment with pioglitazone reduces both hepatic and myocardial steatosis in patients with T2DM.[95] In another example of the role of FFA on the myocardium, there is a significant correlation between the development of NAFLD and abnormalities in left ventricular energy metabolism.[96,97] In diabetic patients with NAFLD, fatty liver and elevated hepatic transaminases coexist with myocardial insulin resistance and coronary dysfunction.[98] This is consistent with a report that intramyocardial lipid accumulation in obese individuals precedes left ventricular hypertrophy and closely correlates with elevated plasma FFA levels and peripheral vascular resistance.[99]

SUMMARY: AN INTEGRATED VIEW OF INSULIN RESISTANCE, LIPOTOXICITY, AND NON-ALCOHOLIC STEATOHEPATITIS

Fig. 5 summarizes the wide metabolic defects caused by insulin resistance and FFA-induced lipotoxicity. When lipid supply surpasses the metabolic ability to adapt, the insult will lead in different organs (liver, skeletal muscle, pancreatic beta-cells, vascular bed) to individual metabolic adaptation but to similar cellular stress responses: lipid-peroxidation, ER stress, mitochondrial dysfunction, alteration of lysosomal membranes, ROS formation, activation of protein kinases, and activation of inflammatory pathways. It is well established that the development of NAFLD and NASH are closely linked to the excess flow of FFA, although the molecular mechanisms and multiple factors implicated remain unclear. The presence of hepatic steatosis suggests that the liver behaves as a "metabolic sensor" that is immersed in this energy-rich environment. In the end, its ability to adapt appears to collapse and the liver is subject to FFA-induced "lipotoxicity," NASH, and eventual cirrhosis. Lifestyle and pharmacologic and surgical (bariatric surgery) interventions may reverse lipotoxicity, although much more needs to be learned in reference to the best long-term approach. Understanding the role of insulin resistance and lipotoxicity in NASH as part of a broader metabolic disorder is likely to assist practitioners in the successful management of these challenging patients.

REFERENCES

1. Cusi K. Lessons learned from studying families genetically predisposed to type 2 diabetes mellitus. Curr Diab Rep 2009;9:200–7.
2. Cusi K, DeFronzo R. Non-insulin dependent diabetes mellitus. In: Jefferson LS, Cherrington AD, editors. "The endocrine pancreas and regulation of metabolism," handbook of physiology. Oxford University Press; 2001. p. 1115–68, Chapter 37.
3. Gallagher D, Visser M, Sepulveda D, et al. How useful is body mass index for comparison of body fatness across age, sex, and ethnic groups? Am J Epidemiol 1996;143:228–39.
4. Deurenberg P, Yap M, van Staveren W. Body mass index and percent body fat: meta analysis among different ethnic groups. Int J Obes Relat Metab Disord 1998;22:1164–71.
5. Gastaldelli A, Cusi K, Pettiti M, et al. Relationship between hepatic/visceral fat and hepatic insulin resistance in nondiabetic and type 2 diabetic subjects. Gastroenterology 2007;133:496–506.
6. Belfort R, Harrison SA, Brown K, et al. A placebo-controlled trial of pioglitazone in subjects with nonalcoholic steatohepatitis. N Engl J Med 2006;355:2297–307.
7. Bray G. Obesity: the disease. J Med Chem 2006;49:4001–7.

8. Hamilton M, Hamilton D, Zderic T. Role of low energy expenditure and sitting in obesity, metabolic syndrome, type 2 diabetes, and cardiovascular disease. Diabetes 2007;45:2655–67.
9. Jeffrey R, Harnack L. Evidence implicating eating as a primary driver for the obesity epidemic. Diabetes 2007;56:2673–6.
10. Yach D, Stuckler S, Brownell D. Epidemiological and economic consequences of the global epidemics of obesity and diabetes. Nat Med 2006;12:62–6.
11. Wyatt SB, Winters KP, Dubbert PM. Overweight and obesity: prevalence, consequences, and causes of a growing public health problem. Am J Med Sci 2006; 331:166–74.
12. Runge C. Economic consequences of the obese. Diabetes 2007;56:2668–72.
13. Christakis N, Fowler J. The spread of obesity in a large social network over 32 years. N Engl J Med 2007;357:370–9.
14. Gregor M, Hotamisligil G. Thematic review series: adipocyte biology. Adipocyte stress: the endoplasmic reticulum and metabolic disease. J Lipid Res 2007;48: 1905–14.
15. Kolak M, Westerbacka J, Velagapudi VR, et al. Adipose tissue inflammation and increased ceramide content characterize subjects with high liver fat content independent of obesity. Diabetes 2007;56:1960–8.
16. Bajaj M, Suraamornkul S, Piper P, et al. Decreased plasma adiponectin concentrations are closely related to hepatic fat content and hepatic insulin resistance in pioglitazone-treated type 2 diabetic patients. J Clin Endocrinol Metab 2004;89: 200–6.
17. Burgert TS, Taksali SE, Dziura J, et al. Alanine aminotransferase levels and fatty liver in childhood obesity: associations with insulin resistance, adiponectin, and visceral fat. J Clin Endocrinol Metab 2006;91:4287–94.
18. Targher G. Associations between plasma adiponectin concentrations and liver histology in patients with nonalcoholic fatty liver disease. Clin Endocrinol 2006; 64:679–83.
19. Kim J, van de Wall E, Laplante M, et al. Obesity-associated improvements in metabolic profile through expansion of adipose tissue. J Clin Invest 2007;2621–31.
20. Wild S, Roglic G, Green A, et al. Global prevalence of diabetes: estimates for the year 2000 and projections for 2030. Diabetes Care 2004;27:1047–53.
21. Paolisso G, Tataranni P, Foley J, et al. A high concentration of fasting plasma non-esterified fatty acids is a risk factor for the development of NIDDM. Diabetologia 1995;38:1213–7.
22. Charles M, Eschwege E, Thibult N, et al. The role of non-esterified fatty acids in the deterioration of glucose tolerance in Caucasian subjects: results of the Paris Prospective Study. Diabetologia 1997;40:1101–6.
23. Edelstein SL, Knowler WC, Bain RP, et al. Predictors of progression from impaired glucose tolerance to NIDDM: an analysis of six prospective studies. Diabetes 1997;46:701–10.
24. Ali R, Cusi K. New diagnostic and treatment approaches in nonalcoholic fatty liver disease (NAFLD). An Med 2009;41:265–78.
25. Randle P, Garland P, Hales C, et al. The glucose fatty acid cycle. Its role in insulin sensitivity and the metabolic disturbances of diabetes mellitus. Lancet 1963;1: 785–9.
26. Cusi K, Maezono K, Osman A, et al. Insulin resistance differentially affects the PI 3-kinase- and MAP kinase-mediated signaling in human muscle. J Clin Invest 2000;105:311–20.

27. Dresner A, Laurent D, Marcucci M, et al. Effects of free fatty acids on glucose transport and IRS-1 associated phophatidylinositol 3-kinase activity. J Clin Invest 1999;103:253–9.
28. Kashyap SR, Belfort R, Berria R, et al. Discordant effects of a chronic physiological increase in plasma FFA on insulin signaling in healthy subjects with or without a family history of type 2 diabetes. Am J Physiol Endocrinol Metab 2004;287: E537–46.
29. Belfort R, Mandarino L, Kashyap S, et al. Dose-response effect of elevated plasma free fatty acid on insulin signaling. Diabetes 2005;54:1640–8.
30. Schmitz-Peiffer C, Biden T. Protein kinase C function in muscle liver, and beta-cells and its therapeutic implications for type 2 diabetes. Diabetes 2008;57: 1774–83.
31. McGarry J. Banting lecture 2001: dysregulation of fatty acid metabolism in the etiology of type 2 diabetes. Diabetes 2002;51:7–18.
32. Rachek L, LeDoux S, Wilson G. Palmitate induced mitochondrial deoxyribonucleic acid damage and apoptosis in L6 rat skeletal muscle cells. Endocrinology 2006;148:293–9.
33. Richardson DK, Kashyap S, Bajaj M, et al. Lipid infusion decreases the expression of nuclear encoded mitochondrial genes and increases the expression of extracellular matrix genes in human skeletal muscle. J Biol Chem 2005;280:10290–7.
34. Pessayre D, Fromenty B. NASH: a mitochondrial disease. J Hepatol 2005;42: 928–40.
35. Cusi K, Kashyap S, Gastaldelli A, et al. Effects on insulin secretion and action of a 48-hour reduction of plasma FFA with acipimox in non-diabetic subjects genetically predisposed to type 2 diabetes. Am J Physiol Endocrinol Metab 2007, in press.
36. Santomauro A, Boden G, Silva M, et al. Overnight lowering of free fatty acids with acipimox improves insulin resistance and glucose tolerance in obese diabetic and nondiabetic subjects. Diabetes 1999;48:1836–41.
37. Kahn SE, Haffner SM, Heise MA, et al. Glycemic durability of rosiglitazone, metformin, or glyburide monotherapy. N Engl J Med 2006;355:2427–43.
38. Unger R. Lipotoxicity in the pathogenesis of obesity-dependent NIDDM. Genetic and clinical implications. Diabetes 1995;44:861–70.
39. Nolan CJ, Madiraju MSR, Delghingaro-Augusto V, et al. Fatty acid signaling in the β-cell and insulin secretion. Diabetes 2006;55(Suppl 2):S16–23.
40. Delghingaro-Augusto V, Nolan C, Gupta D, et al. Islet beta cell failure in the 60% pancreatectomised obese hyperlipidaemic Zucker fatty rat: severe dysfunction with altered glycerolipid metabolism without steatosis or a falling beta cell mass. Diabeteologia 2009. Doi:10.1007/s00125-009-1317-8.
41. Zhou Y, Grill V. Long-term exposure of rat pancreatic islets to fatty acids inhibits glucose-induced insulin secretion and biosynthesis through a glucose fatty acid cycle. J Clin Invest 1994;93:870–6.
42. Bollheimer L, Skelly R, Chester M, et al. Chronic exposure to free fatty acid reduces pancreatic beta cell insulin content by increasing basal insulin secretion that is not compensated for by a corresponding increase in proinsulin biosynthesis translation. J Clin Invest 1998;101:1094–101.
43. Boden G, Chen X, Rosner J, et al. Effects of a 48-h fat infusion on insulin secretion and glucose utilization. Diabetes 1995;44:1239–42.
44. Kashyap S, Belfort R, Gastaldelli A, et al. A sustained increase in plasma free fatty acids impairs insulin secretion in nondiabetic subjects genetically predisposed to develop type 2 diabetes. Diabetes 2003;52:2461–74.

45. Mathew M, Tay C, Belfort R, et al. A 48-hour elevation in plasma FFA, but not hyperglycemia, impairs insulin secretion in lean Mexican-American subjects genetically predisposed to T2DM [abstract]. Diabetes 2007;56(s1):A674.
46. Mathew M, Kumar P, Ali R, et al. Insulin secretion in patients with impaired glucose tolerance (IGT) is readily susceptible to FFA-induced lipotoxicity [abstract]. Diabetes 2008;57(Suppl 1):A153.
47. Martin M, Relwani R, Cui MH, et al. Elevated FFA impair glucose effectiveness by increasing net gluconeogenesis. Diabetes 2009;58(Suppl 1):1477.
48. Adiels M, Taskinen M-R, Boren J. Fatty liver, insulin resistance, and dyslipidemia. Curr Diab Rep 2008;8:60–4.
49. Wang S, Swamy A, Kamat A, et al. Hepatic steatosis is associated with mitochondrial dysfunction in obese and diabetic rats [abstract]. Diabetes 2008; 57(Suppl 1):A1501.
50. Choi S, Diehl A. Hepatic triglyceride synthesis and nonalcoholic fatty liver disease. Curr Opin Lipidol 2008;19:295–300.
51. Gentile CL, Pagliassotti MJ. The role of fatty acids in the development and progression of nonalcoholic fatty liver disease. J Nutr Biochem Apr 18, 2008; 19:567–76.
52. Boden G, She P, Mozzoli M. Free fatty acids produce insulin resistance and activate the proinflammatory nuclear factor-kB pathway in rat liver. Diabetes 2005;54: 3458–65.
53. Anderwald C, Brunmair B, Stadlbauer K, et al. Effects of free fatty acids on carbohydrate metabolism and insulin signalling in perfused rat liver. Eur J Clin Invest 2007;37:774–82.
54. Park E, Wong V, Guan X, et al. Salicylate prevents hepatic insulin resistance caused by short-term elevation of free fatty acids in vivo. J Endocrinol 2007; 195:323–31.
55. Shoelson S, Lee J, Goldfine A. Inflammation and insulin resistance. J Clin Invest 2006;116:1793–801.
56. Goldfine A, Fonseca V, Jablonski K, et al. The anti-inflammatory drug salsalate improves glycemia in type 2 diabetes. Diabetes 2009;59(Suppl 1):115.
57. Savage DB, Choi CS, Samuel VT, et al. Reversal of diet-induced hepatic steatosis and hepatic insulin resistance by antisense oligonucleotide inhibitors of acetyl-CoA carboxylases 1 and 2. J Clin Invest 2006;116:817–24.
58. Elsharkawy A, Mann D. Nuclear factor-kappaB and the hepatic inflammation-fibrosis-cancer axis. Hepatology 2007;46:590–7.
59. Samuel VT, Liu Z-X, Wang A, et al. Inhibition of protein kinase Ce prevents hepatic insulin resistance in nonalcoholic fatty liver disease. J Clin Invest 2007;117: 739–45.
60. Roden M, Stingl H, Chandramouli V, et al. Effects of free fatty acid elevation on postabsorptive endogenous glucose production and gluconeogenesis in humans. Diabetes 2000;49:701–7.
61. Boden G, Cheung P, Stein TP, et al. FFA cause hepatic insulin resistance by inhibiting insulin suppression of glycogenolysis. Am J Physiol Endocrinol Metab 2002; 283:E12–9.
62. Mathew M, Darland C, Kumar P, et al. Effect of obesity on insulin secretion in response to a 48-hour physiological increase in plasma FFA in Mexican-American subjects genetically predisposed to type 2 diabetes [abstract]. Diabetes 2008; 56(Suppl 1):A389.
63. Caldwell S, Chang Y, Nakamoto R, et al. Mitochondria in nonalcoholic fatty liver disease. Clin Liver Dis 2004;8:595–617.

64. Greenfield V, Cheung O, Sanyal A. Recent advances in nonalcoholic fatty liver disease. Curr Opin Gastroenterol 2008;24:320–7.
65. Li Z, Berk M, McIntyre T, et al. The lysosomal-mitochondrial axis in free fatty acid-induced hepatic lipotoxicity. Hepatology 2008;47:1495–503.
66. Donnelly KL, Smith CI, Schwarzenberg SJ, et al. Sources of fatty acids stored in liver and secreted via lipoproteins in patients with nonalcoholic fatty liver disease. J Clin Invest 2005;115:1343–51.
67. Barrows BR, Parks EJ. Contributions of different fatty acid sources to very low-density lipoprotein-triacylglycerol in the fasted and fed states. J Clin Endocrinol Metab 2006;91:1446–52.
68. Minheira K, Young S, Villanueva C, et al. Blocking VLDL secretion causes hepatic steatosis but does not affect peripheral lipid stores or insulin sensitivity in mice. J Lipid Research 2008;49:2038–44.
69. Lee, Yan JS, Ng RK, et al. Polyunsaturated fat in the methionine-choline-deficient diet influences hepatic inflammation but not hepatocellular injury. J Lipid Res 2007;48:1885–96.
70. Araya J, Rodrigo R, Videla L, et al. Increase in long-chain polyunsaturated fatty acid n - 6/n - 3 ratio in relation to hepatic steatosis in patients with nonalcoholic fatty liver disease. Clin Sci (Lond) 2004;106:635–43.
71. Allard J, Aghdassi E, Mohammed S, et al. Nutritional assessment and hepatic fatty acid composition in nonalcoholic fatty liver disease (NAFLD): a cross-sectional study. J Hepatol 2008;48:300–7.
72. Stefan N, Peter A, Cegan A, et al. Low hepatic stearoyl-CoA desaturase 1 activity is associated with fatty liver and insulin resistance in obese humans. Diabetologia 2008;51:648–56.
73. Puri P, Baillie R, Wiest M, et al. A lipidomic analysis of nonalcoholic fatty liver disease. Hepatology 2007;46:1081–90.
74. Listenberger L, Han X, Lewis S, et al. Triglyceride accumulation protects against fatty acid-induced lipotoxicity. Proc Natl Acad Sci U S A 2003;100: 3077–82.
75. Qiu W, Federico L, Naples M, et al. Phosphatase and tensin homolog (PTEN) regulates hepatic lipogenesis, microsomal triglyceride transfer protein, and the secretion of apolipoprotein B-containing lipoproteins. Hepatology 2008;48: 1799–809.
76. Vinciguerra M, Veyrat-Durebex C, Moukil MA, et al. PTEN down-regulation by unsaturated fatty acids triggers hepatic steatosis via an NF-kappaBp65/mTOR-dependent mechanism. Gastroenterology 2008;134:268–80.
77. Wu X, Zhang L, Gurley E, et al. Prevention of free fatty acid-induced hepatic lipotoxicity by 18beta-glycyrrhetinic acid through lysosomal and mitochondrial pathways. Hepatology 2008;47:1905–15.
78. Mark N, deAlwis W, Day C. Genes and nonalcoholic fatty liver disease. Curr Diab Rep 2008;8:156–63.
79. Kadowaki T, Yamauchi T. Adiponectin and adiponectin receptors. Endocr Rev 2005;26:439–51.
80. Tiikkainen M, Hakkinen A-M, Korsheninnikova E, et al. Effects of rosiglitazone and metformin on liver fat content, hepatic insulin resistance, insulin clearance, and gene expression in adipose tissue in patients with type 2 diabetes. Diabetes 2004;53:2169–76.
81. Baranova A, Gowder SJ, Schlauch K, et al. Gene expression of leptin, resistin, and adiponectin in the white adipose tissue of obese patients with nonalcoholic fatty liver disease and insulin resistance. Obes Surg 2006;16:1118–25.

82. Kelley D, Mandarino L. Fuel selection in human skeletal muscle in insulin resistance. A reexamination. Diabetes 2000;49:677–83.
83. Cusi K. Nonalcoholic fatty liver disease in type 2 diabetes mellitus. Curr Opin Endocrinol Diabetes Obes 2009;16:141–9.
84. Szendreodi J, Chmelik M, Schmid AI, et al. Defective hepatic energy homeostasis predicts hepatic insulin resistance in type 2 diabetes. Diabetes 2009;58(Suppl 1): 1473.
85. Targher G, Arcaro G. Nonalcoholic fatty liver disease and increased risk of cardiovascular disease. Atherosclerosis 2007;191:235–40.
86. Targher G, Bertolini L, Rodella S, et al. Nonalcoholic fatty liver disease is independently associated with an increased incidence of cardiovascular events in type 2 diabetic patients. Diabetes Care 2007;30:2119–21.
87. Steinberg H, Baron A. Vascular function, insulin resistance and fatty acids. Diabetologia 2002;45:623–34.
88. Tay C, Belfort R, Mathew M, et al. A 2-day lipid or combined lipid-glucose infusion reproduce in healthy subjects the metabolic abnormalities seen in the metabolic syndrome [abstract]. Diabetes 2006;55(Suppl 1):A66.
89. Kashyap S, Belfort R, Cersosimo E, et al. Low-dose lipid infusion induces endothelial activation independent of its metabolic effects. J Cardiometabolic Research, in press.
90. Mathew M, Tay E, Belfort R, et al. A prolonged elevation of plasma FFA induces vascular inflammatory markers in lean and obese healthy nondiabetic subjects [abstract]. Diabetes 2008;57(Suppl 1):A587.
91. Kim F, Tysseling K, Rice J, et al. Free fatty acid impairment of nitric oxide production in endothelial cells is mediated by IKKb. Arterioscler Thromb Vasc Biol 2005; 25:989–94.
92. McGavock J, Victor R, Unger R, et al. Adiposity of the heart, revisited. Ann Intern Med 2006;144:517–24.
93. Reingold JS, McGavock JM, Kaka S, et al. Determination of triglyceride in the human myocardium by magnetic resonance spectroscopy: reproducibility and sensitivity of the method. Am J Physiol Endocrinol Metab 2005;289:E935–9.
94. McGavock J, Lingvay I, Zib I, et al. Cardiac steatosis in diabetes mellitus. Circulation 2007;116(10):1170–5.
95. Zib I, Jacob A, Lingvay I, et al. Effect of pioglitazone therapy on myocardial and hepatic steatosis in insulin-treated patients with type 2 diabetes. J Investig Med 2007;55(5):230–6.
96. Perseghin G, Lattuada G, De Cobelli F, et al. Increased mediastinal fat and impaired ventricular energy metabolism in young men with newly found fatty liver. Hepatology 2008;47:51–8.
97. Jonker J, Rijzewijk L, Vean der Meer R, et al. Hepatic steaotosis is associated with myocardial insulin resistance and decreased myocardial high-energy-phosphate metabolism in uncomplicated T2DM. Diabetes 2009;58(Suppl 1):1484.
98. Lautamäki R, Borra R, Iozzo P, et al. Liver steatosis coexists with myocardial insulin resistance and coronary dysfunction in patients with type 2 diabetes. Am J Physiol Endocrinol Metab 2006;291:E282–90.
99. Kankaanpaa M, Lehto H-R, Parkka J, et al. Myocardial triglyceride content and epicardial fat mass in human obesity: relationship to left ventricular function and serum free fatty acid levels. J Clin Endocrinol 2006;91:4689–95.

Apoptosis and Cytokines in Non-Alcoholic Steatohepatitis

Wing-Kin Syn, MBChB, MRCP[a,b,*], Steve S. Choi, MD[a], Anna Mae Diehl, MD[a]

KEYWORDS

- Apoptosis • Cytokines • Inflammation • Fibrosis
- Non-alcoholic steatohepatitis

Non-alcoholic fatty liver disease (NAFLD) is now the leading cause of chronic liver disease in the United States.[1] It is closely associated with the metabolic syndrome, which is a constellation of insulin resistance, central obesity, hypertension, and dyslipidemia.[2] Histologically, NAFLD may range from simple steatosis to steatohepatitis and cirrhosis.[3,4] Individuals with simple steatosis rarely develop significant disease, whereas nearly 20% of those with non-alcoholic steatohepatitis (NASH) progress to end-stage liver disease.[5,6] Evidence that cirrhosis and hepatocellular carcinoma are more likely to develop in individuals with NASH rather than those with simple steatosis, suggests that NASH is a more serious form of liver injury.[5,7,8]

The "two-hit" hypothesis is a widely accepted paradigm to explain the progression of NAFLD from simple steatosis (fatty liver) to NASH.[8] The first hit involves dysregulated hepatic lipid accumulation (steatosis). Second hit(s) include oxidative, metabolic, and cytokine stresses that overwhelm hepatocyte survival mechanisms, leading to hepatocyte cell death (apoptosis). Indeed, NASH differs from simple steatosis mainly in the degree of hepatocyte injury and apoptosis.[9,10] We have previously proposed that hepatocyte apoptosis is the critical "third hit" that drives the progression from NASH to cirrhosis.[11] Hepatocyte apoptosis triggers regenerative mechanisms to replace dead hepatocytes.[12] However, aberrant repair response may occur in some individuals, resulting in the activation of hepatic stellate cells to myofibroblasts and the hepatic recruitment of proinflammatory, profibrogenic immune cells.

Funding: RO1 DK053792 to Anna Mae Diehl.
[a] Department of Medicine, Division of Gastroenterology, GSRB1, Suite 1073, 595 LaSalle Street, Durham, NC 27710, USA
[b] Centre for Liver Research, Institute of Biomedical Research, University of Birmingham B15 2TT, UK
* Corresponding author. Department of Medicine, Division of Gastroenterology, GSRB1, Suite 1073, 595 LaSalle Street, Durham, NC 27710, USA
E-mail address: wsyn@doctors.org.uk (W-K. Syn).

Clin Liver Dis 13 (2009) 565–580
doi:10.1016/j.cld.2009.07.003
1089-3261/09/$ – see front matter

In this article, we discuss the role of apoptosis and the impact of putative cytokines in the progression of NAFLD.

APOPTOSIS

Programmed cell death or apoptosis is a vital component of normal cellular turnover and development. It is an ATP-dependent process characterized by cell shrinkage, chromatin condensation (pyknosis), membrane blebbing, and budding.[13,14] When appropriately regulated, the process of apoptosis and clearance of apoptotic bodies is limited to specific cells, and is not associated with an inflammatory reaction.[15–17] In contrast, apoptosis occurring in adult tissues in response to noxious insults is typically dysregulated, prolonged,[18] and inflammatory in nature. Adding to the insult, it may ultimately promote fibrosis.[19–21]

Apoptosis is mediated by either the extrinsic (death receptor) pathway or the intrinsic (mitochondrial) organelle-based pathway.[22] Both pathways converge on a similar execution pathway, which is initiated by the cleavage of caspase-3.[14,23] Activation of caspases occurs through the cleavage of aspartate residues and requires caspase activity. This proteolytic cascade amplifies the apoptotic signaling pathway and leads to rapid cell death.

In the liver, apoptosis is typically triggered by ligation of surface death receptors,[24] including Fas (CD95), tumor necrosis factor (TNF) receptor 1, and TNF-related apoptosis-inducing ligand receptors 1 and 2 (TRAIL-R1 and -R2).[24,25] Expression of Fas/CD95 is enhanced in patients with viral hepatitis, alcoholic hepatitis, chronic biliary disease, and acute liver failure.[26] The binding of ligand to its cognate receptor results in the recruitment of cytoplasmic adaptor molecules, Fas-associated protein with death domain and TNF-receptor superfamily, member 1A (TNFRSF1A)–associated via death domain, and the subsequent activation of caspase-8.[27–29] Caspase-8, in turn, activates caspase-3, committing the cell to the final, common pathway of apoptosis.[14] This pathway was demonstrated when mice that were administered anti-Fas antibodies went on to develop massive hepatocyte apoptosis and die from fulminant hepatic failure.[30]

APOPTOSIS AND INFLAMMATION

The link between apoptosis and inflammation was demonstrated in skin and peritoneal experiments as mice injected subcutaneously with anti-Fas antibody developed a robust local inflammatory infiltrate,[31] and inoculation of Fas-L–expressing tumor cells into the murine peritoneal cavity resulted in an interleukin (IL) 1β–mediated neutrophilic infiltration.[32]

Relevant to the liver, inflammation is the critical stage in the progression from steatosis to steatohepatitis.[33] The number of inflammatory cells is minimal in simple steatosis, but is significantly upregulated in individuals with steatohepatitis.[34,35] This increase in inflammatory infiltrate is mirrored by the degree and extent of hepatocyte apoptosis.[9,36] Recent studies have supported this by showing that hepatocyte apoptosis may directly or indirectly promote inflammation.[37–40] Infection with *Listeria monocytogenes* triggered hepatocyte apoptosis and release of neutrophil chemoattractants.[41] Subsequent work demonstrated that macrophage inflammatory protein–2 (MIP-2) and IL-8 regulate hepatic neutrophil infiltration.[42] The use of cathepsin B knock-out mice and pharmacologic inhibitors by Canbay and colleagues[43] demonstrated that apoptosis induced by bile-duct ligation is associated with the production of proinflammatory chemokines CXCL1 and MIP-2. Similar observations were noted with experiments using Fas-L agonists.[39,44] The inflammatory infiltrate was composed predominantly of neutrophils; immune recruitment was mediated largely by CXCL1. When investigators inhibited apoptosis using the caspase inhibitor zDEVD-fmk, they noted a corresponding reduction in CXCL1 and MIP-2 production, as well as in the severity of hepatic inflammation.

Ligation of TNF-R1/CD120a triggers nuclear factor κB (NF-κB) activation and upregulation of proinflammatory cytokines and adhesion molecules.[25] In the galactosamine/endotoxin shock model, TNF-α–mediated caspase-3 activation triggered parenchymal cell apoptosis and neutrophil transmigration,[38,45] while supplementation with the caspase-inhibitor abrogated cellular apoptosis, neutrophil transmigration, and neutrophil-related injury. These studies lend support to the concept that cellular apoptosis is a signal for inflammatory cell recruitment.[38]

Tissue inflammation may similarly ensue during the clearance of apoptotic bodies.[15] Apoptotic bodies are typically rapidly phagocytosed by neighboring cells with the process being noninflammatory, a hallmark of physiologic apoptosis.[16] In contrast, the engulfment of apoptotic bodies by monocytes or Kupffer cells (liver resident macrophages) during liver injury is associated with the upregulation of the death ligands CD95, TRAIL, and TNF-α.[46–48] Complementing this, the depletion of Kupffer cells by gadolinium chloride is associated with impaired apoptotic body engulfment, reduced expression of the chemoattractant MIP-2, and amelioration of liver injury.[49]

Experimental evidence for this "apoptosis-inflammation" axis is supported by findings of hepatocyte apoptosis in patients with alcoholic steatohepatitis[50] and in patients with NASH.[9,51,52] In both, hepatocyte apoptosis correlates strongly with clinical and histologic disease severity. Additionally, the colocalization of apoptotic hepatocytes with polymorphonuclear cells suggests an apoptosis-dependent immune cell recruitment.[53]

APOPTOSIS AND FIBROSIS

The nexus between apoptosis and fibrosis was initially explored by Canbay and coworkers.[20] Mice treated with bile-duct ligation to induce chronic liver injury and fibrosis expressed increased amounts of α–smooth muscle actin, transforming growth factor β (TGF-β), collagen α 1(I), and tissue inhibitor of metalloproteinase 1, compared with sham-operated and Fas-deficient (lpr) mice.[54] Phagocytosis of apoptotic bodies by macrophages stimulated the production of TGF-β, a key profibrogenic cytokine,[47,49] whereas treatment with gadolinium chloride to induce macrophage depletion reduced amounts of TGF-β, collagen α 1 (I), and α–smooth muscle actin after bile-duct ligation. In a similar fashion, engulfment of apoptotic bodies by primary or immortalized hepatic stellate cells was shown to trigger their own activation and promote fibrosis.[48] Both processes could be inhibited pharmacologically with antagonists to PI3-K (LY294002) and p38 mitogen-activated protein kinase (SB203580). Phagocytosis of apoptotic bodies by hepatic stellate cells was confirmed by recent in vivo data in three different models of liver fibrosis.[19] The engulfment of apoptotic bodies triggered nicotinamide adenine dinucleotide phosphate oxidase activation and superoxide production. In turn, these reactive oxygen species stimulated further apoptosis and enhanced fibrosis.[55,56]

Further evidence for a link between apoptosis and fibrosis is derived from caspase inhibition studies in animals. The administration of the pan-caspase inhibitor IDN-6556 to rodents subjected to bile-duct ligation resulted in the attenuation of hepatocyte apoptosis, injury, inflammation, and fibrosis.[57] Similar observations were recorded in animals treated with an antagonist to cathepsin B (R-3032).[43]

APOPTOSIS IN NON-ALCOHOLIC FATTY LIVER DISEASE

Hepatic steatosis occurs as a result of abnormal lipid handling by the liver,[58–61] which sensitizes the liver to injury and inflammation.[8] Obese *ob/ob* mice harbor a homozygous mutation in the leptin gene and are unable to synthesize leptin.[62] They develop spontaneous hepatic steatosis and, when injected with anti-Fas antibody, exhibit massive liver injury.[63] Similarly, mice fed the carbohydrate diet for 8 weeks develop macrovesicular steatosis and upregulate expression of the death receptor, Fas.[64] Treatment with Jo2 (anti-Fas antibody) enhanced hepatocyte apoptosis, hepatic injury, chemokine production (CXCL1 and MIP-2), and infiltration of neutrophils. HepG2 cells cultured in the presence of free fatty acids also developed cellular steatosis, upregulated Fas expression, and were vulnerable to the Fas-L.

NASH, a more advanced lesion than simple steatosis, is characterized by increased hepatocyte injury and apoptosis.[9] The same is true in alcoholic steatohepatitis.[50,52,65] Livers obtained from individuals with alcoholic steatohepatitis and livers obtained from individuals with NASH both show enhanced caspase-3 and -7 activation, as well as Fas and TNF-R1 expression. Using immunohistochemical approaches, Ribeiro and coworkers[66,67] noted that individuals with NASH upregulated expression of NF-κB, a transcription factor that promotes the expression of proinflammatory cytokines, death receptors, and death ligands, such as TNF-α. When compared with normal individuals, those with NASH had higher serum levels of TNF-α.[68–70] However, studies using the TNF-R1 knock-out mice indicated that TNF-α was not always critical for the development of NASH.[71–73] Rather, other molecules signaling through the TNF-R superfamily could be involved. For example, livers from patients with excessive alcohol intake show greater induction of TRAIL. When exposed to free fatty acids, hepatocyte-derived cell lines upregulate TRAIL receptors.[74]

Mice fed the methionine-choline–deficient diet are commonly used in the study of NASH because they exhibit histologic similarities to human disease.[75–77] Eight weeks of methionine-choline–deficient treatment result in increased hepatocyte apoptosis by terminal deoxynucleotidyl transferase–mediated deoxyuridine triphosphate nick-end labeling (TUNEL) staining and active-caspase-3 assays (Witek RP and colleagues, Hepatology, in press), with the onset of apoptosis commensurate to the development of steatohepatitis.[75] In the latter study, investigators noted a sustained upregulation of hepatic p53 tumor suppressor gene. P53 activation was directly associated with *Bcl-XL* suppression, Bid cleavage, caspase-3 activation, and p21 induction. Interestingly, p53 is also known to regulate TRAIL-R expression, and its expression is enhanced in patients with NASH[78] and in obese *ob/ob* mice.[79]

Oxidative stress is one of the second hits believed to mediate the progression to NASH.[8,33] When the amount of free radicals (reactive oxygen species) overwhelm buffering capacity, DNA mutations, peroxidation of membranes, and generation of additional free radicals can occur.[80] At low levels, ROS may activate NF-κB to induce synthesis of proinflammatory cytokines and death-receptor expression.[81,82] In a recent study, rats fed the Lieber-DeCarli high-fat diet (71% of energy from fat) for 6 weeks expressed increased rates of hepatocyte apoptosis that mirrored necroinflammatory changes and oxidative stress.[83] The investigators noted higher phosphorylated Jun-N-terminal kinase (JNK) and Bax (proapoptotic protein) compared with controls. JNK activation has been shown to regulate cellular apoptosis,[83–85] possibly through the regulation of the Bcl-2 family. In addition, JNK1 has been shown to promote the development of murine NASH.[77]

The identification of apoptosis as a critical mediator of inflammation and fibrosis in liver disease is important because it may help lead to the design of future drug therapy and development of noninvasive biomarkers (**Fig. 1**). In this respect, we observed a significant reduction in hepatic fibrosis when genetically obese, diabetic *db/db* mice were treated with a pan-caspase inhibitor (Witek RP and colleagues, Hepatology, in press), while Wieckowska and colleagues[10] measured serum cytokeratin-18

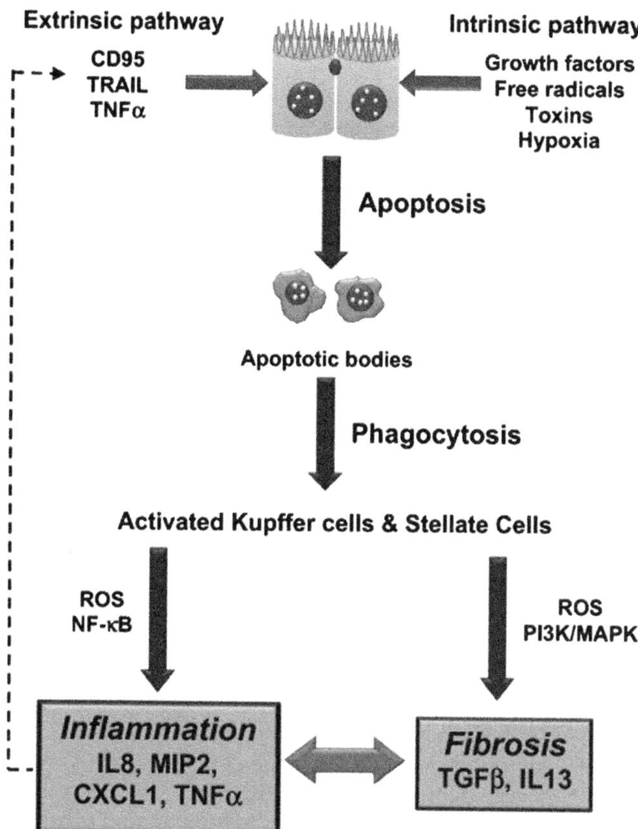

Fig. 1. Hepatocyte apoptosis during liver injury leads to inflammation and fibrosis. During liver injury, ligation of surface death receptors by Fas-L, TNF-α, or TRAIL (extrinsic apoptosis pathway) promotes hepatocyte apoptosis through recruitment of cytoplasmic adaptor molecules and activation of caspase-8. Caspases amplify the apoptotic signaling cascade and commit the hepatocyte to the final execution (apoptosis) pathway (activated caspase-3). The organelle-based (intrinsic apoptosis pathway), non–receptor-mediated apoptosis pathway involves various stimuli (growth factors, cytokines, free radicals, hypoxia, viral infections, and toxins) that disrupt the mitochondrial permeability transition pore and cause the loss of the mitochondrial transmembrane potential. These changes lead to the release of proapoptotic proteins, which initiate the mitochondrial-apoptosis pathway. Clearance of apoptotic bodies occurs through phagocytosis by resident macrophages (Kupffer cells) and hepatic stellate cells. Engulfment of apoptotic bodies is associated with increased ROS-production and activation of transcription factors NF-κB. In turn, this leads to enhanced production of proinflammatory cytokines (TNF-α) and chemokines (MIP-2, IL-8). TNF-α may further drive the extrinsic apoptosis pathway through a feed-forward, paracrine loop. Phagocytosis of apoptotic bodies also induces the production of the profibrogenic cytokines TGF-β and IL-13 via the PI3K and mitogen-activated protein kinase pathways.

fragments (a caspase-3–cleavage product) in human subjects and demonstrated a strong correlation with histologic severity.

CYTOKINES IN STEATOHEPATITIS

In recent decades, investigators have defined the critical roles of proinflammatory cytokines in the pathogenesis of alcoholic steatohepatitis.[50,86] It was noted that patients with severe alcoholic steatohepatitis exhibited high serum levels of TNF-α,[87–89] which correlated with clinical severity. Similar cytokine changes were observed in animal models of alcoholic injury.[90,91] Given that NASH and alcoholic steatohepatitis share common histopathologic features, it is conceivable that similar immunopathogenic mechanisms may be involved in the development of NASH.[86]

Tumor Necrosis Factor α

TNF-α impairs insulin action in vitro and in vivo[92–95] and individuals with insulin resistance show higher serum levels of TNF-α. Administration of TNF-α to individuals also results in impaired insulin sensitivity.[96] The mechanisms responsible for TNF-α effects appear to be related to the sustained activation of inflammatory kinases, such as JNK and inhibitor of K-kinase β (IKKβ).[97] JNK activation inhibits the phosphorylation of insulin receptor substrate 1[98,99] while IKKβ activity leads to the activation of NF-κB and the induction of additional proinflammatory cytokines.[100] Conversely, neutralization of TNF-α improved hepatic insulin resistance in *ob/ob* mice through reductions in JNK and IKKβ activities.[101,102] Similarly, probiotic therapy reduced injury and inflammation in *ob/ob* mice, likely via the downregulation of JNK and IKKβ. TNF-α also modulates the expression of sterol regulatory element binding proteins (SREBP), which are transcription factors involved in regulating enzymes of lipid synthesis.[103] Levels of SREBP-1c are elevated in *ob/ob* mice.[104] Exogenous TNF-α promotes the expression of SREBP-1c[105] while neutralizing antibodies to TNF-α decreases expression of SREBP-1c.

TNF-α expression is upregulated in obesity[106] and serum TNF-α levels are increased in patients with NASH.[68] Gene expression in adipose tissue and liver are similarly enhanced in NASH, and correlated with the stage of disease.[107] More recently, TNF-α polymorphisms have also been noted in individuals with NAFLD compared with the control population.[108,109] Indeed, treatment with metformin and pentoxifylline, drugs that antagonize TNF-α, improve NASH.[110,111] Similar changes in serum and tissue TNF-α levels are observed in animal models of obesity[112] and NASH.[113] Moreover, mice genetically deficient in TNF-R1 are resistant to NASH by the methionine-choline–deficient and high-carbohydrate diets.[71,73] Specifically, TNF-R–deficient mice exhibit reduced Kupffer cell activation and fibrogenesis, suggesting a role of TNF-α in modulating hepatic stellate cell activation.[102,114] More recent work by Yamaguchi and colleagues,[115] however, highlight the possibility that TNF-α alone may be insufficient in the development of fibrosis, as treatment of obese and diabetic *db/db* mice with diacylglycerol acyltransferase 1 antisense oligonucleotides resulted in worse fibrosis despite reductions in the amount of steatosis and TNF-α levels.

The effects of TNF-α may in part be a result of its biologic relationship with adiponectin, an adipose tissue–derived protein. *Ob/ob* mice have low levels of adiponectin compared with TNF-α[116] and the injection of adiponectin to *ob/ob* mice reverses NASH and TNF-α levels. Similar changes were observed in KK-Ay mice, another model of NAFLD.[117,118] Individuals with NASH have lower levels of plasma adiponectin compared with controls.[119,120] Importantly, circulating adiponectin levels may inversely correlate with hepatic inflammation,[107,121] while weight reduction has been shown to increase the ratio of adiponectin to TNF-α and improve NASH.[122,123]

LEPTIN AND TH1/TH2 CYTOKINES IN NON-ALCOHOLIC STEATOHEPATITIS

Leptin is a highly conserved cytokine-like hormone secreted not only by the adipose tissue, but also by activated T cells.[124] Leptin binds to the leptin receptor (Ob-R) that stimulates the Janus-kinase signal transduction and activator of transcription (JAK-STAT) signaling pathways.[125]

Leptin receptors are found on immune cells and leptin has been shown to modulate T cell responses and viability.[126,127] Obese *ob/ob* mice are genetically deficient in leptin[128] and spontaneously develop features of the metabolic syndrome and hepatic steatosis. They also develop thymic atrophy and exhibit changes in neurohumoral factors[129] that lead to the selective reduction in hepatic natural killer T (NKT) cells.[130] Restoration of norepinephrine levels in *ob/ob* mice reduced NKT cell apoptosis and increased NKT cell numbers.[131] NKT cells are critical modulators of the innate and adaptive immune response, and produce both proinflammatory (Th1) cytokine (interferon γ [IFN-γ]) and anti-inflammatory, profibrogenic (Th2) cytokines (IL-4, IL-13).[132] Livers from *ob/ob* mice show significant reductions in IL-4 compared with IFN-γ (Th1 polarization).[130] This may explain their relative resistance to fibrosis despite persistent chronic liver injury. The pro-Th1 milieu would also account for their sensitivity to endotoxin-mediated (lipopolysaccharide) hepatotoxicity,[113] one of the putative second hits in the progression of NAFLD. When *ob/ob* mice are corrected for leptin deficiency, they lose weight and develop less hepatic inflammation. However, they also develop fibrosis,[133–135] thus exhibiting features seen in individuals with progressive NASH. Restoration of leptin levels could also promote fibrogenesis through increases in TGF-β secretion by macrophages.[135,136] Similarly, *ob/ob* mice supplemented with norepinephrine develop less injury and lower amounts of proinflammatory cytokines, but express increased TGF-β expression, hepatic stellate cell activation, and fibrosis.[137] Collectively, the current data suggest that the balance of Th1 and Th2 cytokines in the microenvironment may determine disease outcome.

As hepatic NKT cells are a predominant source of Th2 cytokines, IL-4, and IL-13, depletion of NKT numbers would imply a dearth of profibrogenic factors. NKT cells accumulate in chronic viral hepatitis,[138–140] primary biliary cirrhosiss[141,142] and Wilson disease.[143] Indeed, hepatic and circulating NKT cells from individuals with chronic viral hepatitis show enhanced IL-4 and IL-13 production.[138] IL-13 has been shown to activate hepatic stellate cells via IL-13–Ra2[144] and activate macrophages via the alternative pathway.[145] In the trinitrobenzensulfonic acid model of chronic colitis, IL-13 signaling has been found to initiate a cascade of profibrogenic events that involve TGF-β activation and myofibroblast production of collagen[146]; conversely, antagonism of IL-13 signaling ameliorated murine schistosomiasis hepatic fibrosis.[147] Recent work in our laboratory has shown that wild-type mice with intact leptin signaling possess more NKT cells and exhibit greater fibrosis when treated with the methionine-choline–deficient diet for 8 weeks, and αGalCer-activated NKT cells promote hepatic stellate cell activation in vitro (Syn WK, unpublished data, 2009). Explanted livers from patients with NASH cirrhosis also contain up to fourfold more NKT cells than normal human livers (Syn WK, unpublished data, 2009). Further studies will be needed to determine if NKT-associated cytokines, such as IL-4 and IL-13, regulate NASH progression. The identification of such cytokines could potentially provide novel targets for NASH therapy (**Table 1**).

Table 1
Summary of cytokines in NAFLD

Cytokines	Th1 Proinflammatory	Th2 Profibrogenic	Major Source(s) of Cytokines	Other Known Function(s)
IL-4	−	+	Th2 ymphocytes, NKT	Promotes Th2 differentiation
IL-10	−	−/+	Monocytes, Th2 lymphocytes, (Foxp3) Treg, NKT	Downregulates Th1 cytokine expression; suppresses antigen presentation
IL-13	−	+	Th2 lymphocytes, NKT	Induces secretion of TGF-β; alternative macrophage activation; allergic inflammation; IgE secretion
IFN-γ	+	−	Th1 lymphocytes, NK and NKT	Promotes Th1 and suppresses Th2 differentiation; classical macrophage activation; antiviral and antitumor activity
TNF-α	+	−	Macrophage, lymphoid, and other tissues	Inflammatory, apoptotic activity, cell survival, proliferation and differentiation; via NF-κB, mitogen-activated protein kinase, and caspase activity
Leptin	+	+	Adipose tissue, liver, brain, muscle, T cells	Regulate energy balance; T cell survival and response (Th1 vs Th2 cytokines)
TGF-β	−	+	(Foxp3) Treg, immune cells, stellate and epithelial cells	Apoptosis, cell cycle regulation, angiogenesis; suppress lymphocyte activation (immunosuppression)

Abbreviations: +, pro; −, anti.

SUMMARY

NASH develops in a subgroup of individuals with NAFLD, and differs from simple steatosis with regard to the degree of hepatocyte injury and apoptosis. Hepatocyte apoptosis results in the release of factors that promote the recruitment of inflammatory cells and trigger the deposition of type 1 collagen by hepatic myofibroblasts. Studies have shown that the degree of hepatocyte apoptosis may be assessed by serum measurements of cytokeratin-18 fragments (a caspase-3–cleavage product) in human subjects, and the use of caspase inhibitors may ameliorate the amount of fibrosis in vivo. NASH is also characterized by high levels of proinflammatory cytokines, such as TNF-α, which promote hepatic insulin resistance and drive the progression from simple steatosis to NASH. TNF-α may activate downstream kinases that induce further cytokine production in a feed-forward loop, while attenuating the expression and activity of adiponectin. In aggregate, the balance of Th1 (IFN-γ) and Th2 (IL-4, IL-13) cytokines in the microenvironment may play a critical role in shaping disease outcomes.

REFERENCES

1. Angulo P. Nonalcoholic fatty liver disease. N Engl J Med 2002;346:1221–31.
2. Marchesini G, Bugianesi E, Forlani G, et al. Nonalcoholic fatty liver, steatohepatitis, and the metabolic syndrome. Hepatology 2003;37:917–23.
3. Sheth SG, Gordon FD, Chopra S. Nonalcoholic steatohepatitis. Ann Intern Med 1997;126:137–45.
4. Brunt EM, Janney CG, Di Bisceglie AM, et al. Nonalcoholic steatohepatitis: a proposal for grading and staging the histological lesions. Am J Gastroenterol 1999;94:2467–74.
5. Adams LA, Lymp JF, St Sauver J, et al. The natural history of nonalcoholic fatty liver disease: a population-based cohort study. Gastroenterology 2005;129: 113–21.
6. Matteoni CA, Younossi ZM, Gramlich T, et al. Nonalcoholic fatty liver disease: a spectrum of clinical and pathological severity. Gastroenterology 1999;116: 1413–9.
7. Day CP. Natural history of NAFLD: remarkably benign in the absence of cirrhosis. Gastroenterology 2005;129:375–8.
8. Day CP, James OF. Steatohepatitis: a tale of two "hits". Gastroenterology 1998; 114:842–5.
9. Feldstein AE, Canbay A, Angulo P, et al. Hepatocyte apoptosis and fas expression are prominent features of human nonalcoholic steatohepatitis. Gastroenterology 2003;125:437–43.
10. Wieckowska A, Zein NN, Yerian LM, et al. In vivo assessment of liver cell apoptosis as a novel biomarker of disease severity in nonalcoholic fatty liver disease. Hepatology 2006;44:27–33.
11. Jou J, Choi SS, Diehl AM. Mechanisms of disease progression in nonalcoholic fatty liver disease. Semin Liver Dis 2008;28:370–9.
12. Fan Y, Bergmann A. Distinct mechanisms of apoptosis-induced compensatory proliferation in proliferating and differentiating tissues in the Drosophila eye. Dev Cell 2008;14:399–410.
13. Kerr JF, Wyllie AH, Currie AR. Apoptosis: a basic biological phenomenon with wide-ranging implications in tissue kinetics. Br J Cancer 1972;26:239–57.
14. Elmore S. Apoptosis: a review of programmed cell death. Toxicol Pathol 2007; 35:495–516.

15. Savill J, Fadok V. Corpse clearance defines the meaning of cell death. Nature 2000;407:784–8.
16. Kurosaka K, Takahashi M, Watanabe N, et al. Silent cleanup of very early apoptotic cells by macrophages. J Immunol 2003;171:4672–9.
17. Majno G, Joris I. Apoptosis, oncosis, and necrosis. An overview of cell death. Am J Pathol 1995;146:3–15.
18. Thompson CB. Apoptosis in the pathogenesis and treatment of disease. Science 1995;267:1456–62.
19. Zhan SS, Jiang JX, Wu J, et al. Phagocytosis of apoptotic bodies by hepatic stellate cells induces NADPH oxidase and is associated with liver fibrosis in vivo. Hepatology 2006;43:435–43.
20. Canbay A, Higuchi H, Bronk SF, et al. Fas enhances fibrogenesis in the bile duct ligated mouse: a link between apoptosis and fibrosis. Gastroenterology 2002; 123:1323–30.
21. Canbay A, Friedman S, Gores GJ. Apoptosis: the nexus of liver injury and fibrosis. Hepatology 2004;39:273–8.
22. Green DR, Reed JC. Mitochondria and apoptosis. Science 1998;281:1309–12.
23. Thornberry NA. Caspases: key mediators of apoptosis. Chem Biol 1998;5: R97–103.
24. Faubion WA, Gores GJ. Death receptors in liver biology and pathobiology. Hepatology 1999;29:1–4.
25. Locksley RM, Killeen N, Lenardo MJ. The TNF and TNF receptor superfamilies: integrating mammalian biology. Cell 2001;104:487–501.
26. Galle PR, Krammer PH. CD95-induced apoptosis in human liver disease. Semin Liver Dis 1998;18:141–51.
27. Hsu H, Xiong J, Goeddel DV. The TNF receptor 1–associated protein TRADD signals cell death and NF-kappa B activation. Cell 1995;81:495–504.
28. Wajant H. The Fas signaling pathway: more than a paradigm. Science 2002;296: 1635–6.
29. Kischkel FC, Hellbardt S, Behrmann I, et al. Cytotoxicity-dependent APO-1 (Fas/ CD95)–associated proteins form a death-inducing signaling complex (DISC) with the receptor. EMBO J 1995;14:5579–88.
30. Ogasawara J, Watanabe-Fukunaga R, Adachi M, et al. Lethal effect of the anti-Fas antibody in mice. Nature 1993;364:806–9.
31. Biancone L, Martino AD, Orlandi V, et al. Development of inflammatory angiogenesis by local stimulation of Fas in vivo. J Exp Med 1997;186:147–52.
32. Miwa K, Asano M, Horai R, et al. Caspase 1-independent IL-1beta release and inflammation induced by the apoptosis inducer Fas ligand. Nat Med 1998;4: 1287–92.
33. Syn WK, Teaberry V, Choi SS, et al. Similarities and differences in the pathogenesis of alcoholic and nonalcoholic steatohepatitis. Semin Liver Dis 2009; 29:200–10.
34. Lalor PF, Faint J, Aarbodem Y, et al. The role of cytokines and chemokines in the development of steatohepatitis. Semin Liver Dis 2007;27:173–93.
35. Hubscher SG. Histological assessment of nonalcoholic fatty liver disease. Histopathology 2006;49:450–65.
36. Jaeschke H. Inflammation in response to hepatocellular apoptosis. Hepatology 2002;35:964–6.
37. Maher JJ, Scott MK, Saito JM, et al. Adenovirus-mediated expression of cytokine-induced neutrophil chemoattractant in rat liver induces a neutrophilic hepatitis. Hepatology 1997;25:624–30.

38. Lawson JA, Fisher MA, Simmons CA, et al. Parenchymal cell apoptosis as a signal for sinusoidal sequestration and transendothelial migration of neutrophils in murine models of endotoxin and Fas-antibody-induced liver injury. Hepatology 1998;28:761–7.
39. Faouzi S, Burckhardt BE, Hanson JC, et al. Anti-Fas induces hepatic chemokines and promotes inflammation by an NF-kappa B-independent, caspase-3–dependent pathway. J Biol Chem 2001;276:49077–82.
40. Lauber K, Bohn E, Krober SM, et al. Apoptotic cells induce migration of phagocytes via caspase-3–mediated release of a lipid attraction signal. Cell 2003;113:717–30.
41. Rogers HW, Callery MP, Deck B, et al. Listeria monocytogenes induces apoptosis of infected hepatocytes. J Immunol 1996;156:679–84.
42. Ebe Y, Hasegawa G, Takatsuka H, et al. The role of Kupffer cells and regulation of neutrophil migration into the liver by macrophage inflammatory protein-2 in primary listeriosis in mice. Pathol Int 1999;49:519–32.
43. Canbay A, Guicciardi ME, Higuchi H, et al. Cathepsin B inactivation attenuates hepatic injury and fibrosis during cholestasis. J Clin Invest 2003;112:152–9.
44. Chen JJ, Sun Y, Nabel GJ. Regulation of the proinflammatory effects of Fas ligand (CD95L). Science 1998;282:1714–7.
45. Jaeschke H, Fisher MA, Lawson JA, et al. Activation of caspase 3 (CPP32)–like proteases is essential for TNF-alpha–induced hepatic parenchymal cell apoptosis and neutrophil-mediated necrosis in a murine endotoxin shock model. J Immunol 1998;160:3480–6.
46. Kiener PA, Davis PM, Rankin BM, et al. Human monocytic cells contain high levels of intracellular Fas ligand: rapid release following cellular activation. J Immunol 1997;159:1594–8.
47. Geske FJ, Monks J, Lehman L, et al. The role of the macrophage in apoptosis: hunter, gatherer, and regulator. Int J Hematol 2002;76:16–26.
48. Canbay A, Taimr P, Torok N, et al. Apoptotic body engulfment by a human stellate cell line is profibrogenic. Lab Invest 2003;83:655–63.
49. Canbay A, Feldstein AE, Higuchi H, et al. Kupffer cell engulfment of apoptotic bodies stimulates death ligand and cytokine expression. Hepatology 2003;38:1188–98.
50. Ashkenazi A, Dixit VM. Death receptors: signaling and modulation. Science 1998;281:1305–8.
51. Ziol M, Tepper M, Lohez M, et al. Clinical and biological relevance of hepatocyte apoptosis in alcoholic hepatitis. J Hepatol 2001;34:254–60.
52. Natori S, Rust C, Stadheim LM, et al. Hepatocyte apoptosis is a pathologic feature of human alcoholic hepatitis. J Hepatol 2001;34:248–53.
53. Jaeschke H. Neutrophil-mediated tissue injury in alcoholic hepatitis. Alcohol 2002;27:23–7.
54. Miyoshi H, Rust C, Roberts PJ, et al. Hepatocyte apoptosis after bile duct ligation in the mouse involves Fas. Gastroenterology 1999;117:669–77.
55. Garcia-Trevijano ER, Iraburu MJ, Fontana L, et al. Transforming growth factor beta1 induces the expression of alpha1(I) procollagen mRNA by a hydrogen peroxide-C/EBPbeta-dependent mechanism in rat hepatic stellate cells. Hepatology 1999;29:960–70.
56. Nieto N, Friedman SL, Greenwel P, et al. CYP2E1-mediated oxidative stress induces collagen type I expression in rat hepatic stellate cells. Hepatology 1999;30:987–96.

57. Canbay A, Feldstein A, Baskin-Bey E, et al. The caspase inhibitor IDN-6556 attenuates hepatic injury and fibrosis in the bile duct ligated mouse. J Pharmacol Exp Ther 2004;308:1191–6.
58. Diraison F, Moulin P, Beylot M. Contribution of hepatic de novo lipogenesis and reesterification of plasma non esterified fatty acids to plasma triglyceride synthesis during nonalcoholic fatty liver disease. Diabetes Metab 2003;29:478–85.
59. Charlton M, Sreekumar R, Rasmussen D, et al. Apolipoprotein synthesis in nonalcoholic steatohepatitis. Hepatology 2002;35:898–904.
60. Miele L, Grieco A, Armuzzi A, et al. Hepatic mitochondrial beta-oxidation in patients with nonalcoholic steatohepatitis assessed by 13C-octanoate breath test. Am J Gastroenterol 2003;98:2335–6.
61. Musso G, Gambino R, Cassader M. Recent insights into hepatic lipid metabolism in nonalcoholic fatty liver disease (NAFLD). Prog Lipid Res 2009;48:1–26.
62. Friedman JM, Leibel RL, Siegel DS, et al. Molecular mapping of the mouse *ob* mutation. Genomics 1991;11:1054–62.
63. Siebler J, Schuchmann M, Strand S, et al. Enhanced sensitivity to CD95-induced apoptosis in *ob/ob* mice. Dig Dis Sci 2007;52:2396–402.
64. Feldstein AE, Canbay A, Guicciardi ME, et al. Diet associated hepatic steatosis sensitizes to Fas mediated liver injury in mice. J Hepatol 2003;39:978–83.
65. Ribeiro PS, Cortez-Pinto H, Sola S, et al. Hepatocyte apoptosis, expression of death receptors, and activation of NF-kappaB in the liver of nonalcoholic and alcoholic steatohepatitis patients. Am J Gastroenterol 2004;99:1708–17.
66. Ghosh S, May MJ, Kopp EB. NF-kappa B and Rel proteins: evolutionarily conserved mediators of immune responses. Annu Rev Immunol 1998;16:225–60.
67. Green DR. Overview: apoptotic signaling pathways in the immune system. Immunol Rev 2003;193:5–9.
68. Wigg AJ, Roberts-Thomson IC, Dymock RB, et al. The role of small intestinal bacterial overgrowth, intestinal permeability, endotoxaemia, and tumour necrosis factor alpha in the pathogenesis of nonalcoholic steatohepatitis. Gut 2001;48:206–11.
69. Abiru S, Migita K, Maeda Y, et al. Serum cytokine and soluble cytokine receptor levels in patients with nonalcoholic steatohepatitis. Liver Int 2006;26:39–45.
70. Diehl AM, Li ZP, Lin HZ, et al. Cytokines and the pathogenesis of nonalcoholic steatohepatitis. Gut 2005;54:303–6.
71. Dela Pena A, Leclercq I, Field J, et al. NF-kappaB activation, rather than TNF, mediates hepatic inflammation in a murine dietary model of steatohepatitis. Gastroenterology 2005;129:1663–74.
72. Memon RA, Grunfeld C, Feingold KR. TNF-alpha is not the cause of fatty liver disease in obese diabetic mice. Nat Med 2001;7:2–3.
73. Deng QG, She H, Cheng JH, et al. Steatohepatitis induced by intragastric overfeeding in mice. Hepatology 2005;42:905–14.
74. Malhi H, Barreyro FJ, Isomoto H, et al. Free fatty acids sensitise hepatocytes to TRAIL mediated cytotoxicity. Gut 2007;56:1124–31.
75. Farrell GC, Larter CZ, Hou JY, et al. Apoptosis in experimental NASH is associated with p53 activation and TRAIL receptor expression. J Gastroenterol Hepatol 2009;24:443–52.
76. Larter CZ, Yeh MM. Animal models of NASH: getting both pathology and metabolic context right. J Gastroenterol Hepatol 2008;23:1635–48.
77. Schattenberg JM, Singh R, Wang Y, et al. JNK1 but not JNK2 promotes the development of steatohepatitis in mice. Hepatology 2006;43:163–72.

78. Panasiuk A, Dzieciol J, Panasiuk B, et al. Expression of p53, Bax and Bcl-2 proteins in hepatocytes in nonalcoholic fatty liver disease. World J Gastroenterol 2006;12: 6198–202.
79. Yahagi N, Shimano H, Matsuzaka T, et al. P53 involvement in the pathogenesis of fatty liver disease. J Biol Chem 2004;279:20571–5.
80. Mansouri A, Fromenty B, Berson A, et al. Multiple hepatic mitochondrial DNA deletions suggest premature oxidative aging in alcoholic patients. J Hepatol 1997;27:96–102.
81. Cao Q, Mak KM, Lieber CS. Cytochrome P4502E1 primes macrophages to increase TNF-alpha production in response to lipopolysaccharide. Am J Physiol Gastrointest Liver Physiol 2005;289:G95–107.
82. Boden G, She P, Mozzoli M, et al. Free fatty acids produce insulin resistance and activate the proinflammatory nuclear factor-kappaB pathway in rat liver. Diabetes 2005;54:3458–65.
83. Wang Y, Ausman LM, Russell RM, et al. Increased apoptosis in high-fat diet-induced nonalcoholic steatohepatitis in rats is associated with c-Jun NH2-terminal kinase activation and elevated proapoptotic Bax. J Nutr 2008;138: 1866–71.
84. Davis RJ. Signal transduction by the JNK group of MAP kinases. Cell 2000;103: 239–52.
85. Marderstein EL, Bucher B, Guo Z, et al. Protection of rat hepatocytes from apoptosis by inhibition of c-Jun N-terminal kinase. Surgery 2003;134:280–4.
86. Tilg H, Diehl AM. Cytokines in alcoholic and nonalcoholic steatohepatitis. N Engl J Med 2000;343:1467–76.
87. Bird GL, Sheron N, Goka AK, et al. Increased plasma tumor necrosis factor in severe alcoholic hepatitis. Ann Intern Med 1990;112:917–20.
88. McClain CJ, Barve S, Barve S, et al. Tumor necrosis factor and alcoholic liver disease. Alcohol Clin Exp Res 1998;22:248S–52S.
89. McClain CJ, Cohen DA. Increased tumor necrosis factor production by monocytes in alcoholic hepatitis. Hepatology 1989;9:349–51.
90. Iimuro Y, Gallucci RM, Luster MI, et al. Antibodies to tumor necrosis factor alfa attenuate hepatic necrosis and inflammation caused by chronic exposure to ethanol in the rat. Hepatology 1997;26:1530–7.
91. Yin M, Wheeler MD, Kono H, et al. Essential role of tumor necrosis factor alpha in alcohol-induced liver injury in mice. Gastroenterology 1999;117: 942–52.
92. Peraldi P, Spiegelman B. TNF-alpha and insulin resistance: summary and future prospects. Mol Cell Biochem 1998;182:169–75.
93. Wajant H, Pfizenmaier K, Scheurich P. Tumor necrosis factor signaling. Cell Death Differ 2003;10:45–65.
94. Peraldi P, Hotamisligil GS, Buurman WA, et al. Tumor necrosis factor (TNF)-alpha inhibits insulin signaling through stimulation of the p55 TNF receptor and activation of sphingomyelinase. J Biol Chem 1996;271:13018–22.
95. Hotamisligil GS, Peraldi P, Budavari A, et al. IRS-1–mediated inhibition of insulin receptor tyrosine kinase activity in TNF-alpha– and obesity-induced insulin resistance. Science 1996;271:665–8.
96. Plomgaard P, Bouzakri K, Krogh-Madsen R, et al. Tumor necrosis factor–alpha induces skeletal muscle insulin resistance in healthy human subjects via inhibition of Akt substrate 160 phosphorylation. Diabetes 2005;54:2939–45.
97. Shoelson SE, Lee J, Goldfine AB. Inflammation and insulin resistance. J Clin Invest 2006;116:1793–801.

98. Aguirre V, Uchida T, Yenush L, et al. The c-Jun NH(2)-terminal kinase promotes insulin resistance during association with insulin receptor substrate-1 and phosphorylation of Ser(307). J Biol Chem 2000;275:9047–54.
99. Aguirre V, Werner ED, Giraud J, et al. Phosphorylation of Ser307 in insulin receptor substrate-1 blocks interactions with the insulin receptor and inhibits insulin action. J Biol Chem 2002;277:1531–7.
100. Steinberg GR. Inflammation in obesity is the common link between defects in fatty acid metabolism and insulin resistance. Cell Cycle 2007;6:888–94.
101. Uysal KT, Wiesbrock SM, Marino MW, et al. Protection from obesity-induced insulin resistance in mice lacking TNF-alpha function. Nature 1997;389:610–4.
102. Li Z, Yang S, Lin H, et al. Probiotics and antibodies to TNF inhibit inflammatory activity and improve nonalcoholic fatty liver disease. Hepatology 2003;37:343–50.
103. Weber LW, Boll M, Stampfl A. Maintaining cholesterol homeostasis: sterol regulatory element-binding proteins. World J Gastroenterol 2004;10:3081–7.
104. Shimomura I, Bashmakov Y, Horton JD. Increased levels of nuclear SREBP-1c associated with fatty livers in two mouse models of diabetes mellitus. J Biol Chem 1999;274:30028–32.
105. Endo M, Masaki T, Seike M, et al. TNF-alpha induces hepatic steatosis in mice by enhancing gene expression of sterol regulatory element binding protein-1c (SREBP-1c). Exp Biol Med (Maywood) 2007;232:614–21.
106. Kern PA, Saghizadeh M, Ong JM, et al. The expression of tumor necrosis factor in human adipose tissue. Regulation by obesity, weight loss, and relationship to lipoprotein lipase. J Clin Invest 1995;95:2111–9.
107. Crespo J, Cayon A, Fernandez-Gil P, et al. Gene expression of tumor necrosis factor alpha and TNF-receptors, p55 and p75, in nonalcoholic steatohepatitis patients. Hepatology 2001;34:1158–63.
108. Valenti L, Fracanzani AL, Dongiovanni P, et al. Tumor necrosis factor alpha promoter polymorphisms and insulin resistance in nonalcoholic fatty liver disease. Gastroenterology 2002;122:274–80.
109. Tokushige K, Takakura M, Tsuchiya-Matsushita N, et al. Influence of TNF gene polymorphisms in Japanese patients with NASH and simple steatosis. J Hepatol 2007;46:1104–10.
110. Adams LA, Zein CO, Angulo P, et al. A pilot trial of pentoxifylline in nonalcoholic steatohepatitis. Am J Gastroenterol 2004;99:2365–8.
111. Marchesini G, Brizi M, Bianchi G, et al. Metformin in nonalcoholic steatohepatitis. Lancet 2001;358:893–4.
112. Koteish A, Diehl AM. Animal models of steatosis. Semin Liver Dis 2001;21:89–104.
113. Yang SQ, Lin HZ, Lane MD, et al. Obesity increases sensitivity to endotoxin liver injury: implications for the pathogenesis of steatohepatitis. Proc Natl Acad Sci U S A 1997;94:2557–62.
114. Carter-Kent C, Zein NN, Feldstein AE. Cytokines in the pathogenesis of fatty liver and disease progression to steatohepatitis: implications for treatment. Am J Gastroenterol 2008;103:1036–42.
115. Yamaguchi K, Yang L, McCall S, et al. Diacylglycerol acyltranferase 1 anti-sense oligonucleotides reduce hepatic fibrosis in mice with nonalcoholic steatohepatitis. Hepatology 2008;47:625–35.
116. Xu A, Wang Y, Keshaw H, et al. The fat-derived hormone adiponectin alleviates alcoholic and nonalcoholic fatty liver diseases in mice. J Clin Invest 2003;112:91–100.

117. Masaki T, Chiba S, Tatsukawa H, et al. Adiponectin protects LPS-induced liver injury through modulation of TNF-alpha in KK-Ay obese mice. Hepatology 2004;40:177–84.
118. Yamauchi T, Kamon J, Waki H, et al. The fat-derived hormone adiponectin reverses insulin resistance associated with both lipoatrophy and obesity. Nat Med 2001;7:941–6.
119. Hui JM, Hodge A, Farrell GC, et al. Beyond insulin resistance in NASH: TNF-alpha or adiponectin? Hepatology 2004;40:46–54.
120. Musso G, Gambino R, Biroli G, et al. Hypoadiponectinemia predicts the severity of hepatic fibrosis and pancreatic Beta-cell dysfunction in nondiabetic nonobese patients with nonalcoholic steatohepatitis. Am J Gastroenterol 2005;100:2438–46.
121. Kamada Y, Tamura S, Kiso S, et al. Enhanced carbon tetrachloride–induced liver fibrosis in mice lacking adiponectin. Gastroenterology 2003;125:1796–807.
122. Gabriely I, Barzilai N. Surgical removal of visceral adipose tissue: effects on insulin action. Curr Diab Rep 2003;3:201–6.
123. Esposito K, Pontillo A, Di Palo C, et al. Effect of weight loss and lifestyle changes on vascular inflammatory markers in obese women: a randomized trial. JAMA 2003;289:1799–804.
124. Sanna V, Di Giacomo A, La Cava A, et al. Leptin surge precedes onset of autoimmune encephalomyelitis and correlates with development of pathogenic T cell responses. J Clin Invest 2003;111:241–50.
125. Hoteit MA, Anania FA. Treatment of fibrosis in nonalcoholic fatty liver disease. Curr Gastroenterol Rep 2007;9:47–53.
126. Lord GM, Matarese G, Howard JK, et al. Leptin modulates the T-cell immune response and reverses starvation-induced immunosuppression. Nature 1998; 394:897–901.
127. Faggioni R, Jones-Carson J, Reed DA, et al. Leptin-deficient (*ob/ob*) mice are protected from T cell–mediated hepatotoxicity: role of tumor necrosis factor alpha and IL-18. Proc Natl Acad Sci U S A 2000;97:2367–72.
128. Zhang Y, Proenca R, Maffei M, et al. Positional cloning of the mouse obese gene and its human homologue. Nature 1994;372:425–32.
129. Cohen P, Zhao C, Cai X, et al. Selective deletion of leptin receptor in neurons leads to obesity. J Clin Invest 2001;108:1113–21.
130. Guebre-Xabier M, Yang S, Lin HZ, et al. Altered hepatic lymphocyte subpopulations in obesity-related murine fatty livers: potential mechanism for sensitization to liver damage. Hepatology 2000;31:633–40.
131. Li Z, Oben JA, Yang S, et al. Norepinephrine regulates hepatic innate immune system in leptin-deficient mice with nonalcoholic steatohepatitis. Hepatology 2004;40:434–41.
132. Kronenberg M. Toward an understanding of NKT cell biology: progress and paradoxes. Annu Rev Immunol 2005;23:877–900.
133. Saxena NK, Ikeda K, Rockey DC, et al. Leptin in hepatic fibrosis: evidence for increased collagen production in stellate cells and lean littermates of *ob/ob* mice. Hepatology 2002;35:762–71.
134. Ikejima K, Takei Y, Honda H, et al. Leptin receptor–mediated signaling regulates hepatic fibrogenesis and remodeling of extracellular matrix in the rat. Gastroenterology 2002;122:1399–410.
135. Leclercq IA, Farrell GC, Schriemer R, et al. Leptin is essential for the hepatic fibrogenic response to chronic liver injury. J Hepatol 2002;37:206–13.
136. Wang J, Leclercq I, Brymora JM, et al. Kupffer cells mediate leptin-induced liver fibrosis. Gastroenterology 2009 [Epub ahead of print].

137. Commins SP, Marsh DJ, Thomas SA, et al. Norepinephrine is required for leptin effects on gene expression in brown and white adipose tissue. Endocrinology 1999;140:4772–8.
138. de Lalla C, Galli G, Aldrighetti L, et al. Production of profibrotic cytokines by invariant NKT cells characterizes cirrhosis progression in chronic viral hepatitis. J Immunol 2004;173:1417–25.
139. Nuti S, Rosa D, Valiante NM, et al. Dynamics of intra-hepatic lymphocytes in chronic hepatitis C: enrichment for Valpha24+ T cells and rapid elimination of effector cells by apoptosis. Eur J Immunol 1998;28:3448–55.
140. Durante-Mangoni E, Wang R, Shaulov A, et al. Hepatic CD1d expression in hepatitis C virus infection and recognition by resident proinflammatory CD1d-reactive T cells. J Immunol 2004;173:2159–66.
141. Kita H, Naidenko OV, Kronenberg M, et al. Quantitation and phenotypic analysis of natural killer T cells in primary biliary cirrhosis using a human CD1d tetramer. Gastroenterology 2002;123:1031–43.
142. Harada K, Isse K, Tsuneyama K, et al. Accumulating CD57 + CD3 + natural killer T cells are related to intrahepatic bile duct lesions in primary biliary cirrhosis. Liver Int 2003;23:94–100.
143. Kinebuchi M, Matsuura A, Ohya K, et al. Contribution of Va24Vb11 natural killer T cells in Wilsonian hepatitis. Clin Exp Immunol 2005;139:144–51.
144. Shimamura T, Fujisawa T, Husain SR, et al. Novel role of IL-13 in fibrosis induced by nonalcoholic steatohepatitis and its amelioration by IL-13R-directed cytotoxin in a rat model. J Immunol 2008;181:4656–65.
145. Deepak P, Kumar S, Acharya A. Interleukin-13–induced type II polarization of inflammatory macrophages is mediated through suppression of nuclear factor-kappaB and preservation of IkappaBalpha in a T cell lymphoma. Clin Exp Immunol 2007;149:378–86.
146. Fichtner-Feigl S, Young CA, Kitani A, et al. IL-13 signaling via IL-13R alpha2 induces major downstream fibrogenic factors mediating fibrosis in chronic TNBS colitis. Gastroenterology 2008;135:2003–13, 2013, e2001–e2007.
147. Chiaramonte MG, Cheever AW, Malley JD, et al. Studies of murine schistosomiasis reveal interleukin-13 blockade as a treatment for established and progressive liver fibrosis. Hepatology 2001;34:273–82.

Endoplasmic Reticulum Stress and the Unfolded Protein Response

Ashwani Kapoor, MBBS, Arun J. Sanyal, MBBS, MD*

KEYWORDS

• Non-alcoholic fatty liver disease • Non-alcoholic steatohepatitis
• Fatty liver • Unfolded protein response • ER stress
• Eukaryotic initiation factor • Inflammation
• Metabolic syndrome

The endoplasmic reticulum (ER) is a key cellular organelle that is involved in protein homeostasis. Following synthesis, proteins are exported from the ER to various subcellular locations for use or export. This process involves recognition of specific motifs by the molecular transporters required to take the synthesized proteins to their destination. The primary structure of the protein determines both the specific motifs for binding to targets and its' folding, which determines the availability of the motifs for binding to its targets. Therefore, a key function of the ER is to ensure the fidelity of protein synthesis and processing so that they are folded appropriately, which allows them to be transported to their cellular destination. This is accomplished by several energy-requiring steps within the ER which have been reviewed in depth elsewhere.[1]

When the ability of the ER to ensure fidelity of protein synthesis is overwhelmed by increased protein synthetic drive, primary dysfunction of the ER, or lack of ATP, unfolded proteins accumulates within the ER. The unfolded protein response (UPR) is a fundamental cellular process that is triggered by the accumulation of unfolded proteins within the ER, a phenomenon also referred to as the ER stress response.[2] The goal of the UPR is to restore homeostasis and allow the cell to adapt to the stressor event. If homeostasis is not restored, alternate pathways leading to apoptosis are triggered. The UPR has been shown to be involved in both normal physiologic functions and the cellular response to a host of pathologic states. In this article, we

This manuscript is not under consideration for publication elsewhere. It was supported in part by a grant from the National Institutes of Health to Dr. Arun Sanyal, K24 DK 02755-09.
Department of Internal Medicine, Division of Gastroenterology, Hepatology and Nutrition, Virginia Commonwealth University School of Medicine, 1200 East Broad Street, MCV Box 980341, Richmond, VA 23298-0341, USA
* Corresponding author.
E-mail address: asanyal@mcvh-vcu.edu (A.J. Sanyal).

Clin Liver Dis 13 (2009) 581–590
doi:10.1016/j.cld.2009.07.004
1089-3261/09/$ – see front matter. Published by Elsevier Inc.

will review the pathways by which the UPR unfolds and its potential role in the development and progression of non-alcoholic fatty liver disease (NAFLD).

PATHWAYS OF THE UPR

When the normal mechanisms within the ER that ensure fidelity of protein folding are disturbed, unfolded proteins accumulates in the ER. Many known triggers for ER dysfunction lead to disturbances in protein folding in the ER. These include viral infections, glucose deprivation, changes in redox state, increased cholesterol to phospholipid ratio in the ER membrane, and decreased ATP stores.[3–7] The initial response is to correct this by inhibition of protein synthesis and increased degradation of unfolded protein by way of proteasomes. Simultaneously, adaptive genes are activated which improve protein folding and help the cell adapt to the trigger for UPR. Glucose regulated protein 78/BiP is considered the master regulator of the UPR and is a chaperone protein that is resident within the ER. BiP binds intraluminal proteins on one hand and a number of transmembrane mediators of the UPR on the other, thereby anchoring the latter to the ER (**Fig. 1**). When unfolded proteins accumulate within the ER, BiP is preferentially bound to these proteins, which release the previously bound transmembrane mediators from the ER membrane—thereby activating the UPR.[8]

The PKR-like ER Kinase Pathway

The PKR-like ER kinase (PERK) pathway is designed to produce translational arrest of protein synthesis and help further accumulation of unfolded proteins in the ER. PERK is a Ser/Thr transmembrane kinase that is located on the ER membrane.[8] It is anchored to the ER by interaction with another protein BiP, which resides in the lumen of the ER. Upon accumulation of unfolded proteins in the ER, BiP binds to the unfolded proteins, thus releasing PERK in to the cytoplasm and activating PERK in the process.[9]

Upon activation, PERK oligomerizes and phosphorylates its targets. One target is the eukaryotic initiation factor-2α (eIF-2α).[10,11] eIF-2α Phosphorylation produces a general translational arrest of protein synthesis.[10,11] Normally, during initiation of protein synthesis, GTP-eIF 2α binds to the 40 S ribosome and methionine initiator tRNA forming a ternary complex. After initiation, GDP-eIF 2α is released. For GDP-eIF 2α to be recycled, eIF 2B is required. Phosphorylated eIF 2α at serine 51 binds

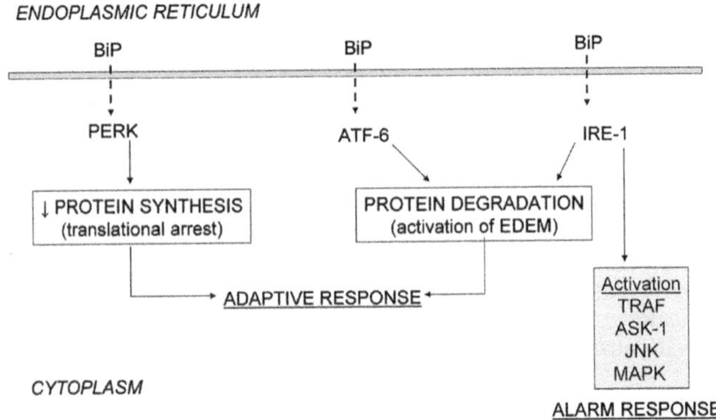

Fig. 1. UPR.

to eIF 2B with high affinity. Thus, eIF 2B cannot recycle GDP-eIF 2α thereby leading to translational arrest.[12]

While the translation of most proteins is arrested by phosphorylation of eIF-2α, some key mRNA paradoxically continue to be translated. Activating transcription factor-4 (ATF4) is such a transcriptional factor and belongs to the bZIP (basic region leucine zipper) family.[10] ATF 4 regulates C/EBP homologous protein (CHOP) promoter by activating it. CHOP can both promote apoptosis and increase expression of the growth arrest and DNA damage 34 (GADD 34), a key survival factor.[13] With recovery from UPR, there is progressive increase in GADD34, which dephosphorylates eIF-2α and returns the system to baseline. Another negative regulator of the PERK arm is $P58^{IPK}$, a heat shock protein 40 family member. It inhibits PERK by inactivating kinase domain of PERK.[14]

Another substrate for PERK is the transcription factor NF-E2-related factor 2 (Nrf2). NrF2 is normally present in the cytosol complexed with Keltch-like ECH-associating protein 1 (Keap-1).[15] Upon phosphorylation, NrF2 dissociates from Keap-1 and translocates to the nucleus. In the nucleus, it binds to the DNA domain called antioxidant response element, which increases transcription of the antioxidant proteins and serves as transcriptional factors that are critical for the cellular response to oxidative stress a known trigger of the UPR.[16] Thus, the PERK pathway represents a major mechanism by which the UPR attempts to restore homeostasis or condemn the cell to death under conditions of ER stress.

The ATF6 Pathway

ATF6 is a bZIP motif-containing transcription factor bound to the ER membrane. ATF 6 has two isoforms, ATF 6α and ATF 6β. Both are ubiquitously expressed. It is activated by its release from BiP, which allows it to translocate to the Golgi system.[17,18] There, it is cleaved by site proteases (S1 and S2 proteases) releasing the active fragments in to the cytoplasm from where it is transported to the nucleus.[19] In the nucleus, the active fragments of ATF6 bind specific sequences in promoter regions, ER stress response elements, of its target genes. A key target of ATF6 is the x-box binding protein-1 (XBP-1).[20]

The Inositol-requiring Enzyme-1 Pathway

Inositol-requiring enzyme (IRE) is an ER resident type I transmembrane protein with a N-terminal ER stress-sensing domain, serine/threonine kinase domain and C-terminal endoribonuclease domain. IRE 1 has two homologs, IRE 1α (present in all cells) and IRE1β (found only in gut).[21] Accumulation of unfolded proteins leads to binding of BiP to such proteins and releasing IRE-1. It is further oligomerized and undergoes autophosphorylation, which leads to its activation.[9]

IRE 1 has RNase activity; this allows it to produce an unconventional cytoplasm splicing of the XBP-1 before messenger RNA (XBP-1 U mRNA) forms spliced XBP-1 (s-XBP-1).[22] sXBP-1 functions as transcription factor and activates transcription of ER chaperones, ER-associated degradation (ERAD) components, by binding to ER stress elements and UPR. This is an important step in the UPR because unspliced XBP-1 protein represses expression of ER chaperones required to direct the unfolded proteins for proteosomal degradation and splicing of XBP-1 is a required step to activate ER degradation enhancing a mannosidases (EDEM), which mediate ERAD of proteins.

ERAD decreases the protein load by degrading unfolded proteins. ERAD is accomplished in four steps. First, mannose residues in the unfolded proteins are recognized by ER degradation-enhancing EDEM proteins. Then it is translocated through translocon sec61 to the cytosol. In the cytosol, unfolded proteins are ubiquitinated by the E1-E2-E3 ubiquitin system, which targets the protein for proteosomal degradation.[23,24]

To date, three types of EDEM proteins, EDEM 1–3, have been identified.[25–27] They all have mannosidase activity but whereas EDEM 1 and EDEM 2 cannot cleave mannose moieties attached to the α1 and α2 positions of glycoproteins, EDEM 3 can perform this function.[25] The relative importance of these forms of EDEM in health and under various disease conditions remain to be clarified.

Alarm Pathways

Another important function of the IRE-1 pathway is the activation of alarm pathways that drive downstream activation of inflammation and apoptosis. This is a critical function of the UPR because if the adaptive responses (inhibition of protein synthesis and increased protein degradation) do not restore homeostasis, the cell is condemned to death. This function is mediated by IRE-1 activation of ASK-1, which further activates a number of key stress response pathways such as mitogen-activated protein kinase (MAP kinase) and c-Jun N terminal kinase (JNK).[28] JNK is a particularly important downstream target of this pathway because it regulates activator protein (AP-1) and NF-κβ activation.[29] These latter transcriptional factors regulate pathways that drive inflammation and worsen insulin resistance.

Another major outcome of the failure of reestablishing homeostasis in the ER and the cell is the activation of apoptotic pathways. All three arms of UPR play roles in inducing apoptosis. Both ATF4, which is downstream of eiF-2α in the PERK pathway and ATF6 activate CHOP, which has proapoptotic activity.[30] IRE-1, by way pf s-XBP-1, also increases the expression of p58, which modulates PERK activity and, therefore, CHOP expression.[31] The IRE-1 pathway can also activate apoptosis by recruiting the adaptor protein TRAF2, which recruits the apoptosis signaling kinase-1 (ASK-1), which, in turn, activates JNK. JNK activates the proapoptotic factor Bim and inhibits the antiapoptotic factor BCL2-family proteins.[32] These trigger caspase activation, which results in apoptosis.[33,34]

EVIDENCE THAT UPR IS ACTIVATED IN NAFLD

Several lines of evidence indicate that the UPR is activated in NAFLD. In early studies, it was noted that feeding increased amounts of saturated fat to rat increased insulin resistance and induced UPR.[35] It was also noted that in animal models of steatohepatitis, mainly induced by a methionine-fed, choline-deficient diet (MCD), there was activation of JNK1 and CHOP—two products that are activated by the UPR.[36] Moreover, hyperhomocysteinemia produced ER stress and activated the UPR in cultured hepatocytes.[37] Finally, NAFLD is associated with several factors known to induce UPR, such as hyperglycemia, mitochondrial injury that depletes ATP, hypercholesterolemia, depletion of phosphatidylcholine, and oxidative stress.[38–40]

We have recently shown that humans with NAFLD show evidence of activated UPR.[41] In this study we examined the expression of the UPR pathways in three groups of subjects: (1) controls with the metabolic syndrome but a normal liver biopsy and liver enzymes, (2) those with biopsy-proven NAFLD, and (3) those with biopsy-proven non-alcoholic steatohepatitis (NASH). Twenty-one subjects with NAFLD and NASH were studied and compared with 17 subjects with normal liver biopsy. The levels of phosphorylated eiF-2α were increased in subjects with NAFLD and NASH compared with controls. Despite this increase, the majority of subjects did not show an increment in ATF4, CHOP, or GADD34 mRNA levels. The levels of ATF4, CHOP, and GADD mRNA were directly proportional to each other. These indicated that, despite activation of the PERK pathway, the downstream elements of the PERK pathway were not activated. These data indicate the activation of the PERK pathway (increased eiF-2α phosphorylation) on one hand and lack of signs to recovery (low levels of GADD 34 mRNA) on the other. Thus, there is evidence of activation of the UPR in subjects with NAFLD and NASH.

BiP mRNA levels, which are widely considered to represent the master indicator of activation of UPR, were increased significantly only in NASH. While there was a trend for increased unspliced XBP-1 mRNA in NASH, the protein levels were not significantly different compared with controls. There was a marked increase in spliced XBP-1 mRNA in a few individuals with NAFLD and a similar number of subjects with NASH. The sXBP-1 mRNA levels were unchanged in the majority of subjects. However, sXBP-1 protein levels were significantly decreased in subjects with NASH, while those in NAFLD were not significantly altered compared with controls. Of note, while there was a progressive increase in EDEM1 mRNA expression from normal to NAFLD to NASH, the subjects with the highest sXBP-1 mRNA had the lowest levels of its downstream target EDEM 1 mRNA only in subjects with NASH. These data indicate that there is a dysregulated expression of the UPR in humans with NASH. This was accompanied by the greatest degree of JNK1 activation. Importantly, while p38 MAP kinase activity was increased in both NAFLD and NASH, JNK1 phosphorylation was only increased in NASH. Moreover, the degree of JNK activation correlated with inflammation and apoptotic activity. The sXBP-1 mRNA correlated with JNK-activity and NAFLD-activity scores.

IMPLICATIONS FOR THE ROLE OF UPR IN DEVELOPMENT OF THE NAFLD PHENOTYPE

Development of a Fatty Liver

Hepatic steatosis results from the accumulation of a variety of lipid within the hepatocytes. While alterations in many different classes of lipids have been noted in livers afflicted by NAFLD, the predominant lipid that accumulates is triacylglycerol (TAG).[38] TAG is derived from esterification of free fatty acids (FFA) within the liver. FFA in hepatocytes comes from either uptake from circulating blood or by de novo lipogenesis (DNL). In NAFLD, fasting–free-fatty acid levels are elevated owing to increased peripheral lipolysis.[42] These have also been shown to contribute substantially to TAG synthesis in subjects with NAFLD.[42] In addition to increased uptake and reesterification of FFA to TAG, subjects with NAFLD have increased DNL.[43]

A key transcriptional factor that regulates the amount of DNL is the sterol regulatory element binding protein-1 (SREBP-1).[44] SREBP-1 has three isoforms (1a, 1c, and 2). SREBP-1c upregulates DNL. It is transcriptionally regulated by the activity of the orphan nuclear receptor liver X receptor (LXR) α.[45] SREBP-1c activity is also increased by hyperinsulinemia, a characteristic feature of the insulin-resistant state.[46] SREBP-1c resides in an inactive form bound to a chaperone protein SREBP cleavage-activating protein in the ER membrane. Activation of SREBP-1c involves cleavage from the ER membrane which releases it to the Golgi and then to the cytoplasm for transport to the nucleus where it binds to the promoter of its target genes that mediate DNL.[47] UPR has been shown to increase SREBP-1c cleavage from the ER. Increased ER membrane cholesterol or decreased phosphatidylcholine, which would increase the cholesterol-to-phospholipid ratio in the ER membrane, would be expected to trigger UPR and activate SREBP-1c. We have previously shown that NAFLD is associated with increased free cholesterol and decreased phosphatidylcholine.[38] Free cholesterol is highly hydrophobic and, a priori, is expected to insert into lipid membranes.

While most cellular free cholesterol resides in the plasma membrane, a small amount is present in the ER and ER function depends closely on maintaining the membrane fluidity, a function of ER membrane cholesterol.[48] While the location of the excess free cholesterol in hepatocytes in NAFLD has not been experimentally verified, it is likely that there is some increase in ER membrane cholesterol, which would be expected to trigger UPR and activation of DNL. Recently, it has been shown that sXBP-1 can also independently trigger maturation of SREBP-1c, thus promoting DNL.[49] These data indicate that UPR may contribute to continued maintenance of the steatotic state by increased DNL. Conversely, the development of steatosis, especially accumulation of free cholesterol, is highly likely to contribute to ER stress and genesis of the UPR.[50]

Development of Steatohepatitis

Steatohepatitis is differentiated from steatosis by the presence of inflammation, cytologic ballooning, and progressive sinusoidal fibrosis. There is also increased apoptotic activity in NASH.[51,52] Over the last decade, there has been intense interest in finding out what specific pathophysiologic processes underlie the development of the specific phenotype of NAFLD (fatty liver versus steatohepatitis). To date, most pathophysiologic processes implicated in the genesis of liver injury and inflammation have been found in NAFLD and NASH; and the differences have mainly been quantitative (eg, oxidative stress).[39,40] Studies indicate that JNK1 activation clearly and remarkably separates subjects with NAFLD from those with NASH. JNK is a well-known activator of apoptosis and inflammation.[32,53] Given the direct relationship between JNK1 activation and apoptosis and inflammation, UPR is likely to play a role in the genesis of cell injury and inflammation. It is worth noting that JNK1 is a promiscuous molecule and is activated by several pathways.[54] While one cannot be certain if UPR is the primary driver of JNK1 activation in NASH, the activation of JNK correlates with sXBP-1 mRNA, a marker of IRE-1 activation suggesting that it does indeed play a role. JNK1 and other stress kinase activity may also contribute to inflammatory responses and worsening insulin resistance.[55,56] These human data have been corroborated by studies demonstrating JNK1 activation in a MCD model of NASH where silencing JNK led to decreased features of steatohepatitis as well as steatosis.[36] Finally, JNK1 activity correlates with apoptotic activity in humans with NASH further supporting a role for this UPR activated molecule in the genesis of cell injury in NASH.[41]

Hepatic fibrosis in NASH results from activation of hepatic stellate cells (HSC) in hepatic sinusoids. HSC are activated by several inflammatory-fibrogenic cytokines.[57] There are no data to indicate that UPR is involved in the activation of HSC in NAFLD or any other liver disease. However, UPR may indirectly affect development of hepatic fibrosis by activating inflammatory pathways in other cells within the liver, resulting in changes in the hepatic microenvironment and, therefore, activating the HSC. This is however speculative and remains to be experimentally verified.

Role of UPR in Progression of NASH to Cirrhosis

It is generally believed that inflammation and apoptosis drive disease progression in NASH and activate profibrogenic pathways that lead to fibrosis and eventually the architectural disruption, which is the hallmark of cirrhosis. The dysregulated activation of UPR may play a role in this process (**Fig. 2**). The adaptive response of the UPR involves inhibition of protein synthesis by way of eiF-2α phosphorylation or increased protein degradation by way of EDEM. While the eiF-2α is phosphorylated in NASH, there is a relative failure to generate EDEM in about 20% of subjects (see description above). This would be expected to decrease the ability to degrade unfolded proteins

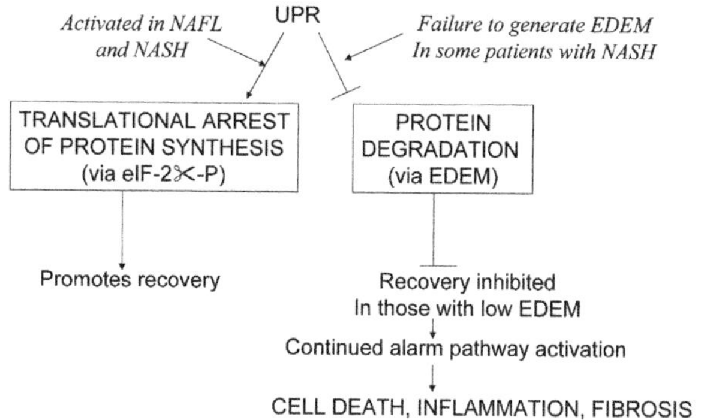

Fig. 2. UPR in human NASH.

and lead to accumulation of unfolded proteins, thereby inhibiting return to baseline. Indeed, the most florid cases of NASH are characterized by accumulation of Mallory bodies in ballooned cells. These Mallory bodies are accumulated heat shock proteins (which are produced in response to oxidative stress) that are ubiquitinylated.[58] Indeed, ubiquitin staining is often used to identify Mallory bodies. If recovery from UPR is retarded, it is more likely to promote inflammatory pathway activation and apoptosis and thereby drive disease progression (see **Fig. 2**). Cross-sectional data from studies support this hypothesis and long-term, follow-up studies are currently under way to confirm this.

In summary, the UPR is a fundamental cellular process that is activated in subjects with NAFLD. In subjects with NASH, there is a dysregulated activation of the UPR with a failure to generate sXBP-1 protein despite adequate sXBP-1 mRNA in about 20% of subjects. This is accompanied by decreased EDEM1 mRNA in these subjects. Failure to generate EDEM1 is also associated with the highest JNK1 activation, NAS score, and apoptosis. These data suggest that UPR plays an important role in the genesis of NASH and may play a role in the progression of NASH to cirrhosis.

REFERENCES

1. Anfinsen CB. Principles that govern the folding of protein chains. Science 1973; 181:223–30.
2. Shamu CE, Cox JS, Walter P. The unfolded-protein-response pathway in yeast. Trends Cell Biol Feb 1994;4:56–60.
3. Brostrom MA, Prostko CR, Gmitter D, et al. Independent signaling of grp78 gene transcription and phosphorylation of eukaryotic initiator factor 2 alpha by the stressed endoplasmic reticulum. J Biol Chem 1995;270:4127–32.
4. Feng B, Yao PM, Li Y, et al. The endoplasmic reticulum is the site of cholesterol-induced cytotoxicity in macrophages. Nat Cell Biol 2003;5:781–92.
5. Gomez E, Powell ML, Bevington A, et al. A decrease in cellular energy status stimulates PERK-dependent eIF2alpha phosphorylation and regulates protein synthesis in pancreatic beta-cells. Biochem J 2008;410:485–93.
6. Su HL, Liao CL, Lin YL. Japanese encephalitis virus infection initiates endoplasmic reticulum stress and an unfolded protein response. J Virol 2002;76: 4162–71.
7. Yacoub Wasef SZ, Robinson KA, Berkaw MN, et al. Glucose, dexamethasone, and the unfolded protein response regulate TRB3 mRNA expression in 3T3-L1

adipocytes and L6 myotubes. Am J Physiol Endocrinol Metab 2006;291: E1274–80.
8. Bertolotti A, Zhang Y, Hendershot LM, et al. Dynamic interaction of BiP and ER stress transducers in the unfolded-protein response. Nat Cell Biol 2000;2:326–32.
9. Liu CY, Schroder M, Kaufman RJ. Ligand-independent dimerization activates the stress response kinases IRE1 and PERK in the lumen of the endoplasmic reticulum. J Biol Chem 2000;275:24881–5.
10. Harding HP, Zhang Y, Bertolotti A, et al. Perk is essential for translational regulation and cell survival during the unfolded protein response. Mol Cell 2000;5: 897–904.
11. Scheuner D, Song B, McEwen E, et al. Translational control is required for the unfolded protein response and in vivo glucose homeostasis. Mol Cell 2001;7: 1165–76.
12. Hinnebusch AG. The eIF-2 alpha kinases: regulators of protein synthesis in starvation and stress. Semin Cell Biol 1994;5:417–26.
13. Novoa I, Zeng H, Harding HP, et al. Feedback inhibition of the unfolded protein response by GADD34-mediated dephosphorylation of eIF2alpha. J Cell Biol 2001;153:1011–22.
14. van Huizen R, Martindale JL, Gorospe M, et al. P58IPK, a novel endoplasmic reticulum stress-inducible protein and potential negative regulator of eIF2alpha signaling. J Biol Chem 2003;278:15558–64.
15. Dinkova-Kostova AT, Holtzclaw WD, Cole RN, et al. Direct evidence that sulfhydryl groups of Keap1 are the sensors regulating induction of phase 2 enzymes that protect against carcinogens and oxidants. Proc Natl Acad Sci U S A 2002;99: 11908–13.
16. Cullinan SB, Zhang D, Hannink M, et al. Nrf2 is a direct PERK substrate and effector of PERK-dependent cell survival. Mol Cell Biol 2003;23:7198–209.
17. Haze K, Okada T, Yoshida H, et al. Identification of the G13 (cAMP-response-element-binding protein-related protein) gene product related to activating transcription factor 6 as a transcriptional activator of the mammalian unfolded protein response. Biochem J 2001;355:19–28.
18. Yoshida H, Okada T, Haze K, et al. ATF6 activated by proteolysis binds in the presence of NF-Y (CBF) directly to the cis-acting element responsible for the mammalian unfolded protein response. Mol Cell Biol 2000;20:6755–67.
19. Ye J, Rawson RB, Komuro R, et al. ER stress induces cleavage of membrane-bound ATF6 by the same proteases that process SREBPs. Mol Cell 2000;6: 1355–64.
20. Yoshida H, Matsui T, Yamamoto A, et al. XBP1 mRNA is induced by ATF6 and spliced by IRE1 in response to ER stress to produce a highly active transcription factor. Cell 2001;107:881–91.
21. Wang XZ, Harding HP, Zhang Y, et al. Cloning of mammalian Ire1 reveals diversity in the ER stress responses. EMBO J 1998;17:5708–17.
22. Yoshida H. Unconventional splicing of XBP-1 mRNA in the unfolded protein response. Antioxid Redox Signal 2007;9:2323–33.
23. Kostova Z, Tsai YC, Weissman AM. Ubiquitin ligases, critical mediators of endoplasmic reticulum-associated degradation. Semin Cell Dev Biol 2007;18(6):770–9.
24. Lippincott-Schwartz J, Bonifacino JS, Yuan LC, et al. Degradation from the endoplasmic reticulum: disposing of newly synthesized proteins. Cell 1988;54:209–20.
25. Hirao K, Natsuka Y, Tamura T, et al. EDEM3, a soluble EDEM homolog, enhances glycoprotein endoplasmic reticulum-associated degradation and mannose trimming. J Biol Chem 2006;281:9650–8.

26. Hosokawa N, Tremblay LO, You Z, et al. Enhancement of endoplasmic reticulum (ER) degradation of misfolded Null Hong Kong alpha1-antitrypsin by human ER mannosidase I. J Biol Chem 2003;278:26287–94.
27. Mast SW, Diekman K, Karaveg K, et al. Human EDEM2, a novel homolog of family 47 glycosidases, is involved in ER-associated degradation of glycoproteins. Glycobiology 2005;15:421–36.
28. Urano F, Wang X, Bertolotti A, et al. Coupling of stress in the ER to activation of JNK protein kinases by transmembrane protein kinase IRE1. Science 2000;287:664–6.
29. Adler V, Schaffer A, Kim J, et al. UV irradiation and heat shock mediate JNK activation via alternate pathways. J Biol Chem 1995;270:26071–7.
30. Wang XZ, Kuroda M, Sok J, et al. Identification of novel stress-induced genes downstream of chop. EMBO J 1998;17:3619–30.
31. Yan W, Frank CL, Korth MJ, et al. Control of PERK eIF2alpha kinase activity by the endoplasmic reticulum stress-induced molecular chaperone P58IPK. Proc Natl Acad Sci U S A 2002;99:15920–5.
32. Davis RJ. Signal transduction by the JNK group of MAP kinases. Cell 2000;103: 239–52.
33. Morishima N, Nakanishi K, Takenouchi H, et al. An endoplasmic reticulum stress-specific caspase cascade in apoptosis. Cytochrome c-independent activation of caspase-9 by caspase-12. J Biol Chem 2002;277:34287–94.
34. Nakagawa T, Zhu H, Morishima N, et al. Caspase-12 mediates endoplasmic-reticulum-specific apoptosis and cytotoxicity by amyloid-beta. Nature 2000; 403:98–103.
35. Wang D, Wei Y, Pagliassotti MJ. Saturated fatty acids promote endoplasmic reticulum stress and liver injury in rats with hepatic steatosis. Endocrinology 2006; 147:943–51.
36. Schattenberg JM, Singh R, Wang Y, et al. JNK1 but not JNK2 promotes the development of steatohepatitis in mice. Hepatology 2006;43:163–72.
37. Ji C, Shinohara M, Kuhlenkamp J, et al. Mechanisms of protection by the betaine-homocysteine methyltransferase/betaine system in HepG2 cells and primary mouse hepatocytes. Hepatology 2007;46:1586–96.
38. Puri P, Baillie RA, Wiest MM, et al. A lipidomic analysis of nonalcoholic fatty liver disease. Hepatology 2007;46:1081–90.
39. Sanyal AJ, Campbell-Sargent C, Mirshahi F, et al. Nonalcoholic steatohepatitis: association of insulin resistance and mitochondrial abnormalities. Gastroenterology 2001;120:1183–92.
40. Seki S, Kitada T, Sakaguchi H. Clinicopathological significance of oxidative cellular damage in non-alcoholic fatty liver diseases. Hepatol Res 2005;33:132–4.
41. Puri P, Mirshahi F, Cheung O, et al. Activation and dysregulation of the unfolded protein response in nonalcoholic fatty liver disease. Gastroenterology 2008;134: 568–76.
42. Donnelly KL, Smith CI, Schwarzenberg SJ, et al. Sources of fatty acids stored in liver and secreted via lipoproteins in patients with nonalcoholic fatty liver disease. J Clin Invest 2005;115:1343–51.
43. Diraison F, Moulin P, Beylot M. Contribution of hepatic de novo lipogenesis and reesterification of plasma non esterified fatty acids to plasma triglyceride synthesis during nonalcoholic fatty liver disease. Diabetes Metab 2003;29: 478–85.
44. Brown MS, Goldstein JL. The SREBP pathway: regulation of cholesterol metabolism by proteolysis of a membrane-bound transcription factor. Cell 1997;89: 331–40.

45. Schultz JR, Tu H, Luk A, et al. Role of LXRs in control of lipogenesis. Genes Dev 2000;14:2831–8.
46. Shimomura I, Bashmakov Y, Horton JD. Increased levels of nuclear SREBP-1c associated with fatty livers in two mouse models of diabetes mellitus. J Biol Chem 1999;274:30028–32.
47. Horton JD, Shah NA, Warrington JA, et al. Combined analysis of oligonucleotide microarray data from transgenic and knockout mice identifies direct SREBP target genes. Proc Natl Acad Sci U S A 2003;100:12027–32.
48. Lange Y, Steck TL. Cholesterol homeostasis and the escape tendency (activity) of plasma membrane cholesterol. Prog Lipid Res 2008;47:319–32.
49. Lee AH, Scapa EF, Cohen DE, et al. Regulation of hepatic lipogenesis by the transcription factor XBP1. Science 2008;320:1492–6.
50. Devries-Seimon T, Li Y, Yao PM, et al. Cholesterol-induced macrophage apoptosis requires ER stress pathways and engagement of the type A scavenger receptor. J Cell Biol 2005;171:61–73.
51. Feldstein AE, Canbay A, Angulo P, et al. Hepatocyte apoptosis and fas expression are prominent features of human nonalcoholic steatohepatitis. Gastroenterology 2003;125:437–43.
52. Ribeiro PS, Cortez-Pinto H, Sola S, et al. Hepatocyte apoptosis, expression of death receptors, and activation of NF-kappaB in the liver of nonalcoholic and alcoholic steatohepatitis patients. Am J Gastroenterol 2004;99:1708–17017.
53. Weston CR, Davis RJ. The JNK signal transduction pathway. Curr Opin Cell Biol 2007;19:142–9.
54. Matsukawa J, Matsuzawa A, Takeda K, et al. The ASK1-MAP kinase cascades in mammalian stress response. J Biochem 2004;136:261–5.
55. Aguirre V, Werner ED, Giraud J, et al. Phosphorylation of Ser307 in insulin receptor substrate-1 blocks interactions with the insulin receptor and inhibits insulin action. J Biol Chem 2002;277:1531–7.
56. White MF. Insulin signaling in health and disease. Science 2003;302:1710–1.
57. Marra F. Hepatic stellate cells and the regulation of liver inflammation. J Hepatol 1999;31:1120–30.
58. Stumptner C, Fuchsbichler A, Lehner M, et al. Sequence of events in the assembly of Mallory body components in mouse liver: clues to the pathogenesis and significance of Mallory body formation. J Hepatol 2001;34:665–75.

Predictors of Steatohepatitis and Advanced Fibrosis in Non-Alcoholic Fatty Liver Disease

Mangesh Pagadala, MD, Claudia O. Zein, MD, MSc, Arthur J. McCullough, MD*

KEYWORDS

- Fatty liver • Liver fibrosis • Serum markers
- Biomarkers • Non-invasive assessment
- Diabetes • Predictors

The prevalence of non-alcoholic fatty liver disease (NAFLD) in the American population is approximately 30% in adults and 10% in children, making it the most common cause of chronic liver disease in the United States.[1,2] Although the majority of patients with NAFLD have a benign clinical course, the development of non-alcoholic steatohepatitis (NASH), with necroinflammation and progressive fibrosis, increases the risk for development of cirrhosis and its complications.[3,4] Among patients with NASH, approximately 28% develop cirrhosis over an 8-year follow-up period.[4,5]

The gold standard for diagnosing and staging NAFLD is liver biopsy. Liver biopsy is associated with costs and risks that make it impractical for generalized use in a condition that affects such a high portion of the population. Furthermore, liver biopsy is also limited by significant sampling error in NAFLD.[6,7] Thus, there is a pressing need for accurate non-invasive predictors of NAFLD that would also allow differentiation of those subjects at higher risk of disease progression. At present, in the clinical setting, some demographic factors, blood tests, and imaging studies can be used to predict a higher risk of disease in patients being evaluated for NAFLD. These predictors, however, are of limited sensitivity and specificity compared with liver biopsy. The development and validation of accurate predictors and scoring systems to identify patients at higher risk for NASH and fibrosis would allow identification of subjects who would benefit the most from liver biopsy and potentially help monitor disease

Department of Gastroenterology and Hepatology, Digestive Disease Institute of the Cleveland Clinic, Cleveland Clinic Lerner College of Medicine, A 31, 9500 Euclid Avenue, Cleveland, OH 44195, USA
* Corresponding author.
E-mail address: mcculla@ccf.org (A. J. McCullough).

Clin Liver Dis 13 (2009) 591–606
doi:10.1016/j.cld.2009.07.011
1089-3261/09/$ – see front matter

progression and response to therapeutic modalities in the future.[8] Nevertheless, it is important to emphasize the importance of establishing the diagnosis of NASH and advanced fibrosis in NAFLD[9,10] (discussed later).

PREDICTORS OF NON-ALCOHOLIC STEATOHEPATITIS

Several demographic, anthropomorphic, clinical, and laboratory factors are associated with NAFLD and with histologic severity of disease. Among these, the factors most reliably associated with the presence of NASH and of advanced fibrosis include older age, insulin resistance (IR)/diabetes mellitus (DM), obesity, and hypertension. However, the potential applicability of these variables in predicting severity of disease in the clinical setting is limited.

Demographic Factors

Race

Ethnic differences in the prevalence of NAFLD are reported, with lower prevalence in African Americans compared with non–African Americans and highest prevalence in Hispanic patients followed by white patients.[1,11] Some studies have reported similar findings regarding steatohepatitis.[12,13] Campos and colleagues[13] observed a higher prevalence of NASH in obese white and Hispanic patients compared with African Americans (35% versus 11%) and higher risk of NASH independent of presence of the metabolic syndrome (odds ratio [OR] 8.4, P = .005). Kallwitz and colleagues[14] also noted lower prevalence of liver steatosis, NASH, and advanced fibrosis in obese patients who were African Americans compared with non-Hispanic white and Hispanic patients. These and other studies suggest that African Americans might be protected from development of NAFLD and disease severity.[15] Variations in visceral adipose tissue distribution and on IR influenced by genetic and physiologic factors may explain these differences.[16–18]

Gender and age

Reports regarding the association between risk for NASH and gender are variable. Some studies report a higher risk for NASH in women,[19,20] others a higher risk in men,[21] and others are unable to demonstrate a definitive association.[13,22,23] Older age also is associated with a higher risk of NASH.[20]

Elements of the Metabolic Syndrome

Insulin resistance and diabetes mellitus

IR is known to play a key role in the pathophysiology of NAFLD.[24–26] In addition, the results of several studies suggest that a higher degree of IR is associated with a higher likelihood of development of steatohepatitis in patients with steatosis.[20,27–29] Patients with NASH have higher homeostasis model assessment (HOMA) score, serum insulin level, and C-peptide level compared with controls.[24] Furthermore, various studies have demonstrated the value of measures of IR as predictors of NASH. In one study, a HOMA index greater than 5.8 was a significant predictor of NASH in obese subjects.[28] Similarly, another series reported the Quantitative Insulin Sensitivity Check Index (QUICKI) model as useful in predicting NASH compared with simple steatosis with an accuracy (area under the curve [AUC]) of 0.70.[20]

It is well established that patients with type 2 DM are at higher risk of NAFLD and of developing NASH and advanced fibrosis compared with non–DM subjects.[21,22,30]

Hypertension

The prevalence of hypertension is significantly higher in patients with NASH compared with those with simple steatosis and several studies have demonstrated that this association is independent of other risk factors.[13,19,31]

Obesity

Obesity, defined by increased body mass index (BMI), and central adiposity in subjects who may or may not fit the definition of obesity by BMI are associated with a higher risk of NASH. Obesity defined by increased BMI is strongly associated with prevalence of NAFLD and with severity of the disease.[20,22,32–38] An association between higher BMI and NASH is demonstrated in several studies. In morbidly obese subjects, the prevalence of NAFLD is as high as 90%, whereas that of NASH is of approximately 30% in the same patient population.[32]

Central obesity, as measured by waist-to-hip ratio, is strongly associated with NAFLD and with severity of disease.[24,34] NASH is reported in individuals with non-obese BMI and central obesity (lean NASH).[24,36] One study in non-obese Asian subjects demonstrated an association between waist-to-hip ratio and increased necroinflammation.[36]

Serum Liver Enzymes

The use of serum liver enzymes is used routinely to screen for chronic liver disease, including NAFLD. Elevated transaminases are the most common blood test abnormality in NAFLD. Although alanine aminotransferase (ALT) or aspartate aminotransferase (AST) tend to be higher in patients with NASH compared with those with simple steatosis, these measures are not of enough specificity and specificity for a reliable diagnosis of NASH in the clinical setting. The sensitivity of elevated ALT for a diagnosis of NASH is approximately 40% to 53% and the specificity approximately 50%.[27] In one series of 354 patients with abnormal liver enzymes, the positive predictive value of abnormal transaminases to diagnose NASH was only 34%.[39] In another study involving a cohort of obese women, the sensitivity of ALT in diagnosing NASH was 42%.[40] These findings are not surprising given that some patients with NASH, even many with fibrosis and cirrhosis, often have normal serum liver enzymes.[41]

Lower cutoff levels for serum ALT for men (>30 U/L) and women (>19 U/L) are proposed.[42] Campos and colleagues[13] recently reported that a cutoff point of greater than 27 U/L for AST and ALT best distinguished NASH from no NASH in a cohort of obese patients who underwent bariatric surgery. Decreasing the upper limit of normal (ULN) of AST from greater than 30 U/L to greater than 19 U/L improved the sensitivity for diagnosing NASH from 42% to 74% in a study by Kunde and colleagues[40] but resulted in significant decrease in specificity.

Some studies have also used the AST/ALT ratio (AAR) to predict probable NASH versus simple steatosis.[20,43] In one study of 80 patients with biopsy-proved NAFLD, an AAR greater than 0.8 predicted NASH with an area under the receiver operating characteristic (AUROC) of 0.763.[20] AAR also predicts advanced fibrosis in this patient population.[19,20]

The predictive accuracy of AST and ALT for diagnosis of NASH is low; however, the use of lower ULNs may be used as a limited screening tool.

Biomarkers

Identification of specific and easily available biomarkers that would allow an accurate diagnosis of NASH or advanced fibrosis in NAFLD patients would be valuable. **Table 1** lists many of the biomarkers tested to date in patients with NAFLD.

Table 1
Biochemical markers as predictors of non-alcoholic steatohepatitis and advanced fibrosis

Reference	Marker	Non-alcoholic Steatohepatitis	Fibrosis	Area Under the Curve
Palekar[20]	HA > 45.3 ng/mL		•	0.88
Suzuki[84]	HA > 46.1 ng/mL		•	0.89
Santos[87]	HA > 24.6 ng/mL		•	0.73
	Laminin > 282 ng/mL		•	0.87
	Type IV collagen > 145 ng/mL		•	0.82
Sakugawa[86]	HA > 50 ng/mL		•	0.80
Hasegawa[58]	TGF-β1	•		NR
Haukeland[55]	TNF-α	•		NR
	CCL2/MCP	•		
Wieckowska[67]	Cytokeratin-18	•		0.93
Garcia-Galiano[101]	IGF-1 < 110 ng/mL	•		NR
Baranova[48]	Decreased adiponectin	•		NR
Hui[53]	Decreased adiponectin	•		0.79
Yoneda[56]	High-sensitivity CRP	•	•	0.83
	Type IV collagen		•	
Musso[82]	Adiponectin		•	NR
Wieckowska[57]	Serum IL-6		•	NR
Dixon[29]	C-peptide > 1324 pmol/L		•	NR

CCL2/MCP, CC chemokine ligand 2/monocyte chemoattractant protein; IGF-1, insulin-like growth factor 1; NR, not reported.

Biomarkers of inflammation

The rationale for identification of potentially useful inflammation biomarkers stems from the well-recognized pro-inflammatory environment that chronically exists in NAFLD and NASH.[44] Tumor necrosis factor α (TNF-α) is a pro-inflammatory cytokine that interferes with insulin signaling and promotes steatosis.[45] Adiponectin, an anti-inflammatory adipokine, prevents the accumulation of lipids in the hepatocytes and enhances their sensitivity to insulin.[44] Increased TNF-α levels and TNF-α/adiponectin ratio are present in NAFLD and NASH compared with controls and levels are higher in subjects with NASH compared with those with simple steatosis.[46,47] In one series of obese patients, those with NASH had lower serum adiponectin than those with mild steatosis.[48] Resistin and leptin also are associated with IR and NAFLD.[49–51] Chitturi and colleagues[51] found higher levels of serum leptin in subjects with NASH compared with gender and BMI-matched controls. Subsequent studies, however, have failed to find an association between serum leptin and NASH.[48,52,53] Recent studies have suggested a potential predictive role for interleukin 6 (IL-6) and of high-sensitivity C-reactive protein (CRP) in NAFLD. CRP is an acute phase reactant that is elevated in chronic inflammatory states and elevated in subjects with central obesity. Results are inconsistent between studies,[54–56] however, and only one study reported higher levels of high-sensitivity CRP in NASH.[56] Increased IL-6 expression is reported in patients with NASH.[57] In the same study, the presence of increased plasma IL-6 correlated with presence of NASH and stage of fibrosis; however, after adjusting for HOMA and BMI, only the association with fibrosis remained significant.

Other inflammation-related biomarkers that have yielded unclear results include TGF-β[20,58] and adipocyte-derived chemokine (CC chemokine ligand 2).[55] Partly because of the few studies and small sample sizes, the helpfulness of these inflammatory biomarkers in the clinical setting for non-invasive diagnosis of NASH is uncertain and needs to be studied further.

Biomarkers of oxidative stress

Oxidative stress plays a role in the liver injury and disease progression in NAFLD. Several pathways can result in the production of reactive oxygen species in NAFLD, including mitochondrial, cytochrome P-450, and nitric oxide synthase pathways.[25,45] The extent of reactive oxygen species production can be quantified. **Table 2** lists the examples of oxidative stress biomarkers that have been studied in NAFLD. Chalasani and colleagues[59] reported higher levels of products of lipid peroxidation in patients with NASH compared with controls. In another study, the total antioxidant response was decreased and total plasma peroxide levels were elevated in those with NASH compared with controls.[60] Serum thioredoxine, a marker of oxidative stress, also seems to be a predictor of the histologic severity in NAFLD.[61] Other studies, however, have not been able to corroborate these findings[62,63] and further studies are needed.

Biomarkers of hepatocyte apoptosis

Hepatocyte apoptosis is an important element in the progression of liver injury in NASH. Apoptosis in NASH is mediated by two distinct pathways, both of which could result in activation of caspase, an intracellular protease. Caspase initiates apoptosis by cleaving major intermediate protein filaments in the liver, including cytokeratin-18. Antibodies against these cleaved products have been demonstrated in early apoptotic cells. Apoptosis is associated with increased fibrogenesis in liver mediated by activation of stellate cells.[64–66] In a recent study, Caspase-3-generated cytokeratin-18 predicted NASH with significant accuracy. In that study, a serum level cutoff of 395 U/L had a positive predictive value for NASH of 99.9% and negative predictive value of 85.7% (AUC of 0.93).[64,67] Studies to prospectively validate the usefulness of this marker in larger and diverse populations are needed.

Table 2
Oxidative stress markers as predictors of steatohepatitis versus controls

Reference	N	Predictors	Serum Levels	*P* value
Horoz[60]	22	TAR	Decreased	$P<.05$
		OSI	Increased	$P<.05$
Chalasani[59]	21	TBAR	Increased	$P<.01$
		Ox-LDL	Increased	$P<.01$
Koruk[102]	18	MDA	Increased	$P<.01$
		NO	Increased	$P = .04$
		GSH	Increased	$P<.01$
		SOD	Decreased	$P = 0.04$

Abbreviations: GSH, glutathione; MDA, malondialdehyde; NO, nitric oxide; OSI, oxidative stress index; ox-LDL, oxidized low-density lipoprotein; TAR, total antioxidant response; TBAR, thiobarbituric acid-reacting substance; SOD, superoxide dimutase.

COMPOSITE PREDICTIVE MODELS TO DIAGNOSE NON-ALCOHOLIC STEATOHEPATITIS

With the goal of improving the accuracy of non-invasive diagnosis of NASH, several groups have combined individual demographic, clinical, laboratory, and biochemical markers associated with severity of disease into predictive models of NASH. Some of these are summarized in **Table 3**.

Although the components of the predictive models differ, transaminases and measurements of IR are frequently found among the included predictors. One of the early models proposed was the HAIR model, devised by Dixon and colleagues.[29] The score was calculated based on the presence of hypertension, ALT greater than 40 IU/L, and IR index greater than 5. The AUC for the combination of all three predictors was 0.90.

Recently, Campos and colleagues[13] generated a clinical scoring system to diagnose NASH in morbidly obese patients. Their logistic regression model included hypertension, type 2 DM, AST greater than or equal to 27 IU/L, ALT greater than or equal to 27 IU/L, sleep apnea, and non-black race as predictors. Their scoring system categorizes morbidly obese patients into low, intermediate, high, or very high risk for NASH.[13]

Several additional models have been generated with the goal of predicting NASH (see **Table 3**).[68–70] Unfortunately, none of these models is apt for clinical applicability yet. The main reason for this is that the accuracy of diagnosis is still insufficient compared with histopathology. Also, most of the models have been generated in distinctive subpopulations (eg, morbidly obese subjects) and, therefore, are not generalizable to the overall NAFLD patient population. Further improvement in model accuracy, likely with the addition of biomarker measurements and prospective validation studies in different patient populations, are still needed.

PREDICTORS OF FIBROSIS IN NON-ALCOHOLIC FATTY LIVER DISEASE

The presence of NASH and the occurrence and progression of liver fibrosis in patients with NAFLD leads to the development of clinically relevant outcomes, including

Table 3
Composite models for diagnosis of non-alcoholic steatohepatitis

Reference	N	Population	Area Under the Curve for Non-alcoholic Steatohepatitis	Predictors
Palekar[20]	80	NAFLD	0.76 (CI: 0.65–0.87)	Age, BMI, female gender, AST, AAR, HA
Zein (NPI)[70]	177	NAFLD	0.87 (CI: 0.81–0.93)[a] 0.85 (CI:0.75–0.95)[b]	Age, female gender, BMI, HOMA, log (AST × ALT)
Dixon (HAIR)[29]	105	Obese	0.90 (CI: NR)	HTN, ALT, IR
Gholam[69]	97	Obese	0.82 (CI: NR)	AST, DM
Campos[13]	200	Obese	NR	HTN, DM, AST, ALT, sleep apnea, and non-black race
Poynard (NASHtest)[68]	257	NAFLD	0.79 (CI: 0.69–0.86)[a] 0.79 (CI: 0.67–0.87)[b]	Combination of 13 parameters[c]

Abbreviations: NPI, NASH predictive Index; NR, not reported; HTN, hypertension.
[a] Training population set.
[b] Validation population set.
[c] Age, sex, height, weight, and serum triglyceride, cholesterol, α_2-macroglobulin, apolipoprotein A1, haptoglobin, GGT, AST, ALT, and total bilirubin.

cirrhosis and all its complications. Thus, identifying subjects with early stages of liver fibrosis, in whom therapeutic interventions would yield optimal benefit and impact outcomes, is important.[71,72] Several groups have worked on identifying predictors and models to predict the presence of fibrosis in NAFLD.

Demographic Factors

Race

Although some studies show a relationship between race and prevalence of NAFLD and NASH, race has not been established as a predictor of advanced fibrosis in NAFLD.[13,19]

Gender and age

Similar to what is observed in other chronic liver diseases, older age (>45 years) is predictive of fibrosis and cirrhosis in NAFLD.[19,20,73,74] Development of metabolic syndrome in older age groups might be partly responsible for this. Some studies have found female gender associated with advanced fibrosis.[3,19,75]

Elements of the Metabolic Syndrome

DM,[29,74,76,77] obesity,[19,22,73,78–80] increased waist-to-hip ratio,[21] and hypertension[29] all are independently associated with advanced fibrosis in NAFLD.

Insulin resistance and diabetes mellitus

Several studies show associations between DM and advanced disease in NAFLD.[3,4,30] Similarly, hyperglycemia, hyperinsulinemia, increased IR based on HOMA or QUICKI scores, and measurements indicating increased β–islet cell function all are independently associated with increased liver fibrosis in patients with NAFLD.[19,29,79]

Hypertension

It has been suggested that the association between more severe hepatic fibrosis and arterial hypertension could be related to angiotensin II's profibrogenic properties via production of increased transforming growth factor-beta (TGF-β), leading to hepatic stellate cell activation.[71] Inheriting a combination of high angiotensin and TGF-β1–producing polymorphisms is associated with advanced hepatic fibrosis in obese patients with NAFLD, supporting the hypothesis that increased angiotensin II in hypertensive patients could result in higher TGF-β1 production and promote hepatic fibrosis.[81]

Serum Liver Enzymes

AST levels and ALT levels and AAR greater than 0.8 are independent markers of advanced fibrosis in NAFLD.[19,20,74] Elevated AST[76] and ALT[73] are associated with liver fibrosis in patients with NAFLD.[69,74] Harrison and colleagues[19] reported AST higher in NAFLD subjects with no fibrosis compared with those with advanced fibrosis. In the same study, subjects with AAR greater than 0.8 had a 9.3 times higher risk of severe fibrosis compared with those with AAR lower than 0.8. Other studies have corroborated the utility of AAR greater than 0.8 in distinguishing early versus advanced fibrosis in subjects with NAFLD.[20,74]

Biomarkers of Fibrosis in Non-alcoholic Fatty Liver Disease

Several potential associations between biomarkers and underlying liver fibrosis in NAFLD have been studied and are listed in **Table 1**. A correlation between severity of hepatic fibrosis and decreased adiponectin is shown in small studies.[82] Similar studies have failed to demonstrate a correlation between TNF-α levels and liver fibrosis in NAFLD.[53,82] Leptin, another cytokine associated with liver fibrosis in animal models, was not related fibrosis in human studies.[51,83]

Increased expression of plasma TGF- β, which activates Kupffer and stellate cells,[71] is described in individuals with NAFLD.[81]

Hyaluronic acid (HA), laminin, and collagen are extracellular matrix components. The serum levels of these components are relatively low in normal conditions. Elevated serum levels of HA are seen during accelerated deposition of collagen in the extracellular matrix due to down-regulation of hyaluronate receptors coupled with decreased sinusoidal endothelial cells clearance.[84,85] Serum HA and serum laminin levels are associated with liver fibrosis in NAFLD. Suzuki and colleagues[84] studied the HA levels in 79 patients with biopsy-confirmed NASH. At a cutoff serum level of 46.1 μg/L the presence of HA positively correlated with advanced fibrosis, and this association persisted after adjusting for age and albumin levels. Two other studies using cutoff levels of 45.3 μg/L and 50 μg/L also found HA a strong predictor of liver fibrosis.[20,86] These studies of HA and liver fibrosis in NAFLD show significant sensitivity and specificity of this biomarker; however, larger studies need to be conducted.

In a small study involving 30 subjects, laminin levels greater than 282 μg/L and type IV collagen levels greater than 145 were predictive of advanced fibrosis (AUC 0.80–0.87).[87] The combination of HA, aminoterminal propeptide-1 of type III collagen, and tissue inhibitor of matrix metalloproteinase 1 (TIMP-1) as a predictor of advanced fibrosis has also been studied in 61 subjects with NAFLD and had good accuracy (AUC 0.90).[88]

Serum ferritin is elevated in patients with NAFLD and has been previously associated with IR and hepatic inflammation. Elevated serum ferritin was associated with severe liver fibrosis in 167 patients with NAFLD,[89] but this has not been confirmed by other studies.[74,75,90]

High-sensitivity CRP, another marker of inflammation, is elevated in NAFLD with advanced fibrosis compared with NAFLD with early fibrosis.[56]

Most of the studies described previously were conducted with small sample sizes. In addition, lack of specificity, given the recognized increase of these markers in systemic disease processes, limits the significance and applicability of these results. Larger studies using markers individually or in combination with other markers are needed.

Composite Models to Diagnose Advanced Fibrosis in Non-alcoholic Fatty Liver Disease

The use of composite models as opposed to using individual markers would increase the validity and improve accuracy in diagnosing NASH and advanced fibrosis in NAFLD. Several studies have created composite predictive models of fibrosis in NAFLD. **Table 4** summarizes several of these.

The BAAT score was created by Ratziu and colleagues[73]; it combines four variables: BMI greater than 28 kg/m^2, ALT greater than 2 ULNs, age greater than 50 years, and serum triglycerides greater than 1.7 mmol/L. Each variable was given a score of 0 or 1. Although total scores of 0 or 4 provide excellent sensitivity (score of 0) or specificity (score of 4), the specificity is limited for lower scores and sensitivity is limited a high scores. Furthermore, the score does not have sufficient accuracy in the significant number of subjects who fall in intermediate scores.

Another proposed scoring system is the NAFLD fibrosis score, which uses age, platelet count, albumin, AAR, DM, and BMI to predict advanced fibrosis in NAFLD

Table 4
Composite models for diagnosis of advanced fibrosis in non-alcoholic fatty liver disease

Reference	Model	N	Population	Area Under the Curve for Advanced Fibrosis	Predictors
Ratziu[73]	BAAT	93	Obese	0.84 (CI: NR)	Age, BMI, ALT, TGL
Angulo[74]		144	NASH	NR	Age, BMI, DM, AAR
Angulo[79]	NAFLD fibrosis score	733	NAFLD	0.88 (CI: 0.85–0.92)[a] 0.82 (CI:0.76–0.88)[b]	Age, BMI, AAR, DM, platelet count, albumin
Harrison[19]	BARD	827	NAFLD	0.81 (CI: NR)	BMI, AAR, DM
Ratziu[80]	Fibro Test	267	NAFLD	0.86 (CI: 0.77-0.91)[a] 0.75 (CI: 0.61–0.83)[b]	α_2-Microglobulin, haptoglobulin, total bilirubin, GGT, apolipoprotein A1
Rosenberg[88]	OELF	61	NAFLD	0.87 (CI: 0.66–1.0)	Age, HA, PIIINP, TIMP-1
Guha[91]	ELF	192	NAFLD	0.90 (CI: 0.84–0.96)	HA, PIIINP, TIMP-1

Abbreviations: PIIINP, aminoterminal peptide of procollagen III; NR, not reported; TGL, triglyceride.
[a] Training population set.
[b] Validation population set.

with good accuracy (AUROC 0.88).[79] As with most composite models for liver fibrosis prediction in NAFLD, a significant limitation is the high proportion of indeterminate cases that would evidently limit clinical applicability. Harrison and colleagues[19] generated a scoring system, using BMI greater than or equal to 28 = 1 point, AAR greater than 0.8 = 2 points, and DM = 1 point, and calculated that a composite score of 2 to 4 was associated with an increased OR of 17 of advanced fibrosis with a negative predictive value of 96%. The AUC for that model was 0.81. FibroTest is a biomarker of liver fibrosis initially used in patients with chronic hepatitis C. The Fibro Test-Fibro SURE panel uses five biochemical markers (α_2-macroglobulin, haptoglobulin, total bilirubin, gamma-glutamyl transpeptidase [GGT], and apolipoprotein A1) to predict liver fibrosis. This panel was studied in patients with NAFLD yielding an AUC for advanced fibrosis of 0.86.[80]

The European Liver Fibrosis study group created a scoring system using age, HA, aminoterminal peptide of procollagen III, and TIMP-1 in 1021 subjects with chronic liver disease, including 61 patients with NAFLD.[88] The AUC for this algorithm was 0.80. Subsequently, the same group simplified the original European liver fibrosis (OELF) model by removing age. This did not alter the diagnostic accuracy of the model or improve its diagnostic performance, however, as compared with the original model.[91]

SUMMARY AND FUTURE DIRECTIONS

As with any disease, the clinical importance of NAFLD is dependent on its prevalence and natural history. Because NAFLD has a worldwide prevalence of approximately 30% and a natural history of significant liver- and cardiac-related morbidity/mortality in the subgroup of NAFLD patients with NASH, NAFLD has become a major clinical disease in need of innovative management strategies. Perhaps most important with these strategies is identifying the subgroup of NASH patients without performing liver biopsy, because of its inherent cost, sampling error, and morbidity. Consequently, surrogates for the liver biopsy are being actively pursued.

The justification for evaluating the biomarkers (discussed previously) is based on sound rationale and an ever-increasing understanding of the pathophysiology of NASH. Therefore, exploring and combining biomarkers that reflect inflammation, oxidative stress, apoptosis, the extracellular matrix, and IR along with the components of the metabolic syndrome are justified.

The ability to diagnose fibrosis in NAFLD seems closer at hand than does the ability to differentiate steatosis from NASH. Although the latter is important, even the current best strategy (measuring apoptosis) needs additional field testing and standardization of measures that can be used across laboratories. Also, as shown in **Table 3**, it is doubtful that any single biomarker will suffice and composite models with additional biomarkers combined with standard laboratory tests and demographics, such as those used in the NASH predictive index, will be necessary.

In contrast, the ability to reliably determine fibrosis in NAFLD without a liver biopsy is within sight. As shown in **Tables 1** and **4**, the enhanced liver fibrosis (ELF)/OELF panel provides a diagnostic accuracy that requires only 14% of patients be biopsied[88,91] and, if used with the simple test,[79] the accuracy is above 90% for severe fibrosis. Lesser degrees of fibrosis will require lesser thresholds obtained from the ROC curves.

Even with these encouraging results of the biomarkers, alternative strategies are being pursued. Genetics may be able to predict patients at risk and their likelihood of response to therapy,[92,93] and surface-enhanced laser desorption/ionization (SELDI)-based proteomics may be equal or more accurate than fibrosis panels.[94] These methods, however, are still in early stages of testing (genetics) or not yet cost effective (proteomics).

Other strategies evaluating liver stiffness with the FibroScan (Echosens, Paris, France)[95,96] or magnetic resonance elastography[96] also may provide measures of fibrosis that may be used alone[97] or in combination with a biomarker panel, as done in recent studies.[98] In addition, there are real-time functional studies being performed using carbon-labeled substrates (methacetin and fatty acids) to quantify lysosomal and mitochondrial function in vivo.[99,100]

The advantage of measures of liver stiffness and hepatic organelle function is not only that they complement the platform of biomarkers but also that they are easily performed and well standardized. They can be incorporated into liver clinics to evaluate disease progression over time and monitor response to therapeutic intervention. With further evaluation, the need for liver biopsy in the management of NAFLD will be minimal in 5 to 6 years.

REFERENCES

1. Browning JD, Szczepaniak LS, Dobbins R, et al. Prevalence of hepatic steatosis in an urban population in the united states: impact of ethnicity. Hepatology 2004; 40(6):1387–95.
2. Schwimmer JB, Deutsch R, Kahen T, et al. Prevalence of fatty liver in children and adolescents. Pediatrics 2006;118(4):1388–93.
3. McCullough AJ. The clinical features, diagnosis and natural history of non-alcoholic fatty liver disease. Clin Liver Dis 2004;8(3):521–33, viii.
4. Matteoni CA, Younossi ZM, Gramlich T, et al. Non-alcoholic fatty liver disease: a spectrum of clinical and pathological severity. Gastroenterology 1999;116(6): 1413–9.

5. Ekstedt M, Franzen LE, Mathiesen UL, et al. Long-term follow-up of patients with NAFLD and elevated liver enzymes. Hepatology 2006;44(4):865–73.
6. Ratziu V, Charlotte F, Heurtier A, et al. Sampling variability of liver biopsy in non-alcoholic fatty liver disease. Gastroenterology 2005;128(7):1898–906.
7. Merriman RB, Ferrell LD, Patti MG, et al. Correlation of paired liver biopsies in morbidly obese patients with suspected non-alcoholic fatty liver disease. Hepatology 2006;44(4):874–80.
8. Wieckowska A, McCullough AJ, Feldstein AE. Noninvasive diagnosis and monitoring of non-alcoholic steatohepatitis: present and future. Hepatology 2007;46(2):582–9.
9. Marchesini G, Bugianesi E, Forlani G, et al. Non-alcoholic fatty liver, steatohepatitis, and the metabolic syndrome. Hepatology 2003;37(4):917–23.
10. Harrison SA, Neuschwander-Tetri BA. Non-alcoholic fatty liver disease and non-alcoholic steatohepatitis. Clin Liver Dis 2004;8(4):861–79, ix.
11. Weston SR, Leyden W, Murphy R, et al. Racial and ethnic distribution of non-alcoholic fatty liver in persons with newly diagnosed chronic liver disease. Hepatology 2005;41(2):372–9.
12. Santos L, Molina EG, Jeffers L, et al. Prevalence of non-alcoholic steatohepatitis among ethnic groups. Gastroenterology 2001;120(5):117 [Abstract].
13. Campos GM, Bambha K, Vittinghoff E, et al. A clinical scoring system for predicting non-alcoholic steatohepatitis in morbidly obese patients. Hepatology 2008;47(6):1916–23.
14. Kallwitz ER, Guzman G, TenCate V, et al. The histologic spectrum of liver disease in African-American, non-hispanic white, and hispanic obesity surgery patients. Am J Gastroenterol 2009;104(1):64–9.
15. Caldwell SH, Harris DM, Patrie JT, et al. Is NASH underdiagnosed among African Americans? Am J Gastroenterol 2002;97(6):1496–500.
16. Perry AC, Applegate EB, Jackson ML, et al. Racial differences in visceral adipose tissue but not anthropometric markers of health-related variables. J Appl Physiol 2000;89(2):636–43.
17. Lovejoy JC, de la Bretonne JA, Klemperer M, et al. Abdominal fat distribution and metabolic risk factors: effects of race. Metabolism 1996;45(9):1119–24.
18. Deurenberg P, Yap M, van Staveren WA. Body mass index and percent body fat: a meta analysis among different ethnic groups. Int J Obes Relat Metab Disord 1998;22(12):1164–71.
19. Harrison SA, Oliver D, Arnold HL, et al. Development and validation of a simple NAFLD clinical scoring system for identifying patients without advanced disease. Gut 2008;57(10):1441–7.
20. Palekar NA, Naus R, Larson SP, et al. Clinical model for distinguishing non-alcoholic steatohepatitis from simple steatosis in patients with non-alcoholic fatty liver disease. Liver Int 2006;26(2):151–6.
21. Ong JP, Elariny H, Collantes R, et al. Predictors of non-alcoholic steatohepatitis and advanced fibrosis in morbidly obese patients. Obes Surg 2005;15(3):310–5.
22. Wanless IR, Lentz JS. Fatty liver hepatitis (steatohepatitis) and obesity: an autopsy study with analysis of risk factors. Hepatology 1990;12(5):1106–10.
23. Abrams GA, Kunde SS, Lazenby AJ, et al. Portal fibrosis and hepatic steatosis in morbidly obese subjects: a spectrum of non-alcoholic fatty liver disease. Hepatology 2004;40(2):475–83.

24. Chitturi S, Abeygunasekera S, Farrell GC, et al. NASH and insulin resistance: insulin hypersecretion and specific association with the insulin resistance syndrome. Hepatology 2002;35(2):373–9.
25. McCullough AJ. Pathophysiology of non-alcoholic steatohepatitis. J Clin Gastroenterol 2006;40(Suppl 1):S17–29.
26. Bugianesi E, McCullough AJ, Marchesini G. Insulin resistance: a metabolic pathway to chronic liver disease. Hepatology 2005;42(5):987–1000.
27. Ruhl CE, Everhart JE. Epidemiology of non-alcoholic fatty liver. Clin Liver Dis 2004;8(3):501–19, vii.
28. Boza C, Riquelme A, Ibanez L, et al. Predictors of non-alcoholic steatohepatitis (NASH) in obese patients undergoing gastric bypass. Obes Surg 2005;15(8): 1148–53.
29. Dixon JB, Bhathal PS, O'Brien PE. Non-alcoholic fatty liver disease: predictors of non-alcoholic steatohepatitis and liver fibrosis in the severely obese. Gastroenterology 2001;121(1):91–100.
30. Younossi ZM, Gramlich T, Matteoni CA, et al. Non-alcoholic fatty liver disease in patients with type 2 diabetes. Clin Gastroenterol Hepatol 2004;2(3):262–5.
31. Cortez-Pinto H, Camilo ME, Baptista A, et al. Non-alcoholic fatty liver: another feature of the metabolic syndrome? Clin Nutr 1999;18(6):353–8.
32. Luyckx FH, Desaive C, Thiry A, et al. Liver abnormalities in severely obese subjects: effect of drastic weight loss after gastroplasty. Int J Obes Relat Metab Disord 1998;22(3):222–6.
33. Park JW, Jeong G, Kim SJ, et al. Predictors reflecting the pathological severity of non-alcoholic fatty liver disease: comprehensive study of clinical and immunohistochemical findings in younger Asian patients. J Gastroenterol Hepatol 2007;22(4):491–7.
34. Marchesini G, Brizi M, Bianchi G, et al. Non-alcoholic fatty liver disease: a feature of the metabolic syndrome. Diabetes 2001;50(8):1844–50.
35. Ruderman N, Chisholm D, Pi-Sunyer X, et al. The metabolically obese, normal-weight individual revisited. Diabetes 1998;47(5):699–713.
36. Singh DK, Sakhuja P, Malhotra V, et al. Independent predictors of steatohepatitis and fibrosis in Asian Indian patients with non-alcoholic steatohepatitis. Dig Dis Sci 2008;53(7):1967–76.
37. Kral JG, Schaffner F, Pierson RN Jr, et al. Body fat topography as an independent predictor of fatty liver. Metabolism 1993;42(5):548–51.
38. Banerji MA, Buckley MC, Chaiken RL, et al. Liver fat, serum triglycerides and visceral adipose tissue in insulin-sensitive and insulin-resistant black men with NIDDM. Int J Obes Relat Metab Disord 1995;19(12):846–50.
39. Skelly MM, James PD, Ryder SD. Findings on liver biopsy to investigate abnormal liver function tests in the absence of diagnostic serology. J Hepatol 2001;35(2):195–9.
40. Kunde SS, Lazenby AJ, Clements RH, et al. Spectrum of NAFLD and diagnostic implications of the proposed new normal range for serum ALT in obese women. Hepatology 2005;42(3):650–6.
41. Mofrad P, Contos MJ, Haque M, et al. Clinical and histologic spectrum of non-alcoholic fatty liver disease associated with normal ALT values. Hepatology 2003;37(6):1286–92.
42. Prati D, Taioli E, Zanella A, et al. Updated definitions of healthy ranges for serum alanine aminotransferase levels. Ann Intern Med 2002;137(1):1–10.

43. Sorbi D, Boynton J, Lindor KD. The ratio of aspartate aminotransferase to alanine aminotransferase: potential value in differentiating non-alcoholic steatohepatitis from alcoholic liver disease. Am J Gastroenterol 1999;94(4): 1018–22.
44. Diehl AM, Li ZP, Lin HZ, et al. Cytokines and the pathogenesis of non-alcoholic steatohepatitis. Gut 2005;54(2):303–6.
45. Marchesini G, Marzocchi R, Agostini F, et al. Non-alcoholic fatty liver disease and the metabolic syndrome. Curr Opin Lipidol 2005;16(4):421–7.
46. Feldstein AE, Werneburg NW, Canbay A, et al. Free fatty acids promote hepatic lipotoxicity by stimulating TNF-alpha expression via a lysosomal pathway. Hepatology 2004;40(1):185–94.
47. Abiru S, Migita K, Maeda Y, et al. Serum cytokine and soluble cytokine receptor levels in patients with non-alcoholic steatohepatitis. Liver Int 2006; 26(1):39–45.
48. Baranova A, Gowder SJ, Schlauch K, et al. Gene expression of leptin, resistin, and adiponectin in the white adipose tissue of obese patients with non-alcoholic fatty liver disease and insulin resistance. Obes Surg 2006;16(9):1118–25.
49. Steppan CM, Lazar MA. Resistin and obesity-associated insulin resistance. Trends Endocrinol Metab 2002;13(1):18–23.
50. Kakuma T, Lee Y, Higa M, et al. Leptin, troglitazone, and the expression of sterol regulatory element binding proteins in liver and pancreatic islets. Proc Natl Acad Sci U S A 2000;97(15):8536–41.
51. Chitturi S, Farrell G, Frost L, et al. Serum leptin in NASH correlates with hepatic steatosis but not fibrosis: a manifestation of lipotoxicity? Hepatology 2002;36(2):403–9.
52. Chalasani N, Crabb DW, Cummings OW, et al. Does leptin play a role in the pathogenesis of human non-alcoholic steatohepatitis? Am J Gastroenterol 2003;98(12):2771–6.
53. Hui JM, Hodge A, Farrell GC, et al. Beyond insulin resistance in NASH: TNF-alpha or adiponectin? Hepatology 2004;40(1):46–54.
54. Hui JM, Farrell GC, Kench JG, et al. High sensitivity C-reactive protein values do not reliably predict the severity of histological changes in NAFLD. Hepatology 2004;39(5):1458–9.
55. Haukeland JW, Damas JK, Konopski Z, et al. Systemic inflammation in non-alcoholic fatty liver disease is characterized by elevated levels of CCL2. J Hepatol 2006;44(6): 1167–74.
56. Yoneda M, Mawatari H, Fujita K, et al. High-sensitivity C-reactive protein is an independent clinical feature of non-alcoholic steatohepatitis (NASH) and also of the severity of fibrosis in NASH. J Gastroenterol 2007;42(7):573–82.
57. Wieckowska A, Papouchado BG, Li Z, et al. Increased hepatic and circulating interleukin-6 levels in human non-alcoholic steatohepatitis. Am J Gastroenterol 2008;103(6):1372–9.
58. Hasegawa T, Yoneda M, Nakamura K, et al. Plasma transforming growth factor-beta1 level and efficacy of alpha-tocopherol in patients with non-alcoholic steatohepatitis: a pilot study. Aliment Pharmacol Ther 2001;15(10):1667–72.
59. Chalasani N, Deeg MA, Crabb DW. Systemic levels of lipid peroxidation and its metabolic and dietary correlates in patients with non-alcoholic steatohepatitis. Am J Gastroenterol 2004;99(8):1497–502.
60. Horoz M, Bolukbas C, Bolukbas FF, et al. Measurement of the total antioxidant response using a novel automated method in subjects with non-alcoholic steatohepatitis. BMC Gastroenterol 2005;5:35.

61. Sumida Y, Nakashima T, Yoh T, et al. Serum thioredoxin levels as a predictor of steatohepatitis in patients with non-alcoholic fatty liver disease. J Hepatol 2003; 38(1):32–8.
62. Solga SF, Alkhuraishe A, Cope K, et al. Breath biomarkers and non-alcoholic fatty liver disease: preliminary observations. Biomarkers 2006;11(2):174–83.
63. Bonnefont-Rousselot D, Ratziu V, Giral P, et al. Blood oxidative stress markers are unreliable markers of hepatic steatosis. Aliment Pharmacol Ther 2006; 23(1):91–8.
64. Feldstein AE, Canbay A, Angulo P, et al. Hepatocyte apoptosis and fas expression are prominent features of human non-alcoholic steatohepatitis. Gastroenterology 2003;125(2):437–43.
65. Canbay A, Friedman S, Gores GJ. Apoptosis: the nexus of liver injury and fibrosis. Hepatology 2004;39(2):273–8.
66. Canbay A, Taimr P, Torok N, et al. Apoptotic body engulfment by a human stellate cell line is profibrogenic. Lab Invest 2003;83(5):655–63.
67. Wieckowska A, Zein NN, Yerian LM, et al. In vivo assessment of liver cell apoptosis as a novel biomarker of disease severity in non-alcoholic fatty liver disease. Hepatology 2006;44(1):27–33.
68. Poynard T, Ratziu V, Charlotte F, et al. Diagnostic value of biochemical markers (NashTest) for the prediction of non alcoholo steato hepatitis in patients with non-alcoholic fatty liver disease. BMC Gastroenterol 2006;6:34.
69. Gholam PM, Flancbaum L, Machan JT, et al. Non-alcoholic fatty liver disease in severely obese subjects. Am J Gastroenterol 2007;102(2):399–408.
70. Zein CO, Edmison JM, Schluchter M, et al. A NASH predictive index (NPI) for use in patients with non-alcoholic fatty liver disease [abstract]. Hepatology 2007;46(4):747A.
71. Bataller R, Brenner DA. Liver fibrosis. J Clin Invest 2005;115(2):209–18.
72. Brunt EM. Non-alcoholic steatohepatitis. Semin Liver Dis 2004;24(1):3–20.
73. Ratziu V, Giral P, Charlotte F, et al. Liver fibrosis in overweight patients. Gastroenterology 2000;118(6):1117–23.
74. Angulo P, Keach JC, Batts KP, et al. Independent predictors of liver fibrosis in patients with non-alcoholic steatohepatitis. Hepatology 1999;30(6):1356–62.
75. Chitturi S, Weltman M, Farrell GC, et al. HFE mutations, hepatic iron, and fibrosis: ethnic-specific association of NASH with C282Y but not with fibrotic severity. Hepatology 2002;36(1):142–9.
76. Tsang SW, Ng WF, Wu BP, et al. Predictors of fibrosis in asian patients with non-alcoholic steatohepatitis. J Gastroenterol Hepatol 2006;21(1 Pt 1):116–21.
77. Younossi ZM, Kleiner DE, Gramlich TL, et al. Application of NIDDK NASH pathologic protocol to patients with non-alcoholic fatty liver disease. Gastroenterology 2000;118(4):974 [Abstract] AASLD.
78. Willner IR, Waters B, Patil SR, et al. Ninety patients with non-alcoholic steatohepatitis: Insulin resistance, familial tendency, and severity of disease. Am J Gastroenterol 2001;96(10):2957–61.
79. Angulo P, Hui JM, Marchesini G, et al. The NAFLD fibrosis score: a noninvasive system that identifies liver fibrosis in patients with NAFLD. Hepatology 2007; 45(4):846–54.
80. Ratziu V, Massard J, Charlotte F, et al. Diagnostic value of biochemical markers (FibroTest-FibroSURE) for the prediction of liver fibrosis in patients with non-alcoholic fatty liver disease. BMC Gastroenterol 2006;6:6.
81. Dixon JB, Bhathal PS, Jonsson JR, et al. Pro-fibrotic polymorphisms predictive of advanced liver fibrosis in the severely obese. J Hepatol 2003;39(6):967–71.

82. Musso G, Gambino R, Biroli G, et al. Hypoadiponectinemia predicts the severity of hepatic fibrosis and pancreatic beta-cell dysfunction in nondiabetic nonobese patients with non-alcoholic steatohepatitis. Am J Gastroenterol 2005;100(11): 2438–46.
83. Angulo P, Alba LM, Petrovic LM, et al. Leptin, insulin resistance, and liver fibrosis in human non-alcoholic fatty liver disease. J Hepatol 2004;41(6):943–9.
84. Suzuki A, Angulo P, Lymp J, et al. Hyaluronic acid, an accurate serum marker for severe hepatic fibrosis in patients with non-alcoholic fatty liver disease. Liver Int 2005;25(4):779–86.
85. Tamaki S, Ueno T, Torimura T, et al. Evaluation of hyaluronic acid binding ability of hepatic sinusoidal endothelial cells in rats with liver cirrhosis. Gastroenterology 1996;111(4):1049–57.
86. Sakugawa H, Nakayoshi T, Kobashigawa K, et al. Clinical usefulness of biochemical markers of liver fibrosis in patients with non-alcoholic fatty liver disease. World J Gastroenterol 2005;11(2):255–9.
87. Santos VN, Leite-Mor MM, Kondo M, et al. Serum laminin, type IV collagen and hyaluronan as fibrosis markers in non-alcoholic fatty liver disease. Braz J Med Biol Res 2005;38(5):747–53.
88. Rosenberg WM, Voelker M, Thiel R, et al. Serum markers detect the presence of liver fibrosis: a cohort study. Gastroenterology 2004;127(6):1704–13.
89. Bugianesi E, Manzini P, D'Antico S, et al. Relative contribution of iron burden, HFE mutations, and insulin resistance to fibrosis in non-alcoholic fatty liver. Hepatology 2004;39(1):179–87.
90. Younossi ZM, Gramlich T, Bacon BR, et al. Hepatic iron and non-alcoholic fatty liver disease. Hepatology 1999;30(4):847–50.
91. Guha IN, Parkes J, Roderick P, et al. Noninvasive markers of fibrosis in non-alcoholic fatty liver disease: validating the european liver fibrosis panel and exploring simple markers. Hepatology 2008;47(2):455–60.
92. Day CO. The potential role of genes in non-alcoholic fatty liver disease. Clin Liver Dis 2004;8:673–91.
93. Baranova A, Schlauch K, Collantes R, et al. Microarray technology in the study of obesity and non-alcoholic fatty liver disease. Liver Int 2005;25:1–6.
94. Younossi ZM, Baranova A, Ziegler K, et al. A genomic and proteomic study of the spectrum of non-alcoholic fatty liver disease. Hepatology 2005;42: 665–74.
95. Roulot D, Dzernichow S, LeClesiau H, et al. Liver stiffness values in apparently healthy subjects: Influence of gender and the metabolic syndrome. J Hepatol 2008;48:606–13.
96. Nobili V, Vizzutti F, Arena U, et al. Accuracy and reproducibility of transient elastography for the diagnosis of fibrosis in pediatric non-alcoholic steatohepatitis. Hepatology 2008;48:442–8.
97. Meng Y, Talwalker JA, Glaser KJ, et al. Assessment of hepatic fibrosis with magnetic resonance elastography. Clin Gastroenterol Hepatol 2007;5: 1207–13.
98. Pinzani M, Vizzutti F, Arena U, et al. Technology insight: noninvasive assessment of liver fibrosis by biochemical scores and elastography. Nat Clin Gastroenterol Hepatol 2008;5:95–106.
99. Goetze O, Selzner N, Fruehauf H, et al. Methacetin breath test as a quantitative liver function test in patients with chronic hepatitis C infection continuous automatic molecular correlation spectroscopy compared to isotopic ratio mass spectroscopy. Aliment Pharmacol Ther 2007;26:705–11.

100. Spahr L, Negro F, Leandro G, et al. Impaired hepatic mitochondrial oxidation using the ^{13}C-methionine breath test in patients with macrovesicular steatosis and patients with cirrhosis. Med Sci Monit 2003;9:6–11.
101. Garcia-Galiano D, Sanchez-Garrido MA, Espejo I, et al. IL-6 and IGF-1 are independent prognostic factors of liver steatosis and non-alcoholic steatohepatitis in morbidly obese patients. Obes Surg 2007;17(4):493–503.
102. Koruk M, Taysi S, Savas MC, et al. Oxidative stress and enzymatic antioxidant status in patients with non-alcoholic steatohepatitis. Ann Clin Lab Sci 2004; 34(1):57–62.

New Imaging Techniques for Non-Alcoholic Steatohepatitis

Jeffrey D. Browning, MD

KEYWORDS

- Fatty liver • Steatohepatitis • Ultrasound
- Computed tomography • Magnetic resonance

Since the initial description of non-alcoholic steatohepatitis (NASH) in 1980,[1] this disease has been increasingly recognized in clinical practice, paralleling the rise in obesity and diabetes mellitus in the general population. At present, NASH is thought to represent the more extreme phenotype of non-alcoholic fatty liver disease (NAFLD), which is currently viewed as a spectrum of liver pathology ranging from the benign accretion of triglycerides in liver (simple hepatic steatosis) to the morbid condition of excess intrahepatic triglycerides in association with a predominantly neutrophilic inflammatory infiltrate and fibrosis (steatohepatitis). Our current understanding of the development and progression of NAFLD is best encapsulated by a multistep process originally proposed by Day and James[2] and subsequently expanded by Wanless and Shiota[3] A prerequisite for the development of NASH is the accumulation of excess triglycerides within hepatocytes, constituting the first step in this model. In some individuals, caused either directly or indirectly by the accumulated triglycerides, hepatocyte necrosis occurs. Such necrosis leads to the release of bulk lipid from the hepatocyte into the interstitium resulting in inflammation, injury to hepatic veins ,and-over time, perivenular fibrosis caused by venous obstruction with secondary collapse, and in severe cases, cirrhosis.

Though a diagnosis of NAFLD is typically inferred from readily available data (eg, history, laboratory, radiographic) defining precisely where along the spectrum of NAFLD a particular patient resides (ie, staging and risk assessment) requires a liver biopsy. Currently, this measure is reserved for those patients who present with clinical

J.D.B. is a Disease Oriented Clinical Scholar for the University of Texas Southwestern Medical Center and is supported by NIH RL1DK081187 and 1K23DK074396.
Department of Internal Medicine and Advanced Imaging Research Center, The University of Texas Southwestern Medical Center, 5323 Harry Hines Boulevard, Dallas, TX 75390-8568, USA
E-mail address: jeffrey.browning@utsouthwestern.edu

Clin Liver Dis 13 (2009) 607–619
doi:10.1016/j.cld.2009.07.002
liver.theclinics.com
1089-3261/09/$ – see front matter

evidence of hepatic steatosis coincident with elevated alanine aminotransferase (ALT). However, ALT levels are a poor discriminator of the presence or absence of steatohepatitis; Mofrad and colleagues[4] demonstrated an equal likelihood of having inflammation, ballooning degeneration, and fibrosis in subjects with NAFLD, regardless of whether the prebiopsy ALT value was normal or abnormal. Since only 20% of individuals with NAFLD are likely to undergo evaluation for an elevated ALT, the current volume of NAFLD-related health care use, despite recent increases, represents a small portion of a looming health care problem.[5,6] It is estimated that 71 million individuals in the United States alone have a fatty liver.[7] Subjecting all of these individuals to liver biopsy to determine the presence or absence of steatohepatitis is impractical; however, equally impractical is making the assumption that those individuals with a normal ALT are unlikely to have significant NAFLD-related liver disease.

As a result, clinicians are in dire need of a noninvasive screening test for NASH to identify at-risk individuals with NAFLD who are candidates for liver biopsy and most likely to benefit from aggressive lifestyle or pharmacologic intervention. Such a test should be (1) inexpensive, (2) easily applied to large populations, and (3) have a high sensitivity. At present, no such test exists. The purpose of this article is to review the strengths and weakness of current clinical and experimental imaging modalities for non-invasive detection of NAFLD, with an emphasis on NASH.

ULTRASOUND

In clinical practice, ultrasound is typically the first-line imaging modality used in the assessment of liver function test abnormalities. In the setting of hepatic steatosis, liver is typically hyperechoic or bright caused by reflection and attenuation of the sound beam by fat.[8] While additional findings can aid in the diagnosis of fatty infiltration of the liver by ultrasound (decreased visualization of hepatic vasculature, loss of diaphragmatic definition, sparing of the gallbladder fossa, and hypoechoic kidneys), the test is qualitative and has difficulty distinguishing between hepatic steatosis and other diffuse parenchymal diseases of the liver. Additionally, ultrasound is insensitive to modest levels of hepatic triglyceride that may be clinically important. Indeed, the majority of individuals identified as having fatty infiltration by ultrasound have greater than 33% of hepatocytes affected histologically and greater than 10% liver fat content by proton magnetic resonance spectroscopy.[9,10] As such, the sensitivity of ultrasound in detecting hepatic steatosis has ranged widely (60%–94%) depending on the population chosen for study.[11–15] Standard ultrasound provides no information to the clinician regarding the presence or absence of steatohepatitis. Though hepatic fibrosis, a component of NASH, may be detected by this imaging modality, the sensitivity is poor, especially in the setting of mild or moderate fibrosis.[11–15]

Duplex Doppler ultrasonography can enhance standard ultrasound by assessing blood flow in the hepatic and portal vasculature. The current paradigm for the progression of NAFLD would suggest that hepatic blood flow is impaired as a consequence of hepatic vein obliteration.[3] Indeed, there are several studies demonstrating changes in the hepatic artery resistance index, phasicity of right hepatic vein blood flow, or velocity of portal vein blood flow that are inversely related to the degree of fatty infiltration of the liver[16–20] with a single study indicating an association of these findings with portal inflammation.[21] In addition, Magalotti and colleagues[22] demonstrated improvement in portal vein velocity and blood flow in subjects with NAFLD after treatment with metformin. However, whether these changes in hepatic vasculature are reflective of anything more than the presence of excess hepatic triglycerides is unclear: steatosis alone is associated with impaired microcirculation in the liver, probably as a result of sinusoidal compression by hepatocytes engorged with triglycerides.[23] Furthermore, many of these indices are difficult to reliably reproduce from center to center and operator to operator, making their utility for noninvasively differentiating simple steatosis from steatohepatitis questionable.[24]

A newer technology that can also supplement traditional ultrasonography is transient or dynamic elastography for the detection of hepatic fibrosis. This technique analyzes the axial propagation of a transient, mechanically generated shear wave through the liver, a process that is related to tissue elasticity or stiffness. Theoretically, elastography could be implemented using a standard ultrasound machine; however, only the proprietary Fibroscan device (EchoSens, Paris, France) has been extensively studied in liver fibrosis to date. Though this technique demonstrates an adequate sensitivity (>80%) for detecting cirrhosis (F4) in a variety of liver diseases (eg, hepatitis C and B, primary biliary cirrhosis, primary sclerosing cholangitis, alcohol) the ability to detect more subtle forms of fibrosis (F1-F3) remains questionable.[25–28] A single study of Japanese subjects with NAFLD demonstrated that advanced fibrosis (≥F3) could be detected using Fibroscan with a sensitivity of 85%.[29] However, consideration must be given to a factor that limits the utility of this technique: adiposity. The shear waves upon which Fibroscan is dependent to assess tissue elasticity are strongly attenuated in tissues, meaning that significant overlying adipose tissue, as is encountered in most patients who have NAFLD, severely limits the diagnostic value. The mean body mass index of the Japanese population studied was 27 kg/m^2, consistent with the known occurrence of metabolic syndrome and its complications in Asian populations at lower degrees of adiposity. As such, the utility of this technique in a typical Western population with NAFLD remains unclear. Indeed, the authors of this study reported failure of the technique in 5% of subjects who were obese. At present, further study is required to determine if Fibroscan is a viable method for differentiating patients who have NAFLD with no fibrosis from those who have minimal or moderate fibrosis (ie, those likely to have NASH). However, based upon data available for staging other forms of liver disease, this seems unlikely.[25–28]

Contrast enhanced ultrasonography is a new imaging modality that has the potential to increase the utility of ultrasound in a variety of diseases. The contrast agents used are microbubbles with an outer shell composed of albumin, galactose, lipid, or polymers, and an inner gas core (air, perfluorocarbon, nitrogen, and so forth) with a typical diameter of 1 to 4 μm.[30] These agents are injected intravenously, with microbubble residence time in the circulation primarily determined by the rate of uptake by immune cells, such as macrophages.[31] Though typically used to assess blood flow and vascular disorders, a delayed imaging technique assessing microbubble uptake by liver was recently applied in a study of Japanese subjects in an attempt to distinguish NAFLD from NASH.[32] Importantly, no subjects with NASH in this study were cirrhotic, with the vast majority (86%) having mild fibrosis (F1-F2) and all having mild to moderate inflammation (Grade 1: 52%; Grade 2: 48%). Ultrasound images of liver were obtained after contrast injection at 5-minute intervals for 50 minutes, with subjects who had NASH demonstrating a marked decrease in contrast material uptake by liver as compared with subjects who had NAFLD and healthy volunteers at the 5- and 20- minute time point (**Figs. 1** and **2**). Using a cut-off value of signal intensity at the 5-minute time point from the receiver operator characteristic curve, sensitivity for the detection of NASH was an astounding 100%. The difference in signal intensity between the groups appeared to be related to fibrosis and the phagocytic activity of Kupffer cells.[31] These data are intriguing, providing a potential method by which patients who have NASH can be identified in a noninvasive manner. At present, this technique could not be implemented in real-time because of the need for signal

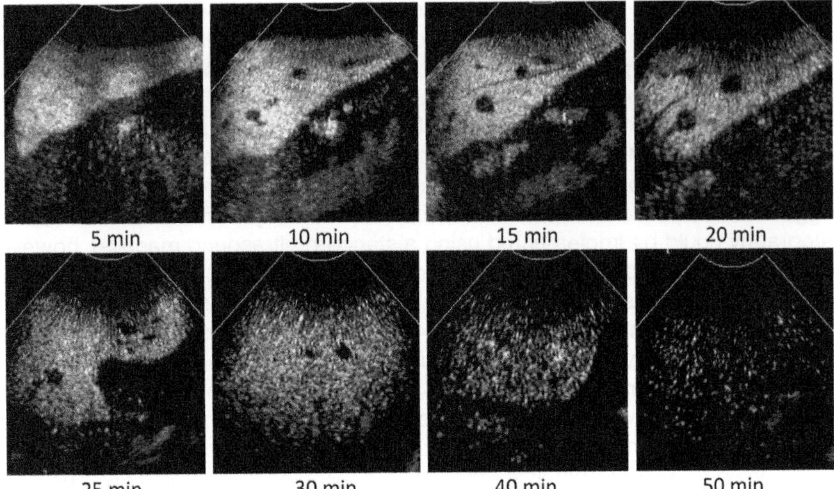

Fig. 1. Ultrasonographic contrast images of liver obtained at 5-minute intervals after injection of Levovist (Schering AG) in a patient who has simple hepatic steatosis. Microbubble uptake is observed for the first 15 minutes followed by washout over the ensuing time period. (*From* Iijima H, Moriyasu F, Tsuchiya K, et al. Decrease in accumulation of ultrasound contrast microbubbles in non-alcoholic steatohepatitis. Hepatology Research 2007;37:722–30; with permission).

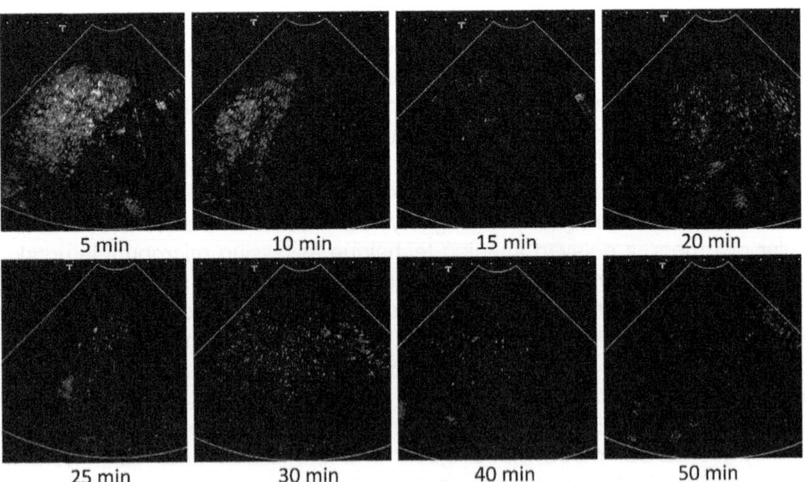

Fig. 2. Ultrasonographic contrast images of liver obtained at 5-minute intervals after injection of Levovist (Schering AG) in a patient who has steatohepatitis. Microbubble uptake is observed only during the initial 5 minutes after injection followed by rapid washout. The maximum intensity is markedly lower than that observed in patients who have simple hepatic steatosis. (*From* Iijima H, Moriyasu F, Tsuchiya K, et al. Decrease in accumulation of ultrasound contrast microbubbles in non-alcoholic steatohepatitis. Hepatology Research 2007;37:722–30; with permission).

intensity analysis in a separate software package. In addition, confirmatory studies are needed in a larger and better characterized population to verify these findings.

CT

Noncontrast single-energy CT can be used to provide qualitative to semiquantitative information regarding the presence of hepatic steatosis. In this technique, the density of liver and spleen in Hounsfield units are typically compared, generating a proportion known as the liver-spleen ratio, or less commonly, as a differential attenuation value. As triglycerides accumulate in the liver, the apparent density of the organ by CT decreases, leading to a reduction in the liver-spleen ratio. This ratio is highly correlated with the presence of fat by histology ($R = 0.77$), with values less than approximately 1.0 being associated with the presence of moderate to severe fatty infiltration.[10] However, as with ultrasonography, parenchymal diseases other than hepatic steatosis can alter the density of liver thereby decreasing the specificity of CT for liver fat. Additionally, the liver-spleen ratio is unable to diagnose NASH. Though CT does provide additional anatomic information beyond the measure of organ density (caudate-to-right lobe ratio, presence of porta hepatis lymphadenopathy, craniocaudal liver span, and the size of the preportal space), a recent study found that these features provide no additional information that is helpful in distinguishing simple hepatic steatosis from steatohepatitis. Finally, the newer, semiexperimental modality of dual-energy CT offers no diagnostic advantage over the standard single-energy technique in NAFLD.[33]

The use of standard iodinated contrast enhancement is typically not used as a diagnostic tool for NAFLD in CT, as it can obscure the presence of hepatic steatosis and provides no benefit in distinguishing bland steatosis from steatohepatitis.[34] However, many studies have used dynamic contrast-enhanced CT in an attempt to stage fibrosis in chronic liver disease.[35–40] In the simplest form, dynamic CT may consist of the acquisition of unenhanced images followed by images acquired in the arterial and venous phase, familiar to most hepatologists as a multiphase or triple-phase scan. A more complex form, known as perfusion CT, involves repeated, rapid scan acquisitions (~1 second interval) at the same location (maximum axial field of view of 20 mm) to determine time-attenuation curves and allow perfusion parameters to be calculated by a variety of methods (eg, moments [tracer dilution analysis], slope [compartmental analysis], deconvolution [linear systems analysis]).[41] Unfortunately, the majority of studies of this methodology have been limited to subjects with known cirrhosis, demonstrating overall reduced liver perfusion in individuals with end-stage liver disease.[35–38,40] In a single study, the perfusion parameters of subjects with noncirrhotic liver disease were no different than the normal control population, indicating that this technique may be unable to adequately resolve early forms of liver injury or fibrosis.[39] There are currently no reports of the use of dynamic CT using standard iodinated contrast agents in NAFLD. However, the known impairment in liver perfusion present in NAFLD, even in the absence of fibrosis, makes the utility of this imaging modality in staging NAFLD questionable.[23] This is highlighted by a recently published study using perfusion CT with xenon gas as the contrast agent in subjects with NASH.[42] In this study, subjects with stage 4 fibrosis showed significant difference in perfusion parameters only when compared with subjects with stage 1 fibrosis and no differences were noted between the noncirrhotic stages of NASH. In addition, the liver perfusion values reported for all subjects who had NASH (eg, 63.4 ± 16.9 and 45.5 ± 10.4 mL/100 mL/min for stage 1 and 4, respectively) were similar to those previously reported for cirrhosis (67 ± 23 mL/100 mL/min) and markedly lower than those previously reported for normal subjects (108 ± 32 mL/100 mL/min).[39,42]

MRI

Unlike ultrasonography and CT, which rely on alterations in an external energy beam (acoustic or X ray, respectively) to generate structural images, the data used to generate MRI are derived from differences in the precessional frequencies of atomic nuclei, most commonly the proton (^1H). For simplicity sake, the proton can be thought of as a spinning magnetic dipole. When placed in a strong magnetic field, as in a clinical imaging system, protons tend to align with and precess about the axis of the field, similar to a top spinning on a tilted axis. The frequency of precession of the protons within the field differs depending upon the environment in which it resides, meaning that a proton within water will precess at a slightly different frequency than one within a fatty acid. These differences in precession frequency can be determined by using an electromagnetic pulse (ie, pulse sequence) to perturb the alignment of the protons within the primary magnetic field followed by measurement of the current induced in a detector coil by the precessing protons. The signal obtained can be resolved into anatomic data for imaging purposes or a frequency spectrum for direct biochemical analysis by way of spectroscopy.

In MRI, a phenomenon known as phase cycling is commonly exploited to diagnose hepatic steatosis using a technique referred to as out-of-phase and in-phase imaging, chemical-shift imaging, phase-shift imaging, phase-cancellation imaging, or two-point Dixon method. After perturbation of the protons in fat and water by an electromagnetic pulse, the signal obtained is a function of the precessional frequency of the protons. Because of the frequency differences between the protons in fat and water, the signals obtained may be either additive (ie, in-phase) or subtractive (ie, out-of-phase) depending upon the duration of time between the electromagnetic pulse and signal acquisition (ie, echo time). Signal loss on the out-of-phase images, as compared with the in-phase images, indicates the presence of fat, allowing for the semiquantitative determination of liver fat. Indeed, the sensitivity for detecting mild to severe hepatic steatosis ranges from 80% to 95%.[43] This technique, however, is incapable of differentiating simple steatosis from steatohepatitis. Other MRI modalities, such as diffusion-weighted and diffusion-tensor imaging, while showing mixed results in staging other forms of chronic liver disease, have not been studied in NAFLD.[44]

MRI can be enhanced by way of the use of contrast agents. Similar to contrast enhanced ultrasound discussed above, superparamagnetic iron oxide contrast agents used in MRI (ie, Endorem, Feridex, Resovist [Bayer Health care]) are avidly taken up by the reticuloendothelial system.[45] In areas of normal liver where macrophages are present and active, uptake of these contrast agents leads to a loss of signal on T_2-weighted images. While a group in France has attempted to use these agents to detect fibrosis, the utility of their technique in detecting mild to moderate fibrosis remains unclear because of the predominance of patients who have cirrhosis studied (93%).[46] Recently, a group in Japan has attempted to optimize the pulse sequences used in conjunction with these contrast agents to allow the noninvasive assessment of not only fibrosis but liver injury in general.[47] These authors found that a marked difference in intensity enhancement was apparent between normal and injured liver after contrast injection when using a moderately long echo time as opposed to heavily T_1- or T_2-weighted images. This methodology was subsequently applied to a group of 19 individuals with mild to moderate fibrosis (stage 0 to 2) and varying NAFLD activity scores, demonstrating a negative correlation between signal attenuation by the contrast agent (%T_2) and severity of NAFLD (**Fig. 3**).[48] A kinetic analysis of the decrease in signal intensity over the 10 minutes following contrast injection was also performed and demonstrated a significant correlation between the

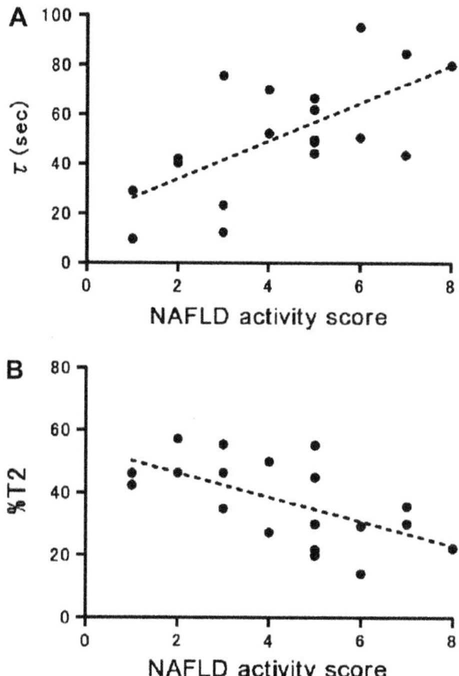

Fig. 3. Relationship between liver biopsy histologic score and the parameters of super paramagnetic iron-oxide enhanced MRI. Depicted are plots of individual NAFLD activity score versus (*a*) monoexponential curve time constant (τ) determined over the 10-minute period following contrast injection (r = 0.66, *P* = .002) and (*b*) contrast induced signal attenuation derived from pre- and postcontrast images (r = -0.58, *P* = .009). (*From* Tomita K, Tanimoto A, Irie R, et al. Evaluating the severity of non-alcoholic steatohepatitis with superparamagnetic iron oxide-enhanced magnetic resonance imaging. J Magn Reson Imaging Dec 2008;28(6):1444–50; with permission).

mono-exponential curve time constant (τ) and NAFLD activity score (see **Fig. 3**). Using cut offs derived from receiver operator curves, the sensitivity of this technique in differentiating definitive NASH from nondefinitive NASH was 88% to 100%, depending upon whether the analysis was performed using signal attenuation or alterations in the kinetic time constant, respectively. Taken together with that presented above for contrast enhanced ultrasonography, these data suggest that contrast agents targeting the reticuloendothelial system in liver hold promise for providing a noninvasive method for identifying patients with NAFLD at highest risk for progressive liver disease. Much more work is needed, however, to fully evaluate the utility and limitations of such contrast-based methodologies.

Gadolinium-based paramagnetic contrast agents are also commonly used in MRI. Gadopentetate dimeglumine (Magnevist [Bayer Health care]) is an extracellular agent while gadobenate dimeglumine (MultiHance [Bracco Diagnostics Inc.]) and gadoxetate (Eovist or Primovist [Bayer Health care]) are agents that are selectively taken up by hepatocytes and excreted into bile. Of these agents, only gadoxetate has been studied in NAFLD. In an animal model of NASH, there is evidence to suggest that the uptake and clearance of this contrast agent diminishes as the grade and stage of liver disease progresses.[49] There have, however, been no studies as yet of gadoxetate in human NAFLD. A group in Belgium has created an E-selectin targeted contrast agent by linking a ligand mimetic with gadopentetate dimeglumine.[50] The selectins, a family of glycoproteins important for the extravasation and migration of neutrophils, are upregrulated by endothelial cells after stimulation by TNF-α, IL-1, and lipopolysaccharide. This experimental agent was able to easily distinguish acute hepatitis in a rodent model of hepatic inflammation (D-galactosamine and lipopolysaccharide coadministration).[50] Whether this agent will be suitable for use in humans remains to be determined.

With magnetic resonance spectroscopy, the signal obtained is analyzed in the frequency domain to determine the molecular composition of the tissue of interest. With this method, planning images are obtained and then a cubic volume of interest (ie, voxel) is chosen within the organ. For proton magnetic resonance spectroscopy, the predominant signals in liver are derived from water and the methyl ($-CH_3$) and methylene ($-CH_2-$) groups of triglycerides (**Fig. 4**). While this technique provides a quantitative measure of liver triglyceride content in agreement with values assessed by histologic and biochemical measures,[51,52] it provides no direct information regarding the presence of inflammation or fibrosis. However, information about the fatty acid composition of triglycerides (ie, saturated or unsaturated) within liver can be obtained because of the different environment, and, hence, different precessional frequency, of protons adjacent to double bonds (see **Fig. 4**). Corbin and colleagues[53] have recently reported that the induction of steatohepatitis in two separate murine models (*ob/ob* mice subjected to lipopolysaccharide injection and C57BL/6j mice placed on a methionine-choline deficient diet) is associated with a significant increase in unsaturated fatty acyl chains as determined by proton magnetic resonance spectroscopy. Though NAFLD is typically associated with decreased levels of polyunsaturated fatty acids,[54] the authors suggest that the inflammatory milieu of steatohepatitis selectively mobilizes these fatty acids from the plasma membrane (a magnetic resonance invisible environment) to the cytosol (a magnetic resonance visible environment).[53] A group in Australian has begun using proton magnetic resonance spectroscopy to study hepatic lipid composition in NAFLD.[54] At present, their spectroscopic technique has been validated but only studied in subjects with spectroscopically, but not biopsy, proven NAFLD. It remains to be determined if hepatic lipid composition assessed non-invasively by proton magnetic resonance spectroscopy will be helpful in differentiating simple steatosis from steatohepatitis in humans.

Phosphorous (^{31}P) is another atomic nuclei that can be studied using magnetic resonance spectroscopy. With this technique, cytosolic concentrations of the components of energy, glucose, and membrane phospholipid metabolism can be quantified, including adenosine triphosphate, inorganic phosphate, phosphomonoesters, and phosphodiesters. However, unlike ^{1}H magnetic resonance spectroscopy, the majority of clinical imaging systems are incapable of phosphorous-based spectroscopic studies without additional hardware and software. Nonetheless, many research groups have examined the utility of phosphorous spectroscopy in assessing liver injury and fibrosis.[55] Because of the heterogeneous nature of many prior reports relating phosphorous spectroscopy parameters to liver disease/injury, a group from Sweden has attempted to refine how these parameters are used.[56] Using a combination of the phosphomonoester and phoshpodiester peaks to calculate the hepatic anabolic charge, the authors demonstrated a sensitivity of 93% for detecting severe fibrosis ($\geq$F3) and 89% for detecting moderate to severe fibrosis ($\geq$F2). Unfortunately, this technique was not specifically applied to differentiate NAFLD from NASH, even though one of the study groups was composed entirely of subjects who had NAFLD of varying severity. In another study using phosphorous

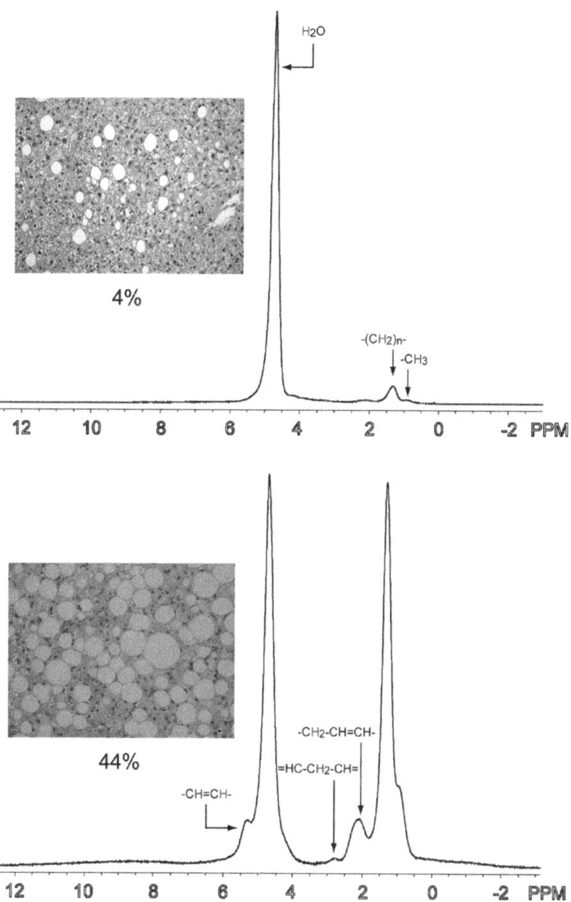

Fig. 4. Hepatic proton magnetic resonance spectra from a patient with and a patient without NAFLD. The top spectrum is from a patient with minimal steatosis histologically, equating to 4% liver fat content spectroscopically. In this spectrum, it can be seen that the signal obtained is derived predominantly from protons in water (H_2O) and the methyl ($-CH_3$) and methylene ($-(CH_2)_n-$) groups of triglycerides. The lower spectrum is from a patient who has severe fatty infiltration of the liver histologically, with a liver fat content of 44% as determined by the proton spectrum. In this patient, an estimate of the degree of unsaturation of the fatty acid components of the triglyceride can be obtained by examining the signals from protons adjacent to double bonds ($-CH_2-HC=CH-$, $-CH=CH-$, $=CH-CH_2-HC=$).

spectroscopy in NAFLD, Cortez-Pinto and colleagues[57] examined the ability of human subjects with biopsy proven NASH to regenerate adenosine triphosphate after a fructose challenge. This study was based upon the observation that an animal model of NAFLD was much more susceptible to ATP depletion as a result of stress or other insult than control animals. Unlike glucose, the metabolism of fructose, which occurs predominantly in liver, is unregulated. The entry of large quantities of fructose into liver can lead to phosphorous trapping and adenosine triphosphate depletion. Indeed, the authors of this study noted a significant decrease in adenosine triphosphate by phosphorous spectroscopy in all subjects after infusion of a fructose bolus. However, while normal subjects were able to recover their preinfusion adenosine triphosphate levels by 60 minutes postinfusion, those who had NASH were not. While intriguing, this study did not assess if this finding was specific to NASH or a universal finding in NAFLD. Additionally, in a follow-up to this study it was found that in vivo phosphorous spectroscopy was significantly hindered by increased adiposity, with measures also showing marked variability over time.[58]

SUMMARY

No imaging modality has yet been proven to reliably differentiate simple hepatic steatosis from steatohepatitis. Though this review has focused on the predominant nonnuclear imaging modalities available to clinicians at the present time, techniques using positron emission tomography and single photon emission computed tomography, though unstudied in the staging of NAFLD, may prove fruitful in the future. The key feature of the techniques outlined in this review that demonstrated the most interesting results have one thing in common: imaging was not performed in a passive manner, but was undertaken as a method to investigate functional differences between simple hepatic steatosis and steatohepatitis based upon the current working model for pathogenesis and progression. Advances in our understanding of the pathophysiologic changes that lead to NAFLD and NASH will allow a logical and focused approach to exploiting current imaging modalities for staging purposes in the future. On the horizon are new contrast agents, especially with regard to MRI. Such contrast agents may take the form of traditional agents capable of peptide targeting, as presented above with the E-selectin targeted gadolinium-based agent. Conversely, a new class of agents is currently being developed that exploits a magnetic resonance phenomenon known as chemical exchange saturation transfer.[59] Such agents have the potential to act as gene reporters and biologic sensors responsive to tissue level environmental changes. An untapped modality for staging liver disease is carbon (^{13}C) magnetic resonance spectroscopy. This technique has a much lower inherent sensitivity as compared with ^{1}H spectroscopy; however, when combined with tracers enriched with ^{13}C the study of complex metabolic pathways is undertaken with ease. Such an approach could allow for targeted study of metabolic derangements thought to be specific for NASH using an in vivo, or even in vitro, approach. Much more work is needed to obtain a reliable, imaging-based predictor of NASH. Advances will necessitate the close collaboration of experts in the field of imaging and hepatology and will likely rely on functional differences in hepatic physiology and metabolism inherent to NASH.

REFERENCES

1. Ludwig J, Viggiano TR, McGill DB, et al. Nonalcoholic steatohepatitis: mayo clinic experiences with a hitherto unnamed disease. Mayo Clin Proc 1980;55(7):434–8.
2. Day CP, James OFW. Steatohepatitis: a tale of two "hits"? Gastroenterology 1998; 114(4):842–5.
3. Wanless IR, Shiota K. The pathogenesis of non-alcoholic steatohepatitis and other fatty liver diseases: a four-step model including the role of lipid release and hepatic venular obstruction in the progression to cirrhosis. Semin Liver Dis 2004;24(1):99–106.
4. Mofrad P, Contos MJ, Haque M, et al. Clinical and histologic spectrum of nonalcoholic fatty liver disease associated with normal ALT values. Hepatology 2003;37(6):1286–92.

5. Browning JD, Szczepaniak LS, Dobbins R, et al. Prevalence of hepatic steatosis in an urban population in the United States: impact of ethnicity. Hepatology 2004; 40(6):1387–95.
6. Weston SR, Leyden W, Murphy R, et al. Racial and ethnic distribution of nonalcoholic fatty liver in persons with newly diagnosed chronic liver disease. Hepatology 2005;41(2):372–9.
7. Szczepaniak LS, Leonard D, Browning JD, et al. Magnetic resonance spectroscopy to measure hepatic triglyceride content: prevalence of hepatic steatosis in the general population. Am J Physiol Endocrinol Metab 2005;288:E462–8 [Epub 2004].
8. Lonardo A, Bellini M, Tondelli E, et al. Nonalcoholic steatohepatitis and the "bright liver syndrome": should a recently expanded clinical entity be further expanded? Am J Gastroenterol 1995;90(11):2072–4.
9. Saadeh S, Younossi ZM, Remer EM, et al. The utility of radiologic imaging in nonalcoholic fatty liver disease. Gastroenterology 2002;123(3):745–50.
10. Longo R, Ricci C, Masutti F, et al. Fatty infiltration of the liver. Quantification by 1H localized magnetic resonance spectroscopy and comparison with computed tomography. Invest Radiol 1993;28(4):297–302.
11. Gosink BB, Lemon SK, Scheible W, et al. Accuracy of ultrasonography in diagnosis of hepatocellular disease. AJR Am J Roentgenol 1979;133(1):19–23.
12. Foster KJ, Dewbury KC, Griffith AH, et al. The accuracy of ultrasound in the detection of fatty infiltration of the liver. Br J Radiol 1980;53(629):440–2.
13. Debongnie JC, Pauls C, Fievez M, et al. Prospective evaluation of the diagnostic accuracy of liver ultrasonography. Gut 1981;22(2):130–5.
14. Saverymuttu SH, Joseph AE, Maxwell JD. Ultrasound scanning in the detection of hepatic fibrosis and steatosis. Br Med J (Clin Res Ed) 1986;292:13–5.
15. Joseph AE, Saverymuttu SH, al-Sam S, et al. Comparison of liver histology with ultrasonography in assessing diffuse parenchymal liver disease. Clin Radiol 1991;43:26–31.
16. Mihmanli I, Kantarci F, Yilmaz MH, et al. Effect of diffuse fatty infiltration of the liver on hepatic artery resistance index. J Clin Ultrasound 2005;33(3):95–9.
17. Oguzkurt L, Yildirim T, Torun D, et al. Hepatic vein Doppler waveform in patients with diffuse fatty infiltration of the liver. Eur J Radiol 2005;54(2):253–7.
18. Balci A, Karazincir S, Sumbas H, et al. Effects of diffuse fatty infiltration of the liver on portal vein flow hemodynamics. J Clin Ultrasound 2008;36(3):134–40.
19. Erdogmus B, Tamer A, Buyukkaya R, et al. Portal vein hemodynamics in patients with nonalcoholic fatty liver disease. Tohoku J Exp Med 2008;215(1):89–93.
20. Uzun H, Yazici B, Erdogmus B, et al. Doppler waveforms of the hepatic veins in children with diffuse fatty infiltration of the liver. Eur J Radiol 2008 [Epub ahead of print].
21. Dietrich CF, Lee JH, Gottschalk R, et al. Hepatic and portal vein flow pattern in correlation with intrahepatic fat deposition and liver histology in patients with chronic hepatitis C. AJR Am J Roentgenol 1998;171(2):437–43.
22. Magalotti D, Marchesini G, Ramilli S, et al. Splanchnic haemodynamics in nonalcoholic fatty liver disease: effect of a dietary/pharmacological treatment. A pilot study. Dig Liver Dis 2004;36(6):406–11.
23. Seifalian AM, Chidambaram V, Rolles K, et al. In vivo demonstration of impaired microcirculation in steatotic human liver grafts. Liver Transpl Surg 1998;4(1):71–7.
24. Lim AK, Patel N, Eckersley RJ, et al. Can Doppler sonography grade the severity of hepatitis C-related liver disease? AJR Am J Roentgenol 2005; 184(6):1848–53.

25. Ziol M, Handra-Luca A, Kettaneh A, et al. Noninvasive assessment of liver fibrosis by measurement of stiffness in patients with chronic hepatitis C. Hepatology 2005;41(1):48–54.
26. Marcellin P, Ziol M, Bedossa P, et al. Non-invasive assessment of liver fibrosis by stiffness measurement in patients with chronic hepatitis B. Liver Int 2009;29(2): 242–7 [Epub 2008 Jul 9].
27. Corpechot C, El Naggar A, Poujol-Robert A, et al. Assessment of biliary fibrosis by transient elastography in patients with PBC and PSC. Hepatology 2006;43(5): 1118–24.
28. Nahon P, Kettaneh A, Tengher-Barna I, et al. Assessment of liver fibrosis using transient elastography in patients with alcoholic liver disease. J. Hepatol 2008; 49(6):1062–8 [Epub 2008 Oct 7].
29. Yoneda M, Mawatari H, Fujita K, et al. Noninvasive assessment of liver fibrosis by measurement of stiffness in patients with nonalcoholic fatty liver disease (NAFLD). Dig Liver Dis 2008;40(5):371–8 [Epub 2007 Dec 20].
30. Lindner JR. Microbubbles in medical imaging: current applications and future directions. Nat Rev Drug Discov 2004;3:527–32.
31. Moriyasu F, Iijima H, Tsuchiya K, et al. Diagnosis of NASH using delayed parenchymal imaging of contrast ultrasound. Hepatol Res 2005;33:97–9.
32. Iijima H, Moriyasu F, Tsuchiya K, et al. Decrease in accumulation of ultrasound contrast microbubbles in nonalcoholic steatohepatitis. Hepatol Res 2007;37: 722–30.
33. Mendler MH, Bouillet P, Le Sidaner A, et al. Dual-energy CT in the diagnosis and quantification of fatty liver: limited clinical value in comparison to ultrasound scan and single-energy CT, with special reference to iron overload. J Hepatol 1998; 28(5):785–94.
34. Jacobs JE, Birnbaum BA, Shapiro MA, et al. Diagnostic criteria for fatty infiltration of the liver on contrast-enhanced helical CT. AJR Am J Roentgenol 1998;171(3): 659–64.
35. Partanen KP. Dynamic CT of liver cirrhosis. Invest Radiol 1984;19(4):303–8.
36. Miles KA, Hayball MP, Dixon AK. Functional images of hepatic perfusion obtained with dynamic CT. Radiology 1993;188(2):405–11.
37. Blomley MJ, Coulden R, Dawson P, et al. Liver perfusion studied with ultrafast CT. J Comput Assist Tomogr 1995;19(3):424–33.
38. Tsushima Y, Blomley JK, Kusano S, et al. The portal component of hepatic perfusion measured by dynamic CT: an indicator of hepatic parenchymal damage. Dig Dis Sci 1999;44(8):1632–8.
39. Van Beers BE, Leconte I, Materne R, et al. Hepatic perfusion parameters in chronic liver disease: dynamic CT measurements correlated with disease severity. AJR Am J Roentgenol 2001;176(3):667–73.
40. Hashimoto K, Murakami T, Dono K, et al. Assessment of the severity of liver disease and fibrotic change: the usefulness of hepatic CT perfusion imaging. Oncol Rep 2006;16(4):677–83.
41. Miles KA, Griffiths MR. Perfusion CT: a worthwhile enhancement? Br J Radiol 2003;76:220–31.
42. Kobayashi M, Suzuki M, Ikeda H, et al. Assessment of hepatic steatosis and hepatic tissue blood flow by xenon computed tomography in nonalcoholic steatohepatitis. Hepatol Res 2009;39(1):31–9 [Epub 2008 Aug 28].
43. Mazhar SM, Shiehmorteza M, Sirlin CB. Noninvasive assessment of hepatic steatosis. Clin Gastroenterol Hepatol 2009;7(2):135–40 [Epub 2008 Dec 6].

44. Bonekamp S, Kamel I, Solga S, et al. Can imaging modalities diagnose and stage hepatic fibrosis and cirrhosis accurately? J Hepatol 2009;50(1):17–35 [Epub 2008 Nov 8].
45. Tanimoto A, Yuasa Y, Shinmoto H, et al. Superparamagnetic iron oxide-mediated hepatic signal intensity change in patients with and without cirrhosis: pulse sequence effects and Kupffer cell function. Radiology 2002;222(3):661–6.
46. Lucidarme O, Baleston F, Cadi M, et al. Non-invasive detection of liver fibrosis: is superparamagnetic iron oxide particle-enhanced MR imaging a contributive technique? Eur Radiol 2003;13(3):467–74 [Epub 2002 Sep 13].
47. Tanimoto A, Mukai M, Kuribayashi S. Evaluation of superparamagnetic iron oxide for MR imaging of liver injury: proton relaxation mechanisms and optimal MR imaging parameters. Magn Reson Med Sci 2006;5(2):89–98.
48. Tomita K, Tanimoto A, Irie R, et al. Evaluating the severity of nonalcoholic steatohepatitis with superparamagnetic iron oxide-enhanced magnetic resonance imaging. J Magn Reson Imaging 2008;28(6):1444–50.
49. Tsuda N, Okada M, Murakami T. New proposal for the staging of nonalcoholic steatohepatitis: evaluation of liver fibrosis on Gd-EOB-DTPA-enhanced MRI. Eur J Radiol; 2008. Doi:10.1016/j.ejrad.2008.1009.1036.
50. Boutry S, Burtea C, Laurent S, et al. Magnetic resonance imaging of inflammation with a specific selectin-targeted contrast agent. Magn Reson Med 2005;53(4): 800–7.
51. Longo R, Pollesello P, Ricci C, et al. Proton MR spectroscopy in quantitative in vivo determination of fat content in human liver steatosis. J Magn Reson Imaging 1995;5(3):281–5.
52. Szczepaniak LS, Babcock EE, Schick F, et al. Measurement of intracellular triglyceride stores by H spectroscopy: validation in vivo. Am J Physiol Endocrinol Metab 1999;276(5 Pt 1):E977–89.
53. Corbin IR, Furth EE, Pickup S, et al. In vivo assessment of hepatic triglycerides in murine nonalcoholic fatty liver disease using magnetic resonance spectroscopy. Biochim Biophys Acta; 2009. Doi:10.1016/j.bbalip.2009.02.014.
54. Puri P, Baillie RA, Wiest MM, et al. A lipidomic analysis of non-alcoholic fatty liver disease. Hepatology 2007;46(4):1081–90.
55. Khan SA, Cox IJ, Hamilton G, et al. In vivo and in vitro nuclear magnetic resonance spectroscopy as a tool for investigating hepatobiliary disease: a review of H and P MRS applications. Liver Int 2005;25(2):273–81.
56. Noren B, Dahlqvist O, Lundberg P, et al. Separation of advanced from mild fibrosis in diffuse liver disease using 31P magnetic resonance spectroscopy. Eur J Radiol 2008;66(2):313–20 [Epub 2007 Jul 23].
57. Cortez-Pinto H, Chatham J, Chacko VP, et al. Alterations in liver ATP homeostasis in human nonalcoholic steatohepatitis: a pilot study. JAMA 1999;282(17): 1659–64.
58. Solga SF, Horska A, Hemker S, et al. Hepatic fat and adenosine triphosphate measurement in overweight and obese adults using 1H and 31P magnetic resonance spectroscopy. Liver Int 2008;28(5):675–81 [Epub 2008 Mar 4].
59. Sherry AD, Woods M. Chemical exchange saturation transfer contrast agents for magnetic resonance imaging. Annu Rev Biomed Eng 2008;10:391–411.

Fatty Liver and Liver Transplantation

Edith Koehler, MD, Kymberly Watt, MD, Michael Charlton, MD, FRCP*

KEYWORDS

- Fatty liver disease • Steatohepatitis • Cirrhosis
- Liver transplantation • Metabolic syndrome • Obesity

Non-alcoholic fatty liver disease (NAFLD) and non-alcoholic steatohepatitis (NASH) are common complications of overnutrition and obesity, affecting up to 30 million people in the United States, of which over 600,000 are likely to have cirrhosis.[1,2] In the setting of worsening epidemics of obesity in developed and developing countries, the global prevalence and impact of NAFLD seems likely to increase. Although only a small minority of patients with NAFLD progress to end-stage liver disease or develop hepatocellular carcinoma (HCC), the large number of patients at risk will translate into major challenges for the liver transplant (LT) community, affecting donors and recipients. Currently 16,000 people are listed for LT; in 2008 approximately 6,000 transplants were performed according to the United States Organ Procurement and Transplantation Network (UNOS http://www.optn.org). The comorbidities and hepatic effects of obesity and NAFLD present important new challenges in the management of LT donors and recipients. This article addresses some of these challenges.

PROGRESSION OF NAFLD TO END-STAGE LIVER DISEASE

There are only a few studies reporting the frequency of NAFLD or NASH as a cause of liver failure. Absent a large prospective natural history study, it is difficult to know the risk of progression obesity to cirrhosis from NASH. There is good evidence that many patients considered to have cryptogenic cirrhosis in fact have NASH as their primary etiology of liver disease.[3,4] Increased oxidation of hepatic fatty acids in cirrhosis[5] leads to loss of steatosis, making a histologic diagnosis of NAFLD difficult in the late stages of disease.[6,7]

Although the Scientific Registry for Transplant Recipients (SRTR) provides accurate nodal data concerning transplant recipients (eg, alive or dead, retransplanted), data involving diagnostic nuances are almost completely lacking. When entering diagnoses for LT recipients at the time of listing, for example, only the primary diagnosis is recorded and, until recently, NASH or NAFLD was not among the 70 available choices. For cryptogenic cirrhosis, a likely alternative primary diagnosis for patients with

---

Department of Gastroenterology and Hepatology, Mayo Clinic and Foundation, Mayo Clinic Transplant Center, CH-10, 200 First Street S.W., Rochester, MN 55905, USA
* Corresponding author.
E-mail address: charlton.michael@mayo.edu (M. Charlton).

Clin Liver Dis 13 (2009) 621–630
doi:10.1016/j.cld.2009.07.010

cirrhosis because of NAFLD, there are no fewer than six appropriate possible choices from the SRTR drop-down list. Although NASH now appears on the drop-down list of primary diagnoses as "cirrhosis fatty liver (NASH)," there are no criteria required for making this selection. An analysis of the SRTR for the frequency of NASH as a primary indication for LT, revealed a 35-fold increase in the frequency of NAFLD as a primary diagnosis between 2001 and 2005. [8] Most or all of that increase, is likely to be attributable to the addition of NAFLD or NASH as a choice on the list of primary diagnoses in 2004. A more reliable index of longitudinal changes in the frequency of NAFLD as an indication for LT is the combined frequency of cryptogenic cirrhosis and NAFLD or NASH. This combination of primary diagnoses has increased from 3.6% to 6.9% in the 5 years between 2001 and 2005—the only indication to have increased in this time frame. This estimate does not include patients with a HCC occurring on a background of cryptogenic cirrhosis or NASH as only the primary diagnosis (HCC in these cases) is recorded by UNOS at the time of listing for LT. A conservative estimate of the frequency of NAFLD as the underlying cause of liver disease among LT recipients would thus be 5% to 10%, equating to 325 to 650 recipients per year, based on current LT volume (http://www.ustransplant.org/). In contrast, the frequency of hepatitis C virus (HCV) as an indication for LT peaked in 2002 at 28% in the United States and has declined every year since (http://www.ustransplant.org/) (**Fig. 1**). It has been projected that NAFLD will be the most common indication for LT in the next 10 to 20 years (**Fig. 2**). **Fig. 1** shows the potential impact of these changing demographics on the relative frequency of NASH as an indication for LT. Unless a safe, effective, and widely prescribed therapy for NAFLD and NASH is identified, liver failure secondary to NASH looks likely to become the most common indication for LT in the United States.

CLINICAL FEATURES OF LIVER FAILURE DUE TO NAFLD AND PRETRANSPLANT CONSIDERATIONS

The clinical features and associations of NAFLD are described in detail elsewhere in this issue. Just as for any patient with liver failure or newly diagnosed cirrhosis, it is important to obtain a detailed history from a patient with NAFLD, particularly with

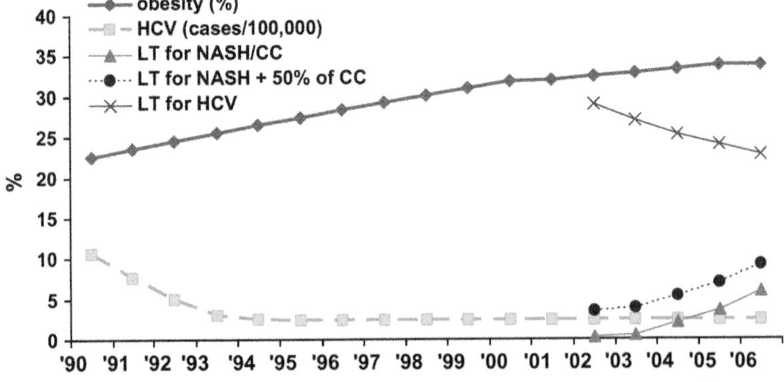

Fig. 1. CDC estimates of incidence of HCV infection and obesity in the United States general population, 1982–2000 (http://www.cec.gov/, plotted with incidence of liver transplant for HCV related cirrhosis and NASH. NASH, non-alcoholic steatohepatitis; CC, cryptogenic cirrhosis; HCV, hepatitis C virus.

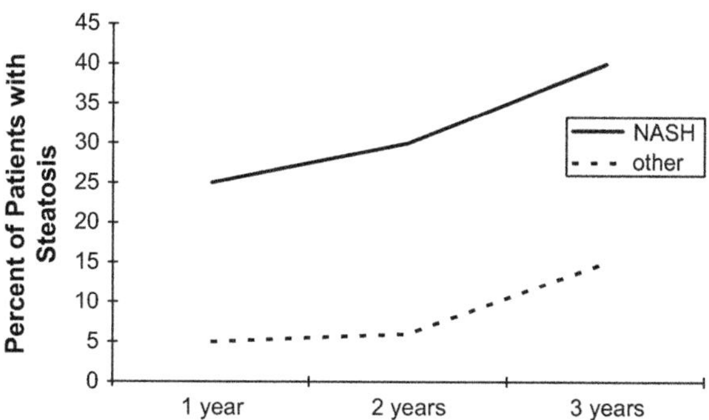

Fig. 2. Percentage of patients with greater than or equal to 33% hepatic steatosis who underwent LT for NASH and other etiologies of liver disease.

regard to previous surgery, drug use, and alcohol consumption. Wilson's disease should be considered and specifically excluded (eg, with 24 hour urinary copper excretion ± tissue copper quantitation) in any patient presenting with evidence of steatosis and liver failure. Hepatocellular failure after bariatric surgery is rare but may occur.[9] Whereas postbariatric surgery hepatic failure is more likely to occur in the setting of preexisting cirrhosis, most patients referred to our transplant unit with postbariatric surgery hepatic failure do not have advanced degrees of fibrosis histologically. The typical picture is of rapidly progressive cholestasis with encephalopathy. Postbariatric surgery hepatic decompensation is probably secondary to the oxidative injury associated with the rapid and large mobilization of peripheral free fatty acids (FFAs) that inevitably occurs following bariatric surgery. Impaired mucosal function with absorption into the portal system of macromolecules, such as inflammatory cytokines and intestinal toxins arising because of changes in the intestinal bacterial flora, has also been proposed.[9] Regardless of cause, hyperalimentation is a cornerstone of treatment (to decrease mobilization of FFA). The benefit of ursodeoxycholic acid and antioxidants such as betaine and N-acetyl cysteine is unknown in this setting but would have a potential physiologic rationale for their use. Patients with cirrhosis due to NASH may describe excessive fatigue, somnolence, or right upper-quadrant pain, potentially suggesting obstructive sleep apnea.[10,11]

In addition to the clinical features of obesity, cirrhosis, and the metabolic syndrome, features of hypopituitarism should be sought in young patients presenting with liver failure due to cryptogenic cirrhosis or NASH.[7,12] Patients with hypopituitarism may develop cirrhosis due to NASH by the second or third decade of life.[12] Patients may, of course, present with complications of cirrhosis and portal hypertension in a manner similar to patients with any other cause of chronic liver disease. Ascites can be relatively difficult to detect clinically in the context of a high body mass index (BMI) because an apron of adipose can preclude accurate examination of the abdominal cavity and the presence of omental adipose can mimic ascites.

In the largest series reported to date, 50% of the patients evaluated for end-stage liver disease secondary to NASH were women.[7] The mean age at the time of evaluation was 54 ± 3 years but appears to occur in a bimodal distribution with patients with panhypopituitarism presenting in the second and third decades of life. Half of patients evaluated for end-stage liver disease secondary to NASH have class II-III obesity (BMI >35), with over one-third of patients having type-2 diabetes, hypercholesterolemia, or hypertriglyceridemia at the time of presentation. A history of previous bariatric surgery (gastric stapling, jejunoileal bypass, and cardiojejunostomy) is also common. One fourth of patients undergoing LT for NAFLD or NASH have HCC diagnosed before transplantation.[7] The prevalence of the MZ phenotype is approximately four- to eight-fold more common (17%) among patients with NASH evaluated for LT than the overall frequency of this phenotype in North America (2%–3.6%).[13,14] It is possible that the combination of NASH and heterozygous alpha$_1$-antitrypsin deficiency are more likely to lead to cirrhotic stages of liver disease than NASH in isolation.

Post-LT Physiology and NAFLD

The prevalence and severity of obesity increases following LT,[15] and is associated with a number of metabolic effects relevant to the development of hepatic steatosis. The prevalence and severity of the metabolic syndrome also increases post-LT.[16] Prosteatotic changes in adipokines have also been described following LT, including increased leptin,[17] decreased adiponectin,[18] and increased tumor necrosis factor.[19] Each of these changes may contribute to recurrent and de novo posttransplant NAFLD and associated insulin resistance.

Levels of oxidative stress, a feature of both animal models of steatohepatitis and humans with NAFLD, are increased post-LT, probably related to calcineurin inhibitors.[20–22] Recent studies have suggested that increased plasma malondialdehyde levels, a marker of oxidative injury, vary with specific immunosuppressive therapies and are specifically worse with cyclosporine than tacrolimus.[23] Each of these effects may have important implications for the natural history of recurrence of NAFLD following LT. Whether calcineurin inhibitor dosing should be minimized or whether tacrolimus should be used as a first line in patients with recurrence of NASH is not known; but there exists a theoretical basis for such an approach to recurrence of NASH following LT.

IMPACT OF NAFLD ON DONOR ORGANS

It is estimated that about a quarter of potential organ donors have hepatic steatosis, the prevalence increasing with age and BMI.[24] Fatty changes in donor liver biopsy have been independently associated with a higher incidence of primary nonfunction.[25] Liver biopsy and ultrasound are often used to quantify steatosis in a potential donor liver, especially in higher risk donors or when the graft appears steatotic macroscopically. As the prevalence of hepatic steatosis increases parallel with the prevalence of obesity and type-2 diabetes, the proportion of donor organs that are unsuitable owing to steatosis may also be expected to increase, owing to the association of primary nonfunction with hepatic steatosis.[25–27] However, livers with microvesicular fat can be used safely for LT, without high rates of primary nonfunction, although there is a significant incidence of poor early graft function, but this did not affect outcome.[28] In addition, graft survival does not appear to depend on the degree of donor steatosis when other contraindications to donor organ use are absent.[29]

Outcomes Following LT for NAFLD or NASH

Reported one and three year patient survival has been 93% and 81%, respectively, following LT for NASH, and are generally comparable to other indications.[7,30] Recurrence of NAFLD is common however.

Histologic recurrence of NAFLD and NASH

In the only prospective histologic analysis reported to date, at 4 months, 60% of transplant recipients with NASH, 4% of transplant recipients with cholestatic disease, 12.5% of transplant recipients with alcoholic disease, and 8% of transplant recipients with HCV developed steatosis grade 2 or higher.[31] At one-year posttransplantation,

60% of transplant recipients with NASH had steatosis grade 2 or higher, with half of these meeting histologic criteria for NASH. Between 5% and 10% of patients undergoing LT for NASH have recurrence that progresses to cirrhosis in long-term follow-up, with graft failure reported in about half of patients with cirrhotic stage recurrence (ie, long-term absolute NASH recurrence associated graft loss rate of 2.5%–5%). A more recent retrospective analysis had similar overall findings but observed no NASH recurrence graft loss.[30] Pretransplant bariatric surgery or a history of panhypopituitarism and post-LT type 2-diabetes mellitus appear to be risk factors for more severe recurrence.

Patients undergoing LT for complications of cryptogenic cirrhosis also seem to be at risk for post-LT NAFLD, with steatosis occurring in about 50% and NASH in 25% of patients in a retrospective study.[32] This frequency was greater than observed in control groups matched for age and weight with pre-LT diagnoses of PBC or alcoholic liver disease.

De novo NAFLD

A single center retrospective report of LT recipients without pre-LT NAFLD described de novo NAFLD in 20%, and de novo NASH in 10%.[33] In multivariate analysis the use of angiotensin-converting enzyme inhibitors (ACE-I) was associated with a reduced risk of developing NAFLD after orthotopic LT (odds ratio, 0.09; 95% CI, 0.010–0.92; $P = .042$). Increase in BMI greater than 10% after orthotopic LT was associated with a higher risk of developing NAFLD (odds ratio, 19.38; 95% CI, 3.50–107.40; $P = .001$). Given the high prevalence of risk factors, it is not surprising that de novo NAFLD is common in the post-orthotopic LT setting, with a significant association with posttransplant weight gain.

The role of protocol liver biopsy

The role of liver biopsy in the diagnosis and management of posttransplant NAFLD or NASH is still evolving. In addition to determining severity of disease, a liver biopsy can also be helpful in determining the effects of medical treatment or change in immunosuppression. Because NASH recurs frequently, can be severe, and cannot be predicted by biochemical profile, protocol, rather than aminotransferase-based, liver biopsies at years one, three, and five postoperatively should be considered.

Treatment of NAFLD Before and After LT

In lieu of a proven efficacious and safe pharmacotherapy for NASH, treatment of NASH should focus on the associated conditions. In obese patients, who make up the majority of patients with NASH, treatment should be centered on weight loss and exercise programs, which are proven efficacious in both adults in children.[34–36] Attainment of an ideal body weight for height is not a prerequisite for improvement in aminotransferases and ultrasonographic evidence of steatosis. Rapid weight loss (eg, secondary to starvation diets or bariatric surgeries) should be avoided as it can exacerbate advanced steatohepatitis and lead to liver failure and/or worsen encephalopathy. A regimen of 140 minutes of exercise per week (eg, 4,000 steps per day of brisk walking) and moderate calorie restriction (25kcal/kg/day) are effective.

For many obese patients sustained weight loss and exercise is, unfortunately, difficult to achieve, particularly in the setting of chronic liver disease. This has lead to a proliferation of empiric and semiempiric studies of pharmacotherapy of NASH. Most studies of pharmacotherapy of NASH have been small, with only a few being randomized with placebo controls. Histologic follow-up is also lacking in many studies of potential treatments of NASH. Improved glycemic control will lower lipid levels in patients with NASH who have type-2 diabetes mellitus (approximately one-third of NASH patients). However, glycemic control in the absence of weight loss will not improve aminotransferases in this patient population.

Metronidazole has been reported to effective in improving steatosis in patients who develop NASH following jejunoileal bypass surgery.[37] As jejunoileal bypass is relatively common among patients undergoing LT due to NASH, presumably due to bacterial overgrowth with translocation of lipopolysaccharide, consideration should be given to: 1) removal of atrophic, redundant loop of jejunum at time of transplantation, and 2) long-term, suppressive antibiotics for treatment of bacterial overgrowth posttransplantation.

Very limited data is available for clofibrate,[38] probuchol (a lipid-lowering agent with antioxidant properties)[39] and gemfibrozil,[40] vitamin E,[41] n-acetyl cysteine,[42] and betaine[43] in NASH. Because of the likely role of increased oxidative stress in the post-LT setting, n-acetyl cysteine and betaine make physiologic sense but there is no conclusive evidence for a beneficial effect for any of these agents to date. Ursodeoxycholic acid, in a randomized, placebo-controlled study, for two years was associated with improvements in liver biochemistries and histology but at a similar frequency to that of the placebo group.[44]

Based on the authors' understanding of the pathogenesis of NAFLD or NASH, insulin sensitization is an appealing approach to treatment. A recent report suggested histologic and biochemical improvement in patients with NASH following therapy with a thiazolidinedione (pioglitazone).[41] Unfortunately, although pioglitazone produces histologic and biochemical improvement in patients with NASH, it can be associated with a significant increase in BMI and possible, although not proven, idiosyncratic hepatotoxicity and is associated with rebound in transaminase elevations on cessation.[45] As peroxisome proliferator-activated receptor (PPAR)-gamma agonists are adipogenic by nature, weight gain is likely to be a class effect of thiazolidinediones, to be enduring, and may negate any histologic benefit in the long term. Combined PPAR-gamma or -alpha agonists appear beneficial in animal models of steatohepatitis.[46] Preliminary results of selective PPAR-alpha agonist in an animal model of NASH have been encouraging, with histologic and biochemical improvement after short courses of PPAR-alpha agonist in methionine and choline deficient mice.[47]

Bariatric Surgery and LT

Post-LT survival among obese patients is comparable to that of leaner patients,[48] although hospital length of stay and complication frequencies are higher.[49] As the prevalence of obesity among LT recipients is increasing, the severity and impact of post-LT obesity is likely to increase also, with an increasing number of patients meeting criteria for consideration of bariatric surgery. Several short-term studies have found a beneficial effect of gastric bypass surgery on NAFLD.[50–52] However, there is scant data on the effects of bariatric surgery before, during, or after LT, including a report describing the beneficial outcome after bariatric surgery in two patients with recurrence of steatohepatitis post-LT.[53] Bariatric surgery has also been employed before transplantation to improve candidacy and, theoretically, post-LT outcomes.[54] It is important to consider some of the potential complications of bariatric surgery in LT recipients. For example, gastric bypass surgery can profoundly affect intestinal drug absorption. If weight-loss surgery is performed pre-LT, thought should be given to sleeve gastrectomy, which preserves access to the gastric fundus (for management of variceal bleeding) and preserves relative absorptive capacity.[55] There is also a risk of hepatic decompensation due to exacerbation of steatohepatitis following bariatric surgery.[9] The role of bariatric surgery in the context of LT continues to evolve.

Choice of immunosuppression

As discussed earlier, many patients with NAFLD have the metabolic syndrome before transplantation. The prevalence of dyslipidemia, hypertension, and insulin resistance all increase following LT because of the effects of immunosuppression. Immunosuppression is an important factor the development and exacerbation of posttransplant metabolic syndrome.[16] Corticosteroids are known to produce insulin resistance, truncal fat deposition, hypertension, and dyslipidemia. Patients with metabolic syndrome posttransplantation have higher risks of developing a major vascular event. Therefore, in an indirect way, immunosuppression can also affect post transplantation outcomes negatively.[16] Tacrolimus may be toxic to beta cells. In addition to increasing oxidative stress and lipid peroxidation, calcineurin inhibitors in general cause hypertension (acute and chronic nephrotoxicity). Sirolimus, in addition to being associated with excess death rates, infections, and hepatic artery thrombosis, is a potent inducer of dyslipidemia. In lieu of randomized studies to determine optimal immunosuppression, steroid avoidance and minimization of calcineurin inhibition should be considered in recipients with NASH. There is increasing evidence that steroid avoidance or minimization of calcineurin inhibitors are safe and reduce the frequency of metabolic complications post-LT.[56–58]

REFERENCES

1. Clark JM, Diehl AM. Nonalcoholic fatty liver disease: an underrecognized cause of cryptogenic cirrhosis. JAMA 2003;289(22):3000–4.
2. Harris MI, Flegal KM, Cowie CC, et al. Prevalence of diabetes, impaired fasting glucose, and impaired glucose tolerance in U.S. adults. The Third National Health and Nutrition Examination Survey, 1988–1994. Diabetes Care 1998;21(4):518–24.
3. Poonawala A, Nair SP, Thuluvath PJ. Prevalence of obesity and diabetes in patients with cryptogenic cirrhosis: a case-control study. Hepatology 2000;32 (4 pt 1):689–92.
4. Booth AM, Caldwell SH, Iezzoni JC. Troglitazone-associated hepatic failure. Am J Gastroenterol 2000;95(2):557–8.
5. Shangraw RE, Jahoor F. Lipolysis and lipid oxidation in cirrhosis and after liver transplantation. Am J Physiol Gastrointest Liver Physiol 2000;278(6):G967–73.
6. Adams LA, Sanderson S, Lindor KD, et al. The histological course of nonalcoholic fatty liver disease: a longitudinal study of 103 patients with sequential liver biopsies. [see comment]. Gastroenterology 2005;42(1):132–8.
7. Charlton M, Kasparova P, Weston S, et al. Frequency of nonalcoholic steatohepatitis as a cause of advanced liver disease. Liver Transpl 2001;7(7):608–14.
8. Angulo P. Nonalcoholic fatty liver disease and liver transplantation. Liver Transpl 2006;12(4):523–34.
9. D'Albuquerque LA, Gonzalez AM, Wahle RC, et al. Liver transplantation for subacute hepatocellular failure due to massive steatohepatitis after bariatric surgery. Liver Transpl 2008;14(6):881–5.
10. Norman D, Bardwell WA, Arosemena F, et al. Serum aminotransferase levels are associated with markers of hypoxia in patients with obstructive sleep apnea. Sleep 2008;31(1):121–6.
11. Newton JL, Jones DE, Henderson E, et al. Fatigue in non-alcoholic fatty liver disease (NAFLD) is significant and associates with inactivity and excessive

daytime sleepiness but not with liver disease severity or insulin resistance. Gut 2008;57(6):807–13.
12. Adams LA, Feldstein A, Lindor KD, et al. Nonalcoholic fatty liver disease among patients with hypothalamic and pituitary dysfunction. Hepatology 2004;39(4): 909–14.
13. Morse JO, Lebowitz MD, Knudson RJ, et al. Relation of protease inhibitor phenotypes to obstructive lung diseases in a community. N Engl J Med 1977;296(21): 1190–4.
14. Webb DR, Hyde RW, Schwartz RH, et al. Serum alpha 1-antitrypsin variants. Prevalence and clinical spirometry. Am Rev Respir Dis 1973;108(4):918–25.
15. Everhart JE, Lombardero M, Lake JR, et al. Weight change and obesity after liver transplantation: incidence and risk factors. Liver Transpl Surg 1998;4(4): 285–96.
16. Laryea M, Watt KD, Molinari M, et al. Metabolic syndrome in liver transplant recipients: prevalence and association with major vascular events. Liver Transpl 2007; 13(8):1109–14.
17. Modan-Moses D, Paret G. Leptin and transplantation: pieces are still missing in the puzzle. [Review] [24 refs]. Isr Med Assoc J 2002;4(3):207–8.
18. Man K, Zhao Y, Xu A, et al. Fat-derived hormone adiponectin combined with FTY720 significantly improves small-for-size fatty liver graft survival. Am J Transplant 2006;6(3):467–76.
19. Boden G. Role of fatty acids in the pathogenesis of insulin resistance and NIDDM. Diabetes 1997;46(1):3–10.
20. Kopp JB, Klotman PE. Cellular and molecular mechanisms of cyclosporin nephrotoxicity. J Am Soc Nephrol 1990;1(2):162–79.
21. Perez de Lema G, Arribas I, Prieto A, et al. Cyclosporin A-induced hydrogen peroxide synthesis by cultured human mesangial cells is blocked by exogenous antioxidants. Life Sci 1998;62(19):1745–53.
22. Vural A, Yilmaz MI, Caglar K, et al. Assessment of oxidative stress in the early posttransplant period: comparison of cyclosporine A and tacrolimus-based regimens. Am J Nephrol 2005;25(3):250–5.
23. Perrea DN, Moulakakis KG, Poulakou MV, et al. Correlation between oxidative stress and immunosuppressive therapy in renal transplant recipients with an uneventful postoperative course and stable renal function. Int Urol Nephrol 2006;38(2):343–8.
24. Koneru B, Dikdan G. Hepatic steatosis and liver transplantation current clinical and experimental perspectives. Transplantation 2002;73(3):325–30.
25. Ploeg RJ, D'Alessandro AM, Knechtle SJ, et al. Risk factors for primary dysfunction after liver transplantation–a multivariate analysis. Transplantation 1993;55(4): 807–13.
26. Marsman WA, Wiesner RH, Rodriguez L, et al. Use of fatty donor liver is associated with diminished early patient and graft survival. Transplantation 1996;62(11): 1246–51.
27. Verran D, Kusyk T, Painter D, et al. Clinical experience gained from the use of 120 steatotic donor livers for orthotopic liver transplantation. Liver Transpl 2003;9(5):500–5.
28. Fishbein TM, Fiel MI, Emre S, et al. Use of livers with microvesicular fat safely expands the donor pool. Transplantation 1997;64(2):248–51.
29. Angele MK, Rentsch M, Hartl WH, et al. Effect of graft steatosis on liver function and organ survival after liver transplantation. Am J Surg 2008;195(2):214–20.
30. Malik SM, deVera ME, Fontes P, et al. Outcome after liver transplantation for NASH cirrhosis. Am J Transplant 2009;9(4):782–93.

31. Maor-Kendler Y, Batts KP, Burgart LJ, et al. Comparative allograft histology after liver transplantation for cryptogenic cirrhosis, alcohol, hepatitis C, and cholestatic liver diseases. Transplantation 2000;70(2):292–7.
32. Contos MJ, Cales W, Sterling RK, et al. Development of nonalcoholic fatty liver disease after orthotopic liver transplantation for cryptogenic cirrhosis. Liver Transpl 2001;7(4):363–73.
33. Seo S, Maganti K, Khehra M, et al. De novo nonalcoholic fatty liver disease after liver transplantation. Liver Transpl 2007;13(6):844–7.
34. Ueno T, Sugawara H, Sujaku K, et al. Therapeutic effects of restricted diet and exercise in obese patients with fatty liver. J Hepatol 1997;27(1):103–7.
35. Coche G, Gottrand F, Sevenet F, et al. Hepatic steatosis in obesity in children. J Radiol 1991;72(4):235–7.
36. Vajro P, Fontanella A, Perna C, et al. Persistent hyperaminotransferasemia resolving after weight reduction in obese children. J Pediatr 1994;125(2): 239–41.
37. Drenick EJ, Fisler J, Johnson D. Hepatic steatosis after intestinal bypass—prevention and reversal by metronidazole, irrespective of protein-calorie malnutrition. Gastroenterology 1982;82(3):535–48.
38. Laurin J, Lindor KD, Crippin JS, et al. Ursodeoxycholic acid or clofibrate in the treatment of non-alcohol-induced steatohepatitis: a pilot study. Hepatology 1996;23(6):1464–7.
39. Merat S, Malekzadeh R, Sohrabi MR, et al. Probucol in the treatment of non-alcoholic steatohepatitis: a double-blind randomized controlled study. J Hepatol 2003;38(4):414–8.
40. Basaranoglu M, Acbay O, Sonsuz A. A controlled trial of gemfibrozil in the treatment of patients with nonalcoholic steatohepatitis. J Hepatol 1999;31(2):384.
41. Belfort R, Harrison SA, Brown KA, et al. A placebo-controlled trial pioglitazone in subjects with non-alcoholic steatohepatitis. N Engl J Med 2006;355(22): 2297–307.
42. Pamuk GE, Sonsuz A. N-acetylcysteine in the treatment of non-alcoholic steatohepatitis. J Gastroenterol Hepatol 2003;18(10):1220–1.
43. Abdelmalek MF, Angulo P, Jorgensen RA, et al. Betaine, a promising new agent for patients with nonalcoholic steatohepatitis: results of a pilot study. Am J Gastroenterol 2001;96(9):2711–7.
44. Lindor KD, Kowdley KV, Heathcote EJ, et al. Ursodeoxycholic acid for treatment of nonalcoholic steatohepatitis: results of a randomized trial. Hepatology 2004; 39(3):770–8.
45. Lutchman G, Modi A, Kleiner DE, et al. The effects of discontinuing pioglitazone in patients with nonalcoholic steatohepatitis. Hepatology 2007;46(2):424–9.
46. Ye JM, Iglesias MA, Watson DG, et al. PPARalpha/gamma ragaglitazar eliminates fatty liver and enhances insulin action in fat-fed rats in the absence of hepatomegaly. Am J Physiol Endocrinol Metab 2003;284(3):E531–40.
47. Ip E, Farrell G, Hall P, et al. Administration of the potent PPARalpha agonist, Wy-14,643, reverses nutritional fibrosis and steatohepatitis in mice. Hepatology 2004;39(5):1286–96.
48. Leonard J, Heimbach JK, Malinchoc M, et al. The impact of obesity on long-term outcomes in liver transplant recipients-results of the NIDDK liver transplant database. Am J Transplant 2008;8(3):667–72.
49. Nair S, Cohen DB, Cohen MP, et al. Postoperative morbidity, mortality, costs, and long-term survival in severely obese patients undergoing orthotopic liver transplantation. Am J Gastroenterol 2001;96(3):842–5.

50. de Almeida SR, Rocha PR, Sanches MD, et al. Roux-en-Y gastric bypass improves the nonalcoholic steatohepatitis (NASH) of morbid obesity. Obes Surg 2006;16(3):270–8.
51. Klein S, Mittendorfer B, Eagon JC, et al. Gastric bypass surgery improves metabolic and hepatic abnormalities associated with nonalcoholic fatty liver disease. Gastroenterology 2006;130(6):1564–72.
52. Barker KB, Palekar NA, Bowers SP, et al. Non-alcoholic steatohepatitis: effect of Roux-en-Y gastric bypass surgery. Am J Gastroenterol 2006;101(2):368–73.
53. Duchini A, Brunson ME. Roux-en-Y gastric bypass for recurrent nonalcoholic steatohepatitis in liver transplant recipients with morbid obesity. Transplantation 2001;72(1):156–9.
54. Takata MC, Campos GM, Ciovica R, et al. Laparoscopic bariatric surgery improves candidacy in morbidly obese patients awaiting transplantation. Surg Obes Relat Dis 2008;4(2):159–64.
55. Butte JM, Devaud N, Jarufe NP, et al. Sleeve gastrectomy as treatment for severe obesity after orthotopic liver transplantation. Obes Surg 2007;17(11):1517–9.
56. Lerut J, Bonaccorsi-Riani E, Finet P, et al. Minimization of steroids in liver transplantation. Transpl Int 2009;22(1):2–19.
57. Klintmalm GB, Washburn WK, Rudich SM, et al. Corticosteroid-free immunosuppression with daclizumab in HCV(+) liver transplant recipients: 1-year interim results of the HCV-3 study. Liver Transpl 2007;13(11):1521–31.
58. Farkas SA, Schnitzbauer AA, Kirchner G, et al. Calcineurin inhibitor minimization protocols in liver transplantation. Transpl Int 2009;22(1):49–60.

NASH and HCC

John M. Page, MD, Stephen A. Harrison, MD, LTC, MC, FACP*

KEYWORDS

- Non-alcoholic fatty liver disease • Non-alcoholic steatohepatitis
- Hepatocellular carcinoma • Cryptogenic cirrhosis
- Hepatic steatosis

Primary liver cancer is the fifth most common malignancy worldwide and the third leading cause of cancer mortality (85%–90%). Hepatocellular carcinoma (HCC) is the predominant cause of primary liver cancer today[1,2] and viral hepatitis and alcohol abuse account for most cases. Non-alcoholic fatty liver disease (NAFLD) is the most common cause of chronic liver disease in the United States, however, encompassing a spectrum of entities marked by hepatic steatosis in the absence of significant alcohol consumption.[3] Although simple steatosis follows a generally benign course, the more aggressive form, non-alcoholic steatohepatitis (NASH), can progress to cirrhosis and result in complications including HCC.[4] A significant number of cases of HCC (15%–50%) remain cryptogenic without known underlying chronic liver disease.[1] Given the association of obesity and diabetes mellitus (DM) with NASH, and cryptogenic cirrhosis (CC), it is increasingly recognized that NASH likely accounts for a substantial portion of cryptogenic HCC.

CHANGES IN DEMOGRAPHIC TRENDS

Although other types of malignancy are generally decreasing in the United States, the incidence of HCC is increasing. Worldwide there are an estimated 500,000 to 1 million new cases each year resulting in 600,000 deaths annually.[5,6] Most cases of HCC occur in the highly endemic areas of Eastern Asia and sub-Saharan Africa where the incidence is over 20 cases per 100,000. Southern European countries are considered at intermediate risk between 5 and 10 cases per 100,000. Traditionally, North America, South America, and Northern Europe have been considered areas of low risk for HCC with fewer than 5 cases per 100,000.[1,5] In all populations, males are disproportionately affected with a two to four times higher rate of HCC than females.

Many areas of high prevalence are now reporting fewer cases of HCC following efforts to vaccinate newborns against the hepatitis B virus (HBV), and efforts in some areas to shift diets away from corn to rice to reduce exposure to the hepatocarcinogen aflatoxin B_1.[1,2] Although the incidence of HCC is decreasing in many

This work received no grant support.
Department of Medicine, Gastroenterology Service, Brooke Army Medical Center, 3851 Roger Brooke Drive, Fort Sam Houston, TX 78234, USA
* Corresponding author.
E-mail address: stephen.harrison@amedd.army.mil (S.A. Harrison).

Clin Liver Dis 13 (2009) 631–647
doi:10.1016/j.cld.2009.07.007
1089-3261/09/$ – see front matter. Published by Elsevier Inc.

high-prevalence areas, it is dramatically increasing in many areas of low prevalence including the United States, where the incidence of HCC has nearly doubled over the past two decades.[1] The increase is most notable among African Americans and whites. Over the 25-year period from 1976 to 2001, although the incidence of HCC among Asians in the United States increased only slightly from 6 to 8 per 100,000, among African Americans the HCC incidence doubled from 2.5 to 5 per 100,000. Over the same period, among whites the incidence of HCC more than doubled from 1 to 2.5 per 100,000.[1] In the United States, however, Asians are still four times as likely and African Americans twice as likely as the white population to have HCC. Furthermore, a recent study has demonstrated that Hispanics have incidence rates second only to those of the Asian population. Hispanic rates of HCC are rising faster than any other demographic, most marked among the native Hispanic population.[7] Recent trends also demonstrate that HCC is now affecting a relatively younger population. Twenty-five years ago, the peak incidence occurred among those 80 to 84 years old. Recently, the peak has shifted to those 70 to 74 years old.[1,2] Mortality rates for all races and both genders have also increased at a similarly significant rate, with HCC being the fastest growing cause of cancer death in the United States male population.[1,2]

The primary risk factor for HCC is cirrhosis, which is present in 70% to 90% of cases.[1] The primary causes of cirrhosis seen in HCC are viral (hepatitis B, hepatitis C); toxic (alcohol, aflatoxin); metabolic (DM, NASH, hereditary hemochromatosis, α_1-antitrypsin deficiency); and immune (autoimmune hepatitis, primary biliary cirrhosis). Although HBV is the most common cause of HCC worldwide, studies demonstrate that in the United States the rates of HCC associated with HBV have been stable. Hepatitis C virus (HCV) remains a major risk factor for HCC in the United States with up to 70% of HCC patients testing positive for antibodies to HCV.[5,8–13] Although several epidemiologic studies have demonstrated that HCV accounts for a significant portion of new United States HCC cases, 15% to 50% of HCC cases occur in patients with CC without other known chronic liver diseases.[1]

INCREASING INCIDENCE OF NAFLD-NASH

NAFLD is the most common cause of abnormal liver enzymes among adults in the United States.[14–16] It is marked by a generalized triglyceride deposition within the hepatic parenchyma that pathologically resembles the macrovesicular steatosis seen in alcoholic liver disease but occurs in subjects without considerable alcohol consumption.[17] The term "non-alcoholic fatty liver disease" originated in 1986 to describe the broad spectrum of related disorders, which includes simple steatosis, steatohepatitis, and its associated advanced fibrosis and cirrhosis.[14,18] The term "non-alcoholic steatohepatitis" was established by Ludwig and coworkers[19] in 1980 to characterize hepatic steatosis with lobular inflammation in the absence of alcohol found in a series of 20 patients evaluated at the Mayo clinic over a 10-year period.[14,19]

In the past, studies estimated the prevalence of NAFLD to be between 10% and 24% of the general population and 57% and 74% of the obese.[20] More recent estimates, however, are that NAFLD affects 30% of the United States population and 90% of the morbidly obese. NASH is now estimated to affect 3% to 6% of the general population and 30% of the morbidly obese.[21] In a study of the prevalence of hepatic steatosis and its relationship to ethnicity, Browning and colleagues[15] used proton magnetic resonance spectroscopy to determine the prevalence of steatosis based on hepatic triglyceride content in 2287 subjects. Almost a third of the subjects were found to have steatosis with a wide variation among different ethnicities. Hepatic steatosis was present in 45% of Hispanics, 33% of whites, and 24% of blacks. A gender difference was only noted among whites, with white men having a higher rate (42%) than white women (24%).

Recent abstract data from a prevalence study of NAFLD-NASH in a primary care setting by Williams and colleagues (Williams CD, Stengel JZ, Asike MI, et al, unpublished data, 2008) demonstrates that both NAFLD and NASH are more prevalent than previously estimated. To date, in this study of 259 adults ages 18 to 70, the overall prevalence of NAFLD by ultrasound criteria was 47.4%. Hispanics had the highest prevalence (55.9%) followed by whites (46.9%) and then African Americans (36.4%). The prevalence of NASH diagnosed by liver biopsy was also higher than previously estimated. Of those diagnosed with NAFLD, 27.8% were found to meet diagnostic criteria for NASH, whereas the overall prevalence of NASH in this entire cohort of patients was 13.2%.

NATURAL HISTORY OF NASH

The natural history of NAFLD is highly variable. Although most patients experience an indolent course, others may progress to cirrhosis and liver-related death. Based on the findings of multiple paired liver biopsy analyses and population studies there is a better understanding of the natural history that leads to the different outcomes among these varied groups; however, many areas remain to be fully elucidated.

Paired liver biopsy data of predominantly NASH patients has shown that over a follow-up period of 2 to 5 years, 18% to 29% of patients improved, 34% to 53% remained stable, and 26% to 37% developed worsening fibrosis with one third of these patients developing rapid progression to advanced fibrosis. Across these paired analyses, 9% developed cirrhosis over this relatively short follow-up period.[3,22–26]

Several population-based studies have also been completed, examining the natural history of patients with simple steatosis.[3] In a follow-up study of a United Kingdom histologic database of patients with simple fatty liver, Teli and colleagues[27] demonstrated the relatively benign course seen in most patients. Forty subjects were evaluated over a mean follow-up period of 11 years (7–16 years). During this period 14 of 40 died, all of non–liver-related causes without clinical evidence of liver disease. Follow-up biopsies were completed in 12 of the 26 remaining living subjects with one patient developing mild fibrosis without progression to steatohepatitis or cirrhosis in any of the other subjects. None of the remaining 14 living patients without follow-up biopsy had laboratory or radiologic evidence of liver disease. In a larger and more recent Danish cohort study of 109 simple fatty liver patients followed for nearly 17 years, similar results were noted. In this study by Dam-Larsen and colleagues,[28] only 1 of 109 patients with simple fatty liver developed cirrhosis and overall the study population achieved the same life expectancy as the general population.

Matteoni and colleagues[4] completed a retrospective review of 132 patients across the full spectrum of fatty liver. The study confirmed the benign course of those with simple steatosis on index biopsy with 4% developing cirrhosis over a follow-up period of up to 18 years compared with 22% of those with fibrosis on index biopsy. This study also highlighted a trend toward increased liver-related deaths among those with fibrosis ($P = 0.08$) compared with the simple steatosis population.[4] Population-based studies have also examined the natural history of patients with NASH. In the series presented by Matteoni and colleagues,[4] NASH follows a more aggressive course with increased rates of cirrhosis (25% versus 3%) and liver-related death (11% versus 2%) compared with fatty liver patients without necrosis.

Two studies have compared the outcomes of cirrhosis in NASH with cirrhosis in HCV. In a prospective cohort study, Hui and colleagues[29] evaluated the long-term morbidity and mortality of 23 Australian NASH patients with cirrhosis. They noted no difference in overall survival between the study population and a comparison group with HCV-related cirrhosis other than a lower incidence of HCC among the NASH population (0 cases versus 8 cases). In a similar study, Sanyal and colleagues[30] compared 152 patients with cirrhosis caused by NASH with 150 matched patients with HCV-related cirrhosis. The investigators noted that although NASH patients with compensated cirrhosis experienced more favorable outcomes than similar patients with HCV, those with decompensated cirrhosis experienced the same poor outcomes experienced by those with HCV. They also noted a lower but not nonexistent risk of developing HCC in those with NASH (10 of 149) compared with those with HCV (25 of 147) with $P<.01$.

In a large community-based cohort study of 420 patients crossing the entire spectrum of NAFLD, Adams and colleagues[31] demonstrated a higher mortality rate (Standardized Mortality Ratio of 1.34) among the study population than the general population. Liver-related death was the third leading cause of death in this NAFLD cohort, occurring in 13% compared with less than 1% of the general population among whom it was only the thirteenth leading cause of death. Overall, 3% of those with NAFLD developed cirrhosis and 2 of 420 developed HCC. These results were recently validated by Rafiq and colleagues[32] in the longest-term follow-up study to date (median follow-up 18.5 years) of patients with biopsy-proved NAFLD. In this retrospective study of 131 of the same patients studied by Matteoni and colleagues[4] a decade ago, the investigators noted a further significantly increased rate of liver-related deaths among patients with NASH (17.5%) compared with those without NASH (3%).

INSULIN RESISTANCE, OBESITY, AND NASH

Although the exact pathophysiologic pathways of NASH are not completely elucidated, it is clear that insulin resistance (IR) plays a key role in its pathogenesis.[15,33–37] In a study of 65 patients with NASH marked by mild to advanced fibrosis, Chitturi and colleagues[38] demonstrated that virtually all subjects (98%) were insulin resistant. This study also noted that IR may be present even in the absence of obesity, occurring also in lean subjects.

Overall, however, anthropometric data from multiple studies demonstrate that patients with NASH have significantly higher body mass indices (BMI), body fat, and more specifically increased central visceral adiposity than matched controls.[39] Elevated BMI has also been linked to increased serum alanine aminotransferase activity used as a surrogate marker for the presence of NAFLD in a large United States population-based study.[40] Central adiposity and serum insulin levels were among the variables accounting for this relationship in the study. Solga and colleagues[41,42] also found a positive correlation between higher caloric intake and inflammation in patients with NASH.

Of note, the national rate of obesity has risen at an alarming pace over the past several decades, increasing overall from 22.9% in 1988 to 1994 to 30.5% in 1999 to 2000.[43,44] This may be partially explained by increased rates of fast food consumption given the findings of a large, long-term prospective study of dietary habits among young adults. Investigators found a significant association between fast food frequency and IR with changes in body weight.[44] Given the current trends in obesity and IR and the fact that they play a major role underlying the development of

NASH, one can expect the incidence of NASH and its liver-related complications likely to increase dramatically over the coming decades.

OBESITY AND HCC

Of equal concern is the finding that not only is obesity a risk factor for NASH, it is also a risk factor for HCC.[45] Two large population studies have demonstrated an association between obesity and liver cancer. Moller and colleagues[46] noted an increased risk of liver cancer (relative risk = 1.9) among obese patients discharged from Danish hospitals. In a more recent prospective United States study, the investigators followed 900,000 subjects for 16 years, controlling for alcohol use and stratifying cancer death risk by BMI. Obese women were found to have an increased risk of death from liver cancer of 1.68 compared with nonobese contemporaries. Obese males had 4.52 times the risk of death from liver cancer compared with nonobese peers. This was the highest increased risk of death from any form of cancer noted among obese patients enrolled in the study.[47] In a prospective study of 771 French patients with well-compensated alcoholic and hepatitis C–related cirrhosis, BMI was found to have a positive linear relationship with incidence of HCC over the follow-up period of up to 7 years. In this study, BMI between 25 and 30 kg/m^2 was associated with a hazard ratio of 2, whereas BMI of 30 kg/m^2 or greater was associated with a hazard ratio of 2.8.[48]

DM AND NASH

In addition to obesity, DM is a key element of the metabolic syndrome characterized by IR. Evidence supports the fact that DM is a risk factor for NAFLD and NASH.[45,49–52] In the previously cited analysis of Dallas Heart Study participants, investigators found that individuals with hepatic steatosis were significantly more likely to be diabetic (18% versus 11%, $P<.001$).[15] Conversely, Neuschwander-Tetri and Caldwell[53] have estimated that 75% of patients with type II DM have some degree of hepatic steatosis. In a large paired liver biopsy study of patients with simple steatosis and NASH, Adams and colleagues[26] determined that DM was a strong independent predictor of higher rates of fibrosis progression. Impaired fasting glucose and DM were also shown to be risk factors for death among patients with NAFLD based on data from a community-based cohort study.[31] Furthermore, DM has been shown to be an independent predictor of liver-related mortality in a recent long-term follow-up study of patients with NAFLD.[32]

DM AND HCC

Very early studies also confirmed a relationship between DM and HCC. Case control studies from as early as 1986 found an increased incidence (up to fourfold) of DM among patients with HCC.[54–56] A 2001 case control study by El-Serag and colleagues[57] of 823 subjects found an increased risk of HCC among diabetics with other risk factors for chronic liver disease including HBV, HCV, and alcoholic cirrhosis. In a subsequent large prospective cohort study of predominantly male veterans, investigators demonstrated that patients with DM were more than twice as likely as controls to develop chronic non-alcoholic liver disease or HCC as shown in **Fig. 1**.[58,59] These results were validated in a large population-based case control study of the Surveillance Epidemiology and End-Results program database demonstrating a 2.87 odds ratio of HCC among older patients with DM without other risk factors for chronic liver disease.[50] In a previously cited prospective study of 771

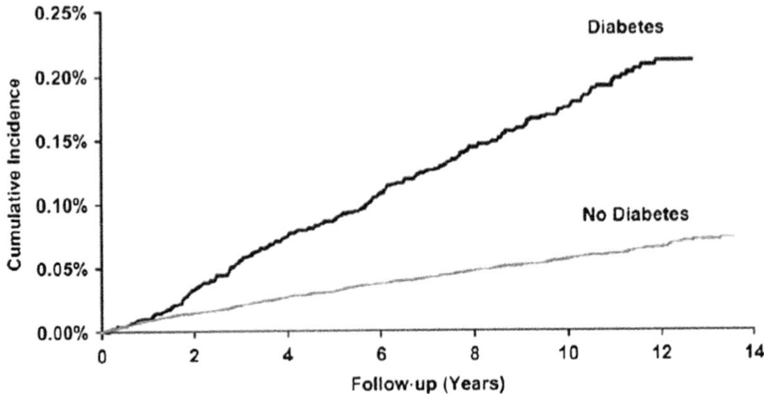

Fig. 1. The cumulative risk of HCC among hospitalized Veterans Administration study population (based on Kaplan-Meier survival analysis). Top line outlines cumulative incidence of HCC at follow-up among patients with DM. Lower line outlines cumulative incidence of HCC at follow-up among patients without DM. The cumulative incidence of HCC was significantly higher among those with DM (*P*<.0001). (*Adapted from* El-Serag HB, Tran T, Everhart JE. Diabetes increases the risk of chronic liver disease and hepatocellular carcinoma. Gastroenterology 2004;126:460–8; with permission).

French patients with well-compensated alcoholic or hepatitis C–related cirrhosis, DM was associated with a 1.6 times increased risk of HCC.[48] DM was also found to be an independent risk factor for HCC arising in the setting of CC.[51] These results are consistent with the findings of multiple other studies involving patients with CC.[45,51,60,61] A systematic review and meta analysis of the literature between 1966 and 2005 also demonstrated a significant association of DM with HCC in 9 of 13 case-controlled studies (pooled odds ratio of 2.5) and 7 of 13 cohort studies (pooled odds ratio of 2.5) as shown in **Fig. 2.**[49]

COMBINED EFFECT OF OBESITY AND DM ON HCC

A synergistic effect of the metabolic factors DM and obesity is evident in relation to HCC incidence. In an Italian case control study of 185 HCC cases without markers

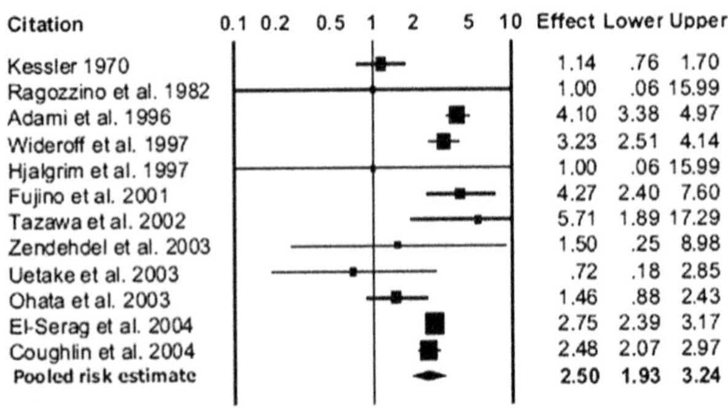

Citation	Effect	Lower	Upper
Kessler 1970	1.14	.76	1.70
Ragozzino et al. 1982	1.00	.06	15.99
Adami et al. 1996	4.10	3.38	4.97
Wideroff et al. 1997	3.23	2.51	4.14
Hjalgrim et al. 1997	1.00	.06	15.99
Fujino et al. 2001	4.27	2.40	7.60
Tazawa et al. 2002	5.71	1.89	17.29
Zendehdel et al. 2003	1.50	.25	8.98
Uetake et al. 2003	.72	.18	2.85
Ohata et al. 2003	1.46	.88	2.43
El-Serag et al. 2004	2.75	2.39	3.17
Coughlin et al. 2004	2.48	2.07	2.97
Pooled risk estimate	**2.50**	**1.93**	**3.24**

Fig. 2. Individual risk ratios with 95% CIs and pooled risk estimates of the association between DM and HCC among 12 cohort studies. (*Adapted from* El-Serag HB, Hampel H, Javadi F. The association between diabetes and hepatocellular carcinoma: a systematic review of epidemiologic evidence. Clin Gastroenterol Hepatol 2006;4:369–80; with permission).

of HBV or HCV, investigators found an increased incidence of HCC among those with obesity defined as BMI of at least 30 kg/m^2 (odds ratio = 3.5) and a similarly increased incidence of HCC among those with DM (odds ratio = 3.5). In those with both obesity and DM, however, the odds ratio of HCC rose to 11.8 compared with nonobese, nondiabetic patients.[62]

Chen and colleagues[63] studied 23,820 Taiwanese residents over a 14-year follow-up period to determine the effects of various metabolic factors on the incidence of HCC, stratified by HBV and HCV seromarkers. BMI over 30 kg/m^2 was independently associated with a twofold increased risk of HCC in those without HBV or HCV and a fourfold increased risk in those with HCV. DM was associated with a relative risk of HCC of 2.27 in those with HBV and 3.52 in those with HCV. Although this study found both elevated BMI and DM independently associated with increased incidence of HCC, the combined effect of both metabolic factors was markedly elevated with a 100-fold increased risk of HCC in HBV or HCV carriers with both obesity and DM.

CC AND HCC

Most cases of HCC occur in the setting of chronic liver disease complicated by cirrhosis and in the United States are secondary to viral hepatitis or alcohol. Less commonly patients develop HCC in the setting of clear metabolic or immune-mediated etiologies.[5] In 15% to 50% of cases of HCC diagnosed in the United States, however, patients have no established risk factors for their underlying cirrhosis and after a thorough investigation are determined to have CC.[1] It has been theorized that CC often represents "burned out" NASH. A significant number of these patients have a phenotype for NASH but the diagnostic histopathologic features of NASH have largely disappeared in the setting of advanced fibrosis and cirrhosis making a diagnosis of the underlying etiology very difficult if not impossible.

To clarify the cause of CC, multiple studies have been performed to clinically characterize and assess risk factors underlying these cases of CC. Caldwell and coworkers[45] completed a study of 70 patients with CC comparing their major risks for liver disease with a group of NASH patients without cirrhosis, a group of patients with cirrhosis secondary to HCV, and a third comparison group with cirrhosis second to primary biliary cirrhosis. Although both obesity (BMI >95th percentile) and DM were significantly more common in the CC group than in those with HCV or primary biliary cirrhosis–associated cirrhosis, the rates of obesity and DM were similar between those with CC and the noncirrhotic NASH comparison population. In a case control study of 49 patients with advanced CC (Child-Pugh score >6), investigators demonstrated significantly higher rates of obesity and DM among subjects compared with age and gender-matched controls with advanced cirrhosis of known etiologies (excluding NASH).[60] Along similar lines, obesity was noted to be an independent risk factor for HCC in patients with CC (odds ratio = 11.1) in a study by Nairet and coworkers.[64] Regimbeau and colleagues[61] demonstrated that CC patients share many characteristic features of NAFLD supporting the theory that NAFLD is a significant risk factor for HCC.

Several studies have also explored the natural history of HCC arising in CC. In a retrospective case control study, Bugianesi and colleagues[51] demonstrated that features suggestive of the metabolic syndrome are observed more frequently in patients with HCC arising in the setting of CC than in matched controls. These features include DM, obesity, dyslipidemia, and IR as shown in **Fig. 3**. In a similar study comparing 27 overweight patients with CC, 10 lean patients with CC, and HCV-related cirrhosis controls, Ratziu and coworkers[65] noted similarly significantly increased rates

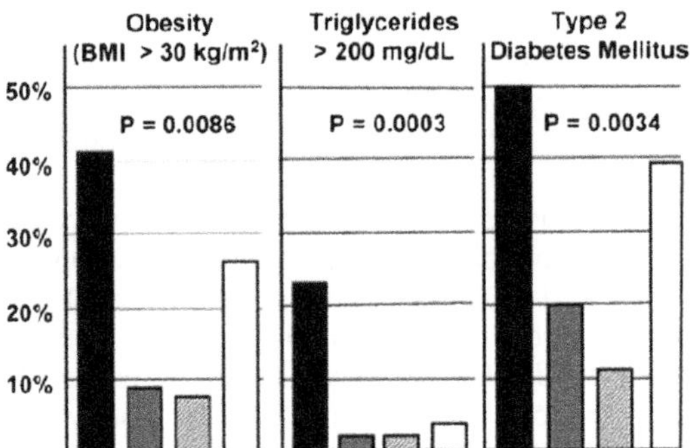

Fig. 3. Prevalence of obesity, hypertriglyceridemia, and diabetes mellitus in patients with HCC second to CC (*dark bars*) versus HCV (*dark gray bars*) versus HBV (*light gray bars*) versus alcohol (*white bars*). *P* values for CC compared with all other etiologies are displayed. BMI, body mass index. (*Adapted from* Bugianesi E, Leone N, Vanni E, et al. Expanding the natural history of non-alcoholic steatohepatitis: from cryptogenic cirrhosis to hepatocellular carcinoma. Gastroenterology 2002;123:134–44; with permission).

of dysmetabolic features among the obese population including DM and hypertriglyceridemia. A higher albeit not significant rate of HCC was also noted among the obese group (30%) compared with the HCV control population (21%) ($P = 0.4$). Also of note, the obese CC patients were diagnosed at a significantly older age than those with HCV cirrhosis (62.1 versus 53.7, $P<.001$). These studies have consistently demonstrated that features consistent with NASH, specifically obesity and DM, occur significantly more frequently in patients with CC than in those with cirrhosis second to alcohol or viral etiologies.

Investigators have also noted unique features of HCC tumors arising in CC. In a surgical series of 210 patients who underwent resection for HCC, Regimbeau and colleagues[61] noted a significantly increased rate of well-differentiated tumors among those with CC (89% versus 64% versus 55%, $P = 0.01$) compared with those with underlying alcohol or viral-related liver disease. These patients were also more likely to have multiple tumors (22%) and large tumors (8.1 cm) compared with those with alcohol (5%, 6 cm) or viral-related HCC (11%, 6.2 cm), although these differences were not statistically significant.

NASH AND HCC

In addition to the numerous studies linking the risk factors for NAFLD to HCC, there have been several studies and numerous case reports that have directly explored the relationship between NAFLD and HCC. In a cohort study of 7326 patients discharged from Danish hospitals over a 16-year period with a diagnosis of fatty liver, investigators evaluated the risk for cancer among patients with NAFLD. The risk for primary liver cancer among NAFLD patients was markedly elevated with a standardized incidence ratio of 4.4.[66]

In a large single center case series of 105 patients with HCC, subgroup analysis of the 30 patients with CC suggested that NAFLD accounted for 47% of the cases of CC and 13% of the cases of HCC. Six of the NAFLD patients had prior histologic confirmation of NASH and eight others had clinical features consistent with NAFLD. Overall, compared with the non-NAFLD subgroup with CC, the NAFLD subgroup featured BMI greater than or equal to 30 (93% versus 13%, $P<.001$); DM (93% versus 25%, $P<.001$); and hyperlipidemia (29% versus 6%, $P<.001$).[67]

There is extensive case literature describing at least 67 cases of HCC arising in the setting of underlying NASH (**Table 1**).[52,68–82] Most cases occur in males (66%). Age at diagnosis ranged from 45 to 82 (mean, 66.7). Most patients were obese (58%) and diabetic (64%). Case data are consistent with the previously cited CC findings of generally large, multiple, well-differentiated tumors.[61] Strikingly, in 33% of cases, HCC seems to have arisen in the absence of cirrhosis.[69,70,72,73,76,79,80,82] In one case, HCC arose in a patient with NASH in the absence of cirrhosis but following a 17-year history of valproic acid use.[76] It is unclear if this represents a case of primary NASH-induced HCC or secondary drug-induced steatohepatitis. Regardless, these cases may compel a more aggressive approach in the future to screening the NASH population for HCC.

In a large series of nine Japanese patients with HCC occurring in the setting of NASH, all but one were diagnosed with the metabolic syndrome. HCC arose in the absence of cirrhosis in 33% of cases. Men comprised 66% and women 33% of the series. Average age of HCC diagnosis was 67.7 years, whereas the median age of HCC diagnosis was 72 years. One patient died following transarterial embolization. There were no recurrences in the other nine patients, however, after an average follow-up of 32 months following resection or radiofrequency ablation. Consistent with previous studies, these investigators noted that age and advanced fibrosis were risk factors for HCC in NASH.[82]

In a large case-controlled study of 34 Japanese NASH patients with HCC, those with HCC were predominantly male (62%); had a median age of 70 years; and 88% had advanced (F3–F4) fibrosis. Older age, low level of AST, low grade of inflammation, and advanced fibrosis were determined to be significant risk factors for developing HCC in NASH. Confirming prior studies, older age and fibrosis had the strongest association with HCC.[83] In a parallel prospective cohort study of 137 NASH patients conducted from 1990 to 2007, the same investigators demonstrated a 5-year cumulative incidence of HCC in NASH of 7.6% and a 5-year survival rate of 82.8% with HCC confirmed as the leading cause of death.[83]

HEPATOCELLULAR CARCINOGENESIS IN THE SETTING OF NASH

Although hepatocarcinogenesis seems to originate in chronic liver damage, the process occurs exponentially in the setting of cirrhosis when the regenerative capacity of the liver is exhausted.[1] It is believed to begin with initiating events leading to cellular DNA damage followed by processes that promote the development of malignant cell lines.[84]

NASH is characterized by IR marked by hyperinsulinemia, which is believed to be a risk factor for colon, endometrial, and pancreatic cancer.[85,86] It may induce HCC by up-regulating multiple growth factors. Insulin induces insulin-like growth factor (IGF)-1, a peptide hormone that stimulates growth through cellular proliferation and inhibition of apoptosis. Insulin also mediates growth by activation of mitogen-activated kinases and phosphorylation of insulin receptor substrate-1 (IRS-1).[84,85,87,88] Human hepatoma cells have been demonstrated to overexpress both IGF-1 and IRS-1.[84] It is also theorized that overexpression of IRS-1 may prevent transforming growth factor-b mediated apoptosis.[84,89] IGF-2 loss of heterozygosity has also been observed to occur in over 60% of HCC cases.[90] This likely coincides with IGF-2 overexpression, observed in HCC, which has been linked to reduced apoptosis and increased cellular proliferation.[91]

There is also evidence that hepatocarcinogenesis in NASH may be partially mediated by increased release of free fatty acids and adipokines secreted by adipose

Table 1
Case reports of HCC in setting of NASH

Case #	Author	Age HCC Dx	Gender	Other Dx	Liver Dz	Tumor #	Size (cm)	Liver Histology	Tx	Follow Up (mo)	Outcome
1	Powell	57	F	DM	4	Multi		Cirrhosis	Surgery	7	Died
2	Cotrim	66	M	OB/DM	4	Single	3	Cirrhosis	PEI	24	Died
3	Zen	72	F	DM	10	Multi	1–1.4	Cirrhosis	NR		NR
4	Orikasa	67	F	DM	NR	Single	2.6	Cirrhosis			NR
5	Shimada	66	F	DM	2.5	Single	1.5	Cirrhosis	Surgery	28	Recurred
6	Yoshioka/ Shimada	69	F		2	Multi	1.5	Cirrhosis	TAE	26	Died
7	Shimada	69	F	OB/DM	0.5	Single	2.5	Cirrhosis	TAI	14	Recurred
8	Shimada	72	M	OB	0	Single	3	Cirrhosis	TAE/PEI	30	Recurred
9	Shimada	63	M	OB	0	Single	2	Cirrhosis	Surgery	48	No recurrence
10	Shimada	56	M	DM	0	Multi	1–6	Cirrhosis	TAE	12	Died
11	Bencheqroun	68	M	OB	0	Unk	Unk	No cirrhosis	Unk	Unk	Unk
12	Mori	76	M	OB/DM	10	Single	1.9	Cirrhosis	RFA	8	No recurrence
13	Bullock	74	M	OB/DM	0	Single	4	No cirrhosis	Surgery	NR	NR
14	Bullock	64	M	OB/DM	0	Single	"large"	No cirrhosis	TAE/Sur	12	No recurrence
15	Cuadrado	74	M	OB/DM	0	Single	NR	No cirrhosis	RFA	12	Recurred
16	Cuadrado	69	M	OB/DM	7	Multi	1/2.2	Cirrhosis	RFA	NR	Transplant
17	Sato	64	M	OB	0	Single	13	No cirrhosis	None	12	Died
18	Ikeda	69	M	OB/DM	NR	Single	4.5	Cirrhosis	TAE/Sur	NR	NR

19	Hai	72	M	OB/DM	0	Single	4	No cirrhosis	Surgery	NR	NR
20	Hai	65	M		NR	Single	6	Cirrhosis	Surgery	NR	NR
21	Ichikawa	66	F	OB	NR	Single	2.5	No cirrhosis	Surgery	14	No recurrence
22	Ichikawa	60	M		NR	Single	1.5	No cirrhosis	Surgery	5	No recurrence
23	Tsutsumi	68	F	NR	26	Single	NR	Cirrhosis	NR	NR	NR
24	Tsutsumi	46	M	NR	26	Single	NR	Cirrhosis	NR	NR	NR
25	Hashizume	74	M	DM	Unk	Single	2.4	Cirrhosis	Surgery	33	No recurrence
26	Hashizume	45	M	OB/DM	Unk	Single	3.5	Cirrhosis	Surgery	22	No recurrence
27	Hashizume	54	M	OB/DM	Unk	Multi	7/1.5	No cirrhosis	Surgry/Chemo	13	No recurrence
28	Hashizume	82	F	OB	Unk	Single	3	No cirrhosis	Surgery	22	No recurrence
29	Hashizume	77	M	OB/DM	Unk	Single	3	Cirrhosis	TAE	11	Died
30	Hashizume	75	M		Unk	Single	3	Cirrhosis	Surgery	NR	No recurrence
31	Hashizume	67	F	DM	Unk	Single	2	Cirrhosis	RFA	NR	No recurrence
32	Hashizume	63	F	OB/DM	Unk	Single	1.5	Cirrhosis	RFA	NR	No recurrence
33	Hashizume	72	M	DM	Unk	Single	4	No cirrhosis	Surgery	50	No recurrence
34–67	Hashimoto	Median	M (21)	OB 62%	NR	Single	NR	F1/2 22%	NR	NR	NR
	Study (N = 34)	70	F (13)	DM 74%				F3/4 88%			

Abbreviations: DM, diabetes mellitus; Dx, diagnosis; NR, not reported; OB, obesity; PEI, percutaneous ethanol injection; RFA, radiofrequencey ablation; TAE, transarterial embolization; TAI, transarterial infusion chemotherapy; Tx, treatment; Unk, unknown.

tissue, which alter the immune response and modulate the release of inflammatory and inhibitory cytokines, such as tumor necrosis factor-α, nuclear factor k –B, and interleukin-6.[1,92–94] This process coincides with reduced release of adiponectin and increased stellate cell activation resulting in increased production of extracellular matrix proteins, growth factors, and further inflammatory cytokines.[1,95]

Further, with respect to NASH, in an insulin-resistant obese mouse model, mitochondrial dysfunction, and hepatic lipid peroxidation have been demonstrated to produce excess production of reactive oxygen species resulting in hepatic hyperplasia and oxidative stress.[85,96] Oxidative stress is theorized to promote carcinogenesis through multiple pathways including induction of mutations in the p53 tumor suppressor gene in a pattern observed in HCC.[85,97] Oxidative stress has been further implicated in blocking expression of transcription factor Nrf1, an activator of hepatic "antioxidant response elements" that regulate gene transcription encoding enzymatic antioxidants. In an animal model, oxidative stress disruption of Nrf1 hepatocyte function resulted in steatohepatitis and spontaneous development of liver cancer.[85,98]

SUMMARY

Although other forms of malignancy in the United States are decreasing, rates of HCC are increasing and have nearly doubled over the past 20 years. Although HBV is the most common cause of HCC worldwide, HCV accounts for a significant portion of new United States HCC cases. Yet, 15% to 50% of HCC cases originate in patients with CC without other known chronic liver diseases.[1] NAFLD is the most common cause of abnormal liver enzymes in the United States, affecting an estimated 30% of the United States population and 90% of the morbidly obese. NASH affects 3% to 6% of the general population and 30% of the morbidly obese, progressing to cirrhosis in up to 20% of cases and to HCC in approximately 7% of cases. Obesity and DM, both risk factors for NASH and CC, are also strongly associated with HCC. Multiple studies support the supposition that NASH accounts for a substantial portion of cryptogenic cases. NASH-induced hepatocarcinogenesis is likely mediated by increased free fatty acid oxidative stress resulting in increased cytokine release in addition to multiple receptor-mediated mechanisms triggering cellular proliferation and inhibiting apoptosis. The increasing prevalence of NASH, in addition to burgeoning rates of obesity and DM, highlight the importance of effective screening for HCC in this population.

REFERENCES

1. El-Serag HB, Rudolph KL. Hepatocellular carcinoma: epidemiology and molecular carcinogenesis. Gastroenterology 2007;132:2537–76.
2. Bosch FX, Ribes J, Cleries R, et al. Epidemiology of hepatocellular carcinoma. Clin Liver Dis 2005;9:191–211.
3. Ong JP, Younossi ZM. Epidemiology and natural history of NAFLD and NASH. Clin Liver Dis 2007;11:1–16.
4. Matteoni CA, Younossi ZM, Gramlich T, et al. Nonalcoholic fatty liver disease: a spectrum of clinical and pathological severity. Gastroenterology 1999;116: 1413–9.
5. Gomaa AI, Khan SA, Toledano MB, et al. Hepatocellular carcinoma: epidemiology, risk factors and pathogenesis. World J Gastroenterol 2008;14:4300–8.
6. Sherman M. Hepatocellular carcinoma: epidemiology, risk factors and screening. Semin Liver Dis 2005;25:143–54.

7. El-Serag HB, Lau M, Eschbach K, et al. Epidemiology of hepatocellular carcinoma in Hispanics in the United States. Arch Intern Med 2007;167:1983–9.
8. Montalto G, Cervello M, Giannitrapani L, et al. Epidemiology, risk factors, and natural history of hepatocellular carcinoma. Ann N Y Acad Sci 2002;963:13–20.
9. Fattovich G, Stroffolini T, Zagni I, et al. Hepatocellular carcinoma in cirrhosis: incidence and risk factors. Gastroenterology 2004;127:S35–50.
10. El-Serag HB, Mason AC. Risk factors for the rising rates of primary liver cancer in the United States. Arch Intern Med 2000;160:3227–30.
11. Hassan MM, Frome A, Patt YZ, et al. Rising prevalence of hepatitis C virus infection among patients recently diagnosed with hepatocellular carcinoma in the United States. J Clin Gastroenterol 2002;35:266–9.
12. Davila JA, Morgan RO, Shaib Y, et al. Hepatitis C infection and the increasing incidence of hepatocellular carcinoma: a population based study. Gastroenterology 2004;127:1372–80.
13. Kulkarni K, Barcak E, El-Serag HB, et al. The impact of immigration on the increasing incidence of hepatocellular carcinoma in the United States. Aliment Pharmacol Ther 2004;20:445–50.
14. Sass DA, Chang P, Chopra KB. Nonalcoholic fatty liver disease: a clinical review. Dig Dis Sci 2005;50:171–80.
15. Browning JD, Szczepaniak LS, Dobbins R, et al. Prevalence of hepatic steatosis in an urban population in the United States: impact of ethnicity. Hepatology 2004;40:1387–95.
16. Clark JM, Brancati FL, Diehl AM. The prevalence and etiology of elevated aminotransferase levels in the United States. Am J Gastroenterol 2003;98:960–7.
17. Bacon BR, Farahvash MJ, Janney CG, et al. Nonalcoholic steatohepatitis: an expanded clinical entity. Gastroenterology 1994;107:1103–9.
18. Schaffner F, Thaler H. Nonalcoholic fatty liver disease. Prog Liver Dis 1986;8:283–98.
19. Ludwig J, Viggiano TR, McDill DB, et al. Nonalcoholic steatohepatitis: Mayo Clinic experiences with a hitherto unnamed disease. Mayo Clin Proc 1980;55:434–8.
20. Angulo P, Lindor KD. Nonalcoholic fatty liver disease. J Gastroenterol Hepatol 2002;17:S186–90.
21. Torres DM, Harrison SA. Diagnosis and therapy of nonalcoholic steatohepatitis. Gastroenterology 2008;134:1682–98.
22. Harrison SA, Torgerson S, Hayashi PH. The natural history of nonalcoholic fatty liver disease: a clinical histopathological study. Am J Gastroenterol 2003;98:2042–7.
23. Ong JP, Younassi ZM. Nonalcoholic fatty liver disease (NAFLD) – two decades later: are we smarter about its natural history? Am J Gastroenterol 2003;98:1915–7.
24. Fassio E, Alvarez E, Dominguez N, et al. Natural history of nonalcoholic steatohepatitis: a longitudinal study of repeat liver biopsies. Hepatology 2004;40:820–6.
25. Lindor KD, Kowdley KV, Heathcote EJ, et al. Ursodeoxycholic acid for treatment of nonalcoholic steatohepatitis: results of a randomized trial. Hepatology 2004;39:770–8.
26. Adams LA, Schuyler S, Lindor KD, et al. The histological course of nonalcoholic fatty liver disease: a longitudinal study of 103 patients with sequential liver biopsies. J Hepatol 2005;42:132–8.
27. Teli MR, James OF, Burt AD, et al. The natural history of nonalcoholic fatty liver: a follow-up study. Hepatology 1995;22:1714–9.

28. Dam-Larsen S, Franzmann M, Andersen IB, et al. Long-term prognosis of fatty liver: risk of chronic liver disease and death. Gut 2004;53:750–5.
29. Hui JM, Kench JG, Chitturi S, et al. Long-term outcomes of cirrhosis in nonalcoholic steatohepatitis compared with hepatitis C. Hepatology 2003;38:420–7.
30. Sanyal AJ, Banas C, Sargent C, et al. Similarities and differences in outcomes of cirrhosis due to nonalcoholic steatohepatitis and hepatitis C. Hepatology 2006;43:682–9.
31. Adams LA, Lymp JF, Sauver JS, et al. The natural history of nonalcoholic fatty liver disease: a population-based cohort study. Gastroenterology 2005;129:113–21.
32. Rafiq N, Bai C, Fang Y, et al. Long term follow-up of patients with nonalcoholic fatty liver. Clin Gastroenterol Hepatol 2009;7:234–8.
33. Bonora E, Kiechl S, Willeit J, et al. Prevalence of insulin resistance in metabolic disorders: the Bruneck Study. Diabetes 1998;47:1643–9.
34. Wanless IR, Lentz JS. Fatty liver hepatitis (steatohepatitis) and obesity: an autopsy study with analysis of risk factors. Hepatology 1990;12:1106–10.
35. Marchesini G, Brizi M, Morselli-Labate AM, et al. Association of nonalcoholic fatty liver disease with insulin resistance. Am J Med 1999;107:450–5.
36. Marchesini G, Brizi M, Bianchi G, et al. Nonalcoholic fatty liver disease a feature of the metabolic syndrome. Diabetes 2001;50:1844–50.
37. Pagano G, Pacini G, Musso G, et al. Nonalcoholic steatohepatitis, insulin resistance and metabolic syndrome: further evidence for an etiologic association. Hepatology 2002;35:367–72.
38. Chitturi S, Abeygunasekera S, Farrell GC, et al. NASH and insulin resistance: insulin hypersecretion and specific association with the insulin resistance syndrome. Hepatology 2002;35:373–9.
39. Chalasani N, Crabb DW, Cummings OW, et al. Does leptin play a role in the pathogenesis of human nonalcoholic steatohepatitis? Am J Gastroenterol 2003;98:2771–6.
40. Ruhl CE, Everhart JE. Determinants of the association of overweight with elevated serum alanine aminotransferase activity in the United States. Gastroenterology 2003;124:71–9.
41. Solga S, Alkhuraishe AR, Clark JM, et al. Dietary composition and nonalcoholic fatty liver disease. Dig Dis Sci 2004;49:1578–83.
42. Capristo E, Miele L, Forgione A, et al. Nutritional aspects in patients with nonalcoholic steatohepatitis (NASH). Eur Rev Med Pharmacol Sci 2005;9:265–8.
43. Flegal KM, Carroll MD, Ogden CL, et al. Prevalence and trends in obesity among U.S. adults 1999–2000. JAMA 2002;288:1723–7.
44. Pereira MA, Kartashov AI, Ebbeling CB, et al. Fast-food habits, weight gain, and insulin resistance (the CARDIA Study): 15 year prospective analysis. Lancet 2005;365:36–42.
45. Caldwell SH, Oelsner DH, Iezzoni JC, et al. Cryptogenic cirrhosis: clinical characterization and risk factors for underlying disease. Hepatology 1999;29:664–9.
46. Moller H, Mellemgaard A, Lindvig K, et al. Obesity and cancer risk: a Danish record-linkage study. Eur J Cancer 1994;30:344–50.
47. Calle EE, Rodriguez C, Walker-Thurmond K, et al. Overweight, obesity, and mortality from cancer in a prospectively studied cohort of U.S. adults. N Engl J Med 2003;348:1625–38.
48. N'Kontchou G, Paries J, Htar MTT, et al. Risk factors for hepatocellular carcinoma in patients with alcoholic or viral C cirrhosis. Clin Gastroenterol Hepatol 2006;4:1062–8.

49. El-Serag HB, Hampel H, Javadi F. The association between diabetes and hepatocellular carcinoma: a systematic review of epidemiologic evidence. Clin Gastroenterol Hepatol 2006;4:369–80.
50. Davila JA, Morgan RO, Shaib Y, et al. Diabetes increases the risk of hepatocellular carcinoma in the United States: a population based case control study. Gut 2005;54:533–9.
51. Bugianesi E, Leone N, Vanni E, et al. Expanding the natural history of nonalcoholic steatohepatitis: from cryptogenic cirrhosis to hepatocellular carcinoma. Gastroenterology 2002;123:134–44.
52. Powell EE, Cooksley WGE, Hanson R, et al. The natural history of nonalcoholic steatohepatitis: a follow up study of forty-two patients for up to 21 years. Hepatology 1989;11:74–80.
53. Neuschwander-Tetri BA, Caldwell SH. Nonalcoholic steatohepatitis: summary of an AASLD single topic conference. Hepatology 2003;37:1202–19.
54. Lawson DH, Gray JM, McKillop C, et al. Diabetes mellitus and primary hepatocellular carcinoma. Q J Med 1986;61:945–55.
55. La Vecchia C, Negri E, Decarli A, et al. Diabetes mellitus and the risk of primary liver cancer. Int J Cancer 1997;73:204–7.
56. Adami HO, Chow WH, Nyren O, et al. Excess risk of primary liver cancer in patients with diabetes mellitus. J Natl Cancer Inst 1996;88:1472–7.
57. El-Serag HB, Richardson PA, Everhart JE. The role of diabetes in hepatocellular carcinoma: a case control study among United States Veterans. Am J Gastroenterol 2001;96:2462–7.
58. El-Serag HB, Tran T, Everhart JE. Diabetes increases the risk of chronic liver disease and hepatocellular carcinoma. Gastroenterology 2004;126:460–8.
59. DiBisceglie AM. What every hepatologist should know about endocrinology: obesity, diabetes and liver disease. Gastroenterology 2004;126:604–6.
60. Poonawala A, Nair SP, Thuluvath PJ. Prevalence of obesity and diabetes in patients with cryptogenic cirrhosis: a case-control study. Hepatology 2000;32: 689–92.
61. Regimbeau JM, Colombat M, Mognol P, et al. Obesity and diabetes as a risk factor for hepatocellular carcinoma. Liver Transpl 2004;10:S69–73.
62. Polesel J, Zucchetto A, Montella M, et al. The impact of obesity and diabetes mellitus on the risk of hepatocellular carcinoma. Ann Oncol 2009;20: 353–8.
63. Chen CL, Yang HI, Yang WS, et al. Metabolic factors and risk of hepatocellular carcinoma by chronic hepatitis B/C infection: a follow-up study in Taiwan. Gastroenterology 2008;135:111–21.
64. Nair S, Mason A, Eason J, et al. Is obesity an independent risk factor for hepatocellular carcinoma? Hepatology 2002;36:150–5.
65. Ratziu V, Bonyhay L, Di Martino V, et al. Survival, liver failure, and hepatocellular carcinoma in obesity-related cryptogenic cirrhosis. Hepatology 2002;35: 1485–93.
66. Sorensen HT, Mellemkjaer L, Jepsen P, et al. Risk of cancer in patients hospitalized with fatty liver: a Danish Cohort Study. J Clin Gastroenterol 2003;36: 356–9.
67. Marrero JA, Fontana RJ, Su GL, et al. NAFLD may be a common underlying liver disease in patients with hepatocellular carcinoma in the United States. Hepatology 2002;36:1349–54.
68. Cotrim HP, Parana R, Braga E, et al. Nonalcoholic steatohepatitis and hepatocellular carcinoma: natural history? Am J Gastroenterol 2000;95:3018–9.

69. Orikasa H, Ohyama R, Tsuka N, et al. Lipid rich clear cell hepatocellular carcinoma arising in nonalcoholic steatohepatitis in a patient with diabetes mellitus. J Submicrosc Cytol Pathol 2001;33:195–200.
70. Zen Y, Katayanagi K, Tsuneyama K, et al. Hepatocellular carcinoma arising in nonalcoholic steatohepatitis. Pathol Int 2001;51:127–31.
71. Shimada M, Hashimoto E, Taniai M, et al. Hepatocellular carcinoma in patients with nonalcoholic steatohepatitis. J Hepatol 2002;37:154–60.
72. Bencheqroun R, Duvoux C, Luciani A, et al. Hepatocellular carcinoma without cirrhosis in a patient with nonalcoholic steatohepatitis. Gastroenterol Clin Biol 2004;28:497–9.
73. Bullock RE, Zaitoun AM, Aithal GP, et al. Association of nonalcoholic steatohepatitis without significant fibrosis with hepatocellular carcinoma. J Hepatol 2004;41: 685–90.
74. Mori S, Yamasaki T, Sakaida I, et al. Hepatocellular carcinoma with nonalcoholic steatohepatitis. J Gastroenterol 2004;39:391–6.
75. Yoshioka Y, Hashimoto E, Yatsuji S, et al. Nonalcoholic steatohepatitis: cirrhosis, hepatocellular carcinoma, and burnt-out NASH. J Gastroenterol 2004;39:1215–8.
76. Sato K, Ueda Y, Ueno K, et al. Hepatocellular carcinoma and nonalcoholic steatohepatitis developing during long-term administration of valproic acid. Virchows Arch 2005;447:996–9.
77. Cuadrado A, Orive A, Garcia-Suarez C, et al. Nonalcoholic steatohepatitis (NASH) and hepatocellular carcinoma. Obes Surg 2005;15:442–6.
78. Ikeda H, Suzuki M, Takahashi H, et al. Hepatocellular carcinoma with silent and cirrhotic nonalcoholic steatohepatitis, accompanying ectopic liver tissue attached to gallbladder. Pathol Int 2006;56:40–5.
79. Hai S, Kubo S, Shuto T, et al. Hepatocellular carcinoma arising from nonalcoholic steatohepatitis: report of two cases. Surg Today 2006;36:390–4.
80. Ichikawa T, Yanagi K, Motoyoshi Y, et al. Two cases of nonalcoholic steatohepatitis with development of hepatocellular carcinoma without cirrhosis. J Gastroenterol Hepatol 2006;21:1865–70.
81. Tsutsumi K, Nakayama H, Sakai Y, et al. Two cases of patients with hepatocellular carcinoma (HCC) that developed in cryptogenic cirrhosis suggestive of nonalcoholic steatohepatitis (NASH) as background liver disease after clinical courses of 26 years. Nippon Shokakibyo Gakkai Zasshi 2007;104:690–7.
82. Hashizume H, Sato K, Takagi H, et al. Primary liver cancers with nonalcoholic steatohepatitis. Eur J Gastroenterol Hepatol 2007;19:827–34.
83. Hashimoto E, Yatsuji S, Tobarki M, et al. Hepatocellular carcinoma in patients with nonalcoholic steatohepatitis. J Gastroenterol 2009;44:S89–95.
84. Harrison SA. Liver disease in patients with diabetes mellitus. J Clin Gastroenterol 2006;40:68–76.
85. Bugianesi E. Nonalcoholic steatohepatitis and cancer. Clin Liver Dis 2007;11: 191–207.
86. Calle EE, Kaaks S. Overweight, obesity and cancer: epidemiological evidence and proposed mechanisms. Nat Rev Cancer 2004;4:579–91.
87. Kaburagi Y, Yamauchi T, Yamamoto-Honda R, et al. The mechanism of insulin-induced signal transduction mediated by the insulin receptor substrate family. Endocr J 1999;46:S25–34.
88. Ish-Shalom D, Christoffersen CT, Vorwerk P, et al. Mitogenic properties of insulin and insulin analogues mediated by the insulin receptor. Diabetologia 1997;40: S25–31.

89. Tanaka S, Mohr L, Schmidt EV, et al. Biological effects of human insulin receptor substrate-1 overexpression in hepatocytes. Hepatology 1997;00:598–604.
90. Yamada T, DeSouza AT, Finkelstein S, et al. Loss of the gene encoding mannose 6-phosphate/insulin-like growth factor ii receptor is an early event in liver carcinogenesis. Proc Natl Acad Sci U S A 1997;94:10351–5.
91. Breuhahn K, Vreden S, Haddad R, et al. Molecular profiling of human hepatocellular carcinoma defines mutually exclusive interferon regulation and insulin-like growth factor ii overexpression. Cancer Res 2004;64:6058–64.
92. Ogata H, Kobayashi T, Chinen T, et al. Deletion of SOCS3 gene in liver parenchymal cells promotes hepatitis-induced hepatocarcinogenesis. Gastroenterology 2006; 131:179–93.
93. Sakurai T, Maeda S, Chang L, et al. Loss of hepatic NF-kappa B activity enhances chemical hepatocarcinogenesis through sustained c-Jun N-terminal kinase 1 activation. Proc Natl Acad Sci U S A 2006;103:10544–51.
94. Luedde T, Beraza N, Kotsikoris V, et al. Deletion of NEMO/IKKgamma in liver parenchymal cells causes steatohepatitis and hepatocellular carcinoma. Cancer Cell 2007;11:119–32.
95. Bataller R, Brenner DA. Liver fibrosis. J Clin Invest 2005;115:209–18.
96. Yang S, Zhu H, Li Y, et al. Mitochondrial adaptations to obesity-related oxidant stress. Arch Biochem Biophys 2000;378:259–68.
97. Hu W, Feng Z, Eveleigh J, et al. The major lipid peroxidation product, trans-4-hydroxy-2-nonenal, preferentially forms DNA adducts at codon 249 of human p53 gene, a unique mutational hotspot in hepatocellular carcinoma. Carcinogenesis 2002;23:1781–9.
98. Xu Z, Chen L, Leung L, et al. Liver-specific inactivation of the Nrf1 gene in adult mouse leads to nonalcoholic steatohepatitis and hepatic neoplasia. Proc Natl Acad Sci U S A 2005;102:4120–5.

Lifestyle Modification as the Primary Treatment of NASH

Brent A. Neuschwander-Tetri, MD*

KEYWORDS

- Insulin resistance • Exercise • Obesity
- Lipotoxicity • *Trans*-fatty acids • High fructose corn syrup

Lifestyle modification, weight loss, exercise—how many times are these interventions recommended to treat non-alcoholic steatohepatitis (NASH) but with uncertainty about the specifics of what to tell patients or unfamiliarity with the data that support these recommendations? This article reviews the rationale and data behind recommending lifestyle changes to prevent and reverse NASH, focusing specifically on changes that lead to increased physical activity in sedentary patients, changes in dietary habits, and decreased calorie consumption to achieve gradual and sustained weight loss in those who are overweight or obese.

In a culture that values avoiding even minimal exertion, such as walking through a parking lot or up a flight of stairs, while surrounding ourselves with an overabundance of inexpensive, delicious, and energy-dense foods, these are not easy changes to make. Ultimately, the success of care providers in helping patients to recognize and overcome these barriers depends on a patient's motivation, but clinicians can be more persuasive and able to bolster this motivation when armed with a conviction based on data that establishes this to be the best course of action for patients with NASH.

LIPOTOXICITY AND NASH

The rationale for recommending exercise and weight loss to patients with NASH can only be understood in the context of the emerging understanding of the role of lipotoxicity in the pathogenesis of this disease. Discussed in more detail in the article by Cusi elsewhere in this issue, lipotoxicity is a term coined by Unger and expanded by others to signify cellular injury caused by excessive free fatty acids and their metabolites, such as phosphatidic acid, lysophosphatidic acid, lysophosphatidyl choline, ceramides, diacylglycerol, and perhaps other intermediaries.[1–3] Some authors have further expanded this term to include triglyceride as a cause of lipotoxicity, but without

Department of Internal Medicine, Division of Gastroenterology and Hepatology, Saint Louis University School of Medicine, 3635 Vista Avenue, St. Louis, MO 63110, USA
* Corresponding author.
E-mail address: tetriba@slu.edu

Clin Liver Dis 13 (2009) 649–665
doi:10.1016/j.cld.2009.07.006
liver.theclinics.com
1089-3261/09/$ – see front matter

evidence that triglyceride droplets themselves are pathogenic, and it may be best to reserve the term for damage caused by fatty acids and their nontriglyceride metabolites.

The commonly accepted but unproved two-hit hypothesis of NASH proposed that the first hit in this disease is the accumulation of excess triglyceride in the liver and the second hit is oxidant stress in this milieu of excess substrate for lipid peroxidation that promotes cellular injury, inflammation, and fibrosis.[4] Although the accumulation of excess lipid in hepatocytes in the form of triglyceride droplets might seem intuitive as the first step in the pathogenesis of NASH,[5] emerging evidence is suggesting that the accumulation of lipid droplets might be only a marker of excessive exposure of hepatocytes to free fatty acids and that their so-called "ectopic storage" as triglyceride under these conditions could actually be protective rather than pathogenic.[6–10] If true, steatosis may only be a marker, albeit a fairly reliable one, for trafficking of excess fatty acids and their metabolites through the liver.

If lipotoxicity is the cause of hepatocellular injury in NASH and steatosis is an "innocent bystander,"[11] then the appropriate goal of therapeutic interventions needs to be prevention of lipotoxicity. This does not mean that steatosis is irrelevant because it is a sensitive marker of excessive fat trafficking through the liver, but the focus of designing therapeutic interventions needs to be on reduction of lipotoxicity. This is primarily achieved by decreasing inappropriate adipose tissue lipolysis and hepatic de novo lipogenesis from excessive carbohydrates, the two major contributors to increased flux of fatty acids through the liver that have been identified in patients with NASH.[9] An important focus of treatment then becomes insulin resistance because this defect at the level of adipose tissue is a major mechanism of inadequate postprandial suppression of lipolysis. Also, the hyperinsulinemia associated with impaired glucose disposal, primarily because of muscle insulin resistance, is a major factor in promoting de novo lipogenesis in the liver.

With this perspective as a background, the following discussion focuses on the role of dietary modifications and exercise in improving adipose and muscle insulin sensitivity and decreasing hepatic de novo lipogenesis.

INSULIN RESISTANCE AND HYPERINSULINEMIA

Insulin resistance, or the inability of insulin to evoke a normal physiologic response at target tissues,[10] is commonly found in patients with NASH.[12] Until β-cell failure develops in patients with insulin resistance, endogenous insulin production increases to compensate for defects in signaling, causing hyperinsulinemia. Both abnormalities, insulin resistance and hyperinsulinemia, may play important roles in the pathogenesis of NASH. Insulin resistance leads to inappropriate lipolysis in adipose tissue, impaired glucose disposal by muscle, and inappropriate glucose production by the liver. The concomitant hyperinsulinemia drives a program of lipogenesis in the liver and downregulates mitochondrial β-oxidation. Together, these metabolic abnormalities seem to be major predisposing factors in the development of NASH.

The flow of fatty acids to the liver is regulated by the rate of adipocyte lipolysis. Once free fatty acids are released from adipocytes, their uptake by the liver is primarily dependent on their concentration in the blood because the liver has no mechanism to shut off fatty acid uptake when its requirements for this source of energy or membrane production are satisfied.[13] The liver can certainly upregulate fatty acid uptake by increasing the expression of fatty acid translocase, also called CD36, and the caveolin-dependent uptake by binding to the fatty acid transporter mAspAT,[13] but it cannot shut off fatty acid uptake.

A focus in understanding hepatocellular injury in NASH moves to adipose tissue and the regulation of lipolysis in adipocytes as a major source of fatty acids. Insulin plays a principal role in shutting off adipocyte lipolysis after a meal; rising postprandial insulin levels signal through the insulin receptor on adipocytes to phosphorylate insulin receptor substrates I and II that activate Akt (protein kinase B) and other downstream signal transduction mediators. In states of insulin resistance when lipolysis is not sufficiently downregulated, the result is continued release of free fatty acids into the blood to be taken up by the liver at a time when the liver is programmed to store energy rather than use fatty acids as a source of energy. In biochemical terms, this means that fatty acids taken up by hepatocytes are not shuttled to the mitochondria for β-oxidation because increased malonyl-CoA levels have inhibited carnitine palmitoyl transferase I. Ideally, the excess fatty acids then enter a path to form triglyceride and are secreted as very low density lipoprotein, but any process that impairs their re-esterification and secretion may favor the accumulation of lipotoxic intermediates.[9]

With this understanding, a rationale is established for treating insulin resistance to prevent inappropriate adipocyte lipolysis. A large body of evidence from the fields of exercise physiology and cardiovascular disease has shown that weight loss and exercise have major beneficial effects on adipocyte insulin signaling. A pharmacologic approach to improving insulin sensitivity is the use of thiazolidinediones, a class of drugs being studied as therapeutic agents for NASH. Recent studies have shown that thiazolidinediones can prevent the activation of adipocyte c-jun kinase, a kinase that when activated can impair adipocyte responsiveness to insulin.[14] Whether this is the primary mechanism underlying the beneficial effects of thiazolidinediones in NASH is yet to be established.

In the insulin-resistant, hyperinsulinemic state, the liver expresses metabolic changes reflecting both insulin resistance with respect to some pathways and excessive signaling with respect to other pathways. One manifestation of hepatic insulin resistance is inappropriate glucose production for a given insulin concentration. This is reflected in two commonly used measures of insulin resistance: the homeostasis model assessment (HOMA) and the quantitative insulin check index. Both measures are based on the product of glucose′ × insulin with the HOMA normalized to a value of 1 by dividing the product by 405 (when glucose is expressed as milligrams per deciliter) and the quantitative insulin check index being a log and inverse transformation of the insuliń́ × glucose product. A high HOMA value or a low quantitative insulin check index value indicates hepatic insulin resistance. Despite the common use of HOMA to assess insulin resistance, the hepatic insulin resistance that it reflects has not been shown to play a role in hepatic lipotoxicity. One study found that the presence of steatosis correlated negatively with exercise fitness, a surrogate for insulin signaling in muscle, and not the HOMA measurement of hepatic insulin sensitivity.[15] Additionally, metformin, a drug that improves hepatic insulin signaling and decreases inappropriate glucose production, has not been shown to improve NASH in most studies,[16–18] although there have been a few reports of benefit.[19–22]

The hyperinsulinemia that results from muscle insulin resistance and impaired glucose disposal most definitely alters hepatic fat metabolism and seems to promote lipotoxicity and triglyceride accumulation. It is interesting to speculate whether these abnormalities would be even more severe if there was not also some degree of coexisting impairment of hepatic insulin signaling pathways in hyperinsulinemic states. In non–insulin-resistant states, exposure of the liver to excessive insulin predisposes to triglyceride accumulation. For example, regional hyperinsulinemia caused by aberrant drainage of insulin-enriched pancreatic venous blood into specific areas causes focal fatty liver[23] and the observation of focal fatty liver around metastases of insulin-secreting tumors[24,25] provide evidence that excess insulin in the absence of insulin resistance and systemic hyperinsulinemia promotes metabolic changes that favor lipid accumulation. Insulin overdose has also been described as a cause of fatty liver with substantial liver enzyme elevations.[26] Most commonly, however, the hyperinsulinemic state is accompanied by insulin resistance, but despite the relative impairment of some insulin signaling pathways, this still alters hepatic fat metabolism to decrease mitochondrial β-oxidation and promote lipogenesis. Interventions that decrease insulin levels by improving peripheral insulin sensitivity at the level of the muscle so that postprandial glucose uptake from the blood is increased favorably alter hepatic lipid trafficking and reduce lipotoxicity.

IMPACT OF EXERCISE ON INSULIN RESISTANCE AND NASH

Although the theoretical basis is strong, only limited data are available to support the recommendation of exercise as an important lifestyle change for patients with NASH (**Table 1**). This is not because major studies have failed to show an effect, but because well-designed studies of exercise that eliminate confounding factors, such as weight loss and dietary changes, have simply not been published. Studies are needed that examine the long-term effects of increased aerobic capacity achieved through regular exercise on measures of hepatic lipotoxicity independent of weight loss in subjects with NASH. It has been shown that the severity of non-alcoholic fatty liver disease (NAFLD) is worse with lower physical fitness,[27] but what is cause and what is effect can only be shown by interventional studies. There are some data that question the role of exercise. One small study of diet and exercise for just 2 weeks showed that whereas caloric restriction reduced liver fat, 2 weeks of minimally exertional exercise did not provide any additive benefit.[28] Another small exercise study found that preventing weight loss caused by exercise with a high-carbohydrate diet prevented the beneficial effects of short-term exercise on insulin resistance in overweight adults.[29] How either of these studies extrapolates to the effects of long-term improved fitness achieved with regular aerobic exercise has not been established. In contrast, a study in rats demonstrated that NAFLD caused by a high-fat diet could be prevented with exercise even if weight gain is maintained.[30] Also, a number of exercise studies in patients with NAFLD with relatively minor amounts of weight loss (<5%) do report improved NASH as described later, a finding that provides some indirect evidence that exercise is important because such small amounts of weight loss typically do not independently improve NASH.

Three observational studies have shown correlations between fitness or sedentary behavior and the risk NAFLD and NASH. In one study, habitual physical activity in 191 employees of a clinic in Italy was assessed using a validated survey and the findings were correlated with liver fat measured by MR spectroscopy.[15] NAFLD was identified in only 2% of those in the top quartile for exercise habits, whereas its prevalence was 11% to 25% in the lower quartiles. Controlling for HOMA or obesity (body mass index) did not affect this association, although visceral adiposity was not specifically measured. In the other two studies, visceral adiposity did seem to be a major determinant of the correlation between fitness or exercise habits and NAFLD, perhaps because visceral fat is a major source of fatty acids delivered to the liver in obesity.[31] Evaluation of a subgroup of male subjects involved in a long-term epidemiologic study in Dallas found that the presence of NAFLD was predicted inversely by fitness and directly by body mass index.[32] Inclusion of waist circumference in the analysis reduced the correlation, again suggesting that preventing visceral obesity through exercise or other means is protective against the development of NAFLD. Because the evidence is correlative rather than causative, an alternate explanation is that visceral obesity impairs fitness, or an independent process leads to NAFLD and visceral adiposity. The third observational study, a component of a large epidemiologic study in Israel, found that leisure time physical activity was associated with reduced abdominal girth and a lower prevalence of NAFLD.[33] The currently available data support recommending exercise, but it would be reassuring to have well-conducted trials to corroborate findings in small and uncontrolled observational studies.

DEFECTS IN MUSCLE THAT COULD IMPAIR THE RESPONSE TO EXERCISE

When patients with NASH are instructed to exercise, an implicit assumption is that most individuals respond similarly to exercise with increased aerobic capacity and experience its associated metabolic benefits. Given the many known and suspected genetic polymorphisms governing the response to exercise, it is now known that this is simply not the case. A number of studies provide evidence that there may be some people who are not able to build muscle and increase aerobic exercise capacity, even with the most earnest attempts to exercise. Much of this investigation is now focusing on mitochondrial biogenesis and function.[34,35] Petersen and coworkers[36,37] evaluated lean, but insulin-resistant, offspring of diabetics and found impaired mitochondrial function, raising the possibility that genetic factors controlling mitochondrial oxidative phosphorylation and ATP production predispose to insulin resistance and the risk of developing diabetes. Others have suggested that mitochondrial function per se is unimpaired in obesity and insulin resistance, but that muscle mitochondrial mass is deficient, suggesting defects in mitochondrial biogenesis.[38] The upstream factors responsible for mitochondrial biogenesis in muscle have been examined in insulin resistance to better understand potential underlying defects. A short episode of exercise in insulin-sensitive but sedentary subjects caused robust increases in PGC-1α, a major transcription factor that regulates expression of mitochondrial genes at the transcript and protein levels, but nearly absent induction in subjects with insulin resistance.[39] AMP-dependent protein kinase (AMPK) may play an upstream regulatory role in PGC-1α expression and its activation was also impaired in these subjects, suggesting defects in AMPK phosphorylation or dephosphorylation are important in regulating PGC-1α activation. Whether insulin resistance is a cause or consequence of these abnormalities remains to be established, but chemically blocking mitochondrial β-oxidation can cause insulin resistance, suggesting that the metabolic and genetic defects that cause impaired PGC-1α expression and resulting mitochondrial biogenesis are the cause and not the consequence of insulin resistance. These intensive metabolic studies performed on relatively few subjects have provided important insights into the underpinnings of insulin resistance and exercise physiology. The relevance of the findings of the studies focusing on the role of PGC-1α has been supported by a large population study in Germany that identified a single nucleotide polymorphism of the gene encoding PGC-1α to be associated with poor response to exercise in terms of increased fitness and improved insulin sensitivity.[40] After 3 hours of endurance exercise per week for 9 months, exercise tolerance was assessed and found to correlate with a specific single nucleotide polymorphism of the PGC-1α gene that was previously shown to be underrepresented in trained athletes. In this study, it was overrepresented in those unable to increase aerobic capacity. The functional significance of this polymorphism has not been demonstrated.

One mechanistic link between insufficient mitochondrial function and insulin resistance is the generation of lipotoxic intermediates that impair insulin signaling. Impaired mitochondrial β-oxidation leads to the accumulation of lipotoxic intermediates capable of activating c-Jun kinase and other serine kinases that impair insulin

Table 1
Effect of lifestyle modification on NASH in studies that included exercise recommendations.

Entry Criteria	Diet	Exercise	N	Age Group	Duration	Control Group	Compliance	F/U Biopsy	F/U Imaging	ALT	Insulin Sensitivity	Comments	Author
Overweight + elevated LFTs	600–800 kcal/day reduction	Told to exercise	39	Adult	2–111 mo	None	17/39 lost > 10% weight	ND	ND	76% → 6% elevated if > 10% weight loss	ND	Retrospective chart review Variable duration HCV not excluded	Palmer[90]
BMI >25+ fatty liver on ultrasound	25 kcal/kg	Jogging 20 min twice daily	15 treated 10 control	Adult	3 mo	No change in usual diet and activities	No dropouts Mean weight loss was 10%	Improved steatosis Nonsignificant trends to improved inflammation and fibrosis. Controls: no changes	ND	Treated: 83 → 27 U/L Control: 73 → 87 U/L	ND	Presence of steatohepatitis not specifically addressed	Ueno[91]
NASH on biopsy	<30% fat <10% saturated fat	Walk/jog 30 min daily	16	Adult	12 wk	None for ALT	All lost weight, mean 5%	ND	ND	61 → 45 U/L	ND	Half received vitamin E with no effect	Kugelmas[92]
BMI >25 + steatosis on biopsy	<30% fat and calorie restricted	150 min aerobic weekly	16	Adult	15 mo	None	Three dropouts 10 maintained weight loss	Improved (only three had biopsies)	ND	77 → 48 U/L	Improvement correlated with weight loss	Study focused on a larger cohort with HCV and NAFLD	Hickman[93]
BMI >95% + ALT >1.5 ULN + steatosis on ultrasound	30 kcal/kg/d	Moderate daily exercise	28	Children	5 mo	None	11/28 lost weight	ND	Liver echogenicity improved in those who lost weight	Normalized in those who lost weight	ND	Half received vitamin E with no effect on ALT or liver echogenicity	Vajro[94]

BMI >25 + NASH on biopsy + Elevated LFTs	Low carbohydrate (40%–45% calories) Low calorie	Exercise recomm-ended	23	Adult	12 mo	None	7 dropouts 15/23 had biopsies 9/23 lost weight (mean 7%)	Improved in those who lost weight	Those with improved biopsy had a trend to decreased visceral fat on CT	Improved only in those who lost weight	Improved only in those who lost weight	Only a minority of subjects lost weight, but those who did improved	Huang[95]
ALT >35 U/L	Caloric restriction	Fitness exercise 20–30 min/day 2–3 times per week	348	Adult	12 mo	None	6% lost > 5% weight 12% started exercising	ND	ND	Improvement associated with: Continuing exercise, >5% weight loss	ND	Only 12% started exercising (>once/wk) which was not associated with improved ALT	Suzuki[49]
Impaired glucose tolerance	<30% fat <10% sat fat	3 h endurance exercise per week	48	Adult	9 mo	Normal glucose tolerance	Mean weight loss 3.2%	ND	Liver fat by MRS: 9.2 → 6.5%	ND	Improved	Large community study focused on preventing diabetes	Schäfer[61]
BMI >95% + ALT >1.5 ULN + steatosis on ultrasound	Low fat, 250 kcal/day deficit	3 h aerobic exercise daily	19	Children	1 mo	No interv ention (N = 38)	Mean weight loss 9%	ND	Ultrasound unchanged	152 → 64 U/L	Improved	Children sent to summer camp for intervention	Wang[96]
NAFLD on biopsy + steatosis on ultrasound+ elevated ALT	Calorie restriction	45 min/day aerobic exercise	90	Children	24 mo	None	4 dropouts Mean weight loss 5 kg	N = 53 biopsies at 2 y: improved in most (see **Fig. 1**)	ND	Improved	Improved	Half received vitamins C and E with no effect	Nobili[54,97]

Abbreviations: F/U, follow-up; HCV, hepatitis C virus; LFT, liver function tests; NAFLD, non-alcoholic fatty liver disease; ND, not done; ULN, upper limit of normal.

signaling by inactivating insulin receptor substrate-1 and other postreceptor mediators of insulin signaling.[41] Of particular relevance to investigators in the field who use mice to study insulin resistance and NASH, the Jackson Laboratory strain of C57BL/6J mice, but not other strains of the C57BL/6J mice, is missing a functional nuclear encoded gene for the mitochondrial protein nicotinamide nucleotide transhydrogenase (Nnt), a defect that predisposes this strain to insulin resistance, and transgenic expression of Nnt in these mice normalizes glucose tolerance and insulin sensitivity.[42,43] Exploiting this serendipitous polymorphism may shed further light on the role of mitochondria in insulin resistance.

IMPACT OF COMBINED EXERCISE AND WEIGHT LOSS ON INSULIN RESISTANCE, NAFLD, AND NASH

Obesity is a major risk factor for insulin resistance. What is not clear is whether it is the obesity per se that predisposes to insulin resistance, or if it is a continuous oversupply of nutrients that causes both obesity and insulin resistance. In favor of the latter is the observation that obese people do not need to lose weight to the point of a healthy body mass index to see substantial improvement in insulin signaling. An overwhelming abundance of data has demonstrated that lifestyle modification that combines exercise and weight loss is effective at improving insulin sensitivity and preventing diabetes.[44–47] Studies have also shown that losing relatively small amounts of weight in the range of 5% to 10% confers significant benefits in terms of NAFLD and NASH.[48–50] Either there is a small fraction of adipose tissue that when lost fixes a lot of problems, or it is the dietary changes themselves that lead to weight loss also lead to improved insulin signaling.

The beneficial effect of weight loss on NAFLD has been reviewed by others and the aggregate message is that weight loss achieved through a calorically restricted balanced diet or bariatric surgery with appropriate postoperative nutritional support does improve NASH.[51–53] Unfortunately, few studies include biopsies as an end point and rigorous large controlled trials have not yet been reported. One recently reported study of lifestyle changes in children with NASH did show substantial histologic benefits, although there was no control group that did not receive lifestyle recommendations (**Fig. 1**).[54] For most people, weight loss is difficult to sustain and the results of weight loss studies tend to focus on small changes occurring over relatively short time periods. Perhaps the most convincing data on the role of weight loss come from studies of the effect of bariatric surgery on NASH. As reviewed elsewhere, bariatric surgery has been shown effectively to reverse steatohepatitis in those who follow the recommended eating restrictions and lose weight.[52,55,56] The importance of maintaining a diet containing essential nutrients has been emphasized by cases of worsening liver disease with fasting or inadequate nutritional support following bariatric surgery.[57–59]

Indirect evidence for the role of exercise and diet on the risk of NAFLD comes from epidemiologic studies. The prospective cohort study of over 50,000 nurses that examined risk factors for insulin resistance and its complications over 6 years demonstrated that time watching television was strongly associated with an increased risk of developing diabetes and walking briskly for 1 hour daily reduced the risk of developing obesity by 24% and diabetes by 34%.[60] A large population intervention study in Germany found that exercise and caloric restriction led to improved liver fat content after 9 months.[61] This occurred with only a 3.2% drop in body mass index, again suggesting that exercise was playing an important role in the beneficial changes.

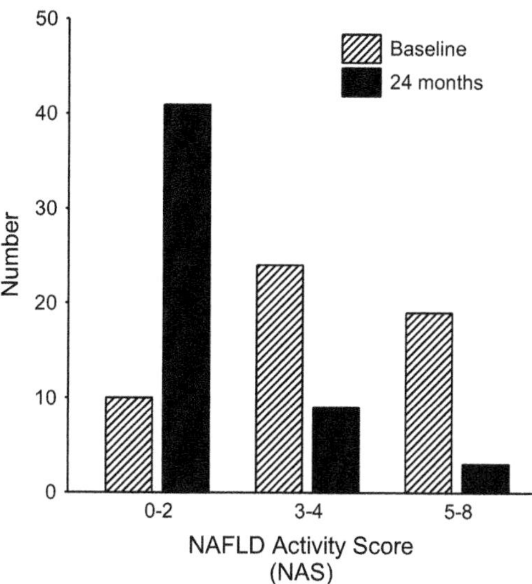

Fig. 1. NAFLD activity score (NAS) of 53 children before and after being treated with caloric restriction and aerobic exercise (45 min/d recommended) for 24 months. The proportion of subjects with a low NAS (0–2) increased from 19% at baseline to 77% after lifestyle change. (*Data from* Nobili V, Manco M, Devito R, et al. Lifestyle intervention and antioxidant therapy in children with non-alcoholic fatty liver disease: a randomized, controlled trial. Hepatology 2008;48:119–28.)

SPECIFIC EATING HABITS AND NASH

Identifying specific foods and food components that increase insulin resistance or promote hepatic lipotoxicity is essential for providing rational recommendations to patients with any of the consequences of insulin resistance. A high-fat diet alone, even in the absence of insulin resistance, obesity, or diabetes, is sufficient to cause transient insulin resistance. Mechanistically, this may be caused by the increase in circulating free fatty acids that are liberated by lipoprotein lipase at the level of adipose tissue, muscle, and perhaps the liver. Fast food is typically high in fat, with some of the larger hamburgers containing more than 100 g of fat, and this is before including the French fries. By comparison, a stick of butter is 92 g of fat. Two common food components deserve special attention: high fructose corn syrup (HFCS) and industrial *trans*-fats.

HFCS

HFCS is a common sweetener in soft drinks and a number of commercially prepared foods. It is produced by breaking down the complex carbohydrates of corn to the monosaccharide glucose, enzymatically converting a portion of the glucose to fructose, and then mixing the fructose and glucose to achieve a desired ratio. Soft drinks are typically sweetened with a solution of 55% fructose, 41% glucose, and 4% residual complex carbohydrates. HFCS has desirable properties for its sweetness, its ease of handling in bulk, and its cost competitiveness compared with other sweeteners. Its regular consumption in large amounts has been associated with the development of insulin resistance and NAFLD, however, in epidemiologic studies and experimental studies.[62–64] Why consuming HFCS should be any different than consuming an isocaloric amount of sucrose, the disaccharide of glucose and fructose that is broken down to the same monosaccharides as HFCS by brush border sucrase-isomaltase, has not been established. One possibility is that the rate of absorption of the monosaccharides is faster than the rate of disaccharide hydrolysis followed by absorption that occurs with sucrose.[63]

Perhaps the biggest problem with HFCS-containing soft drinks is simply the amount of carbohydrate they contain. At around 40 g of carbohydrate per 12-oz serving, a typical can of cola contains the amount of sugar in about 10 sugar cubes. Such comparisons can be useful in discussing dietary habits with patients and especially parents of pediatric patients. High-dose fructose challenges the liver metabolically by depleting hepatic energy reserves because of the rapid first pass uptake of fructose by the liver and phosphorylation by phosphofructokinase.[65,66] Fructose also impairs normal satiety mechanisms, a response that could be particularly problematic when soft drinks are consumed with excessively portioned meals.[67,68]

Trans-fats

Industrial *trans*-fats (ITF) found in partially hydrogenated vegetable oils (vegetable shortening) comprise a relatively new addition to the Western diet that has occurred over the past four to five decades, a time frame that corresponds well with the emergence of NASH as a major liver disease. ITF are inadvertent by-products generated during the process of chemically "hydrogenating" unsaturated fatty acids to saturated fatty acids. Double bonds in natural unsaturated fatty acids occur only in the *cis* configuration and during the industrial process of hydrogenation some are isomerized to the unnatural *trans* configuration rather than being reduced to single bonds.[69–71] Epidemiologic studies identified *trans*-fat consumption as a risk for cardiovascular disease, which has led to a push to eliminate them from foods.[72]

Only a few studies have examined the potential role of dietary ITF as a cause of liver injury, and these suggest that ITF could be a significant but overlooked contributor to the current epidemic of NASH. One study reported a rise in mean ALT from 22 U/L to 97 U/L in just 2 weeks in healthy medical students who ate at least two meals of fast food daily.[73] Although the ITF content of the food consumed was not reported, subjects ate at "well-known" fast food restaurants, a documented source of food rich in ITF.[74] In this hyperalimentation study, subjects increased their caloric intake by 3500 kcal/day and fat intake by 174 g/day, leading to significant weight gain. None became obese, however, and significant aminotransferase elevations preceded weight gain, suggesting that the liver enzyme changes were not a direct reflection of obesity. In another observational study, adipose tissue *trans*-fat content, a marker of dietary ITF exposure, was found to be increased in bariatric surgery patients with NAFLD compared with control patients undergoing surgery for gastroesophageal reflux,[75] a finding that may implicate ITF in the development of NAFLD. To investigate the role of ITF in NASH further, a recent study evaluated *trans*-fat consumption in mice and demonstrated severe steatohepatitis developing after 16 weeks of *trans*-fat feeding.[76] Isocalorically replacing the partially hydrogenated vegetable oil used in this study with lard caused the same degree of obesity and caused only minor steatosis but did not induce steatohepatitis, implicating *trans*-fats as a cause of steatohepatitis in this animal study.

Based on these findings and the epidemiologic studies linking *trans*-fat consumption to cardiovascular disease, dietary recommendations to patients with NASH should include elimination of *trans*-fats from the diet. Despite a growing awareness of their risks, consumption of ITF continues in baked goods, fried food, and a wide variety of other prepared foods.[77–80] Much patient education is needed to achieve elimination of dietary *trans*-fats. In a 2007 survey, 93% of people had heard of *trans*-fats but only 21% could identify three foods with *trans*-fats and only 37% try to buy foods labeled as zero *trans*-fat.[81] Even for those intending to avoid *trans*-fat–containing foods, inadvertent consumption can be significant. Because current Food and Drug Administration labeling standards allow foods with less than 0.5 g *trans*-fats per serving to be labeled as "zero *trans*-fats," editorialists have pointed out that by consuming four to five small, industry-defined, "serving sizes" of zero *trans*-fat food, ITF consumption can easily exceed the recommended daily limit of 2 g.[82] Restaurant food also continues to be a major source of *trans*-fats, especially at a number of large national chain restaurants.

PRACTICAL STRATEGIES FOR ACHIEVING LIFESTYLE MODIFICATIONS IN PATIENTS WITH NASH

If easy paths to success in achieving lifestyle modifications were known, this article would not be needed. Every insulin-resistant person has his or her own challenges, whether they be environmental, dietary, physical, psychologic, genetic, or as is probably seen most commonly, some combination of these factors.[83] **Box 1** provides practical recommendations for lifestyle modification.

When discussing physical activity with patients, the discussion should focus on impediments to increasing physical activity and finding ways for patients to incorporate exercise into their lives on a regular basis indefinitely.[84] It is often helpful to separate the benefits of exercise from weight loss. Because exercise has its own benefits in terms of a sense of well-being and improved insulin responsiveness, being discouraged about lack of weight loss should not be a reason to quit. For adults who were once athletic, the transition back to an active lifestyle may be much easier than for those who have always been sedentary. The minimal goal is to engage in some type of activity that increases the heart rate for 30 to 45 minutes daily. Achieving this goal is no doubt unrealistic for many patients, especially those with physical impediments, but any amount of increased activity is better than none. For many, just starting a regular walking program is significant progress, although it should be

Box 1
Practical recommendations for lifestyle modification

- Exercise goal is 30–45 minutes of activities that increase heart rate at least three times weekly
- Walking is a good start for people completely sedentary, but the goal is to move onto aerobic activities as fitness improves
- Vary exercise activities over time
- Seek a trainer to guide develop and plan to maintain consistency
- Do not think of weight loss as the goal of exercise; the goal of exercise is to change the body's metabolism and improve the sense of well-being
- Limit "screen time" in front of televisions, computers, and video games
- Focus on healthy eating, not dieting
- Eat a protein-containing breakfast daily (eg, meat, cheese, eggs, yoghurt)
- Avoid fasting
- Eliminate sugar-sweetened beverages (sodas, sweetened tea, and so forth)
- Avoid *trans*-fats, including foods labeled as *trans*-fat free but containing hydrogenated or partially hydrogenated vegetable oil

viewed as a prelude to more strenuous activities over time rather than an end in itself. The challenges facing care providers to get their patients to increase physical activity are enormous, and new approaches that overcome impediments are needed.[85]

To most, the idea of dieting to achieve weight loss has many negative connotations because of prior failures and typically invokes the strongly counterproductive psychology of denial. Instead of discussing diets and dieting, the focus needs to be on healthy eating habits, or the positive side of changes in eating habits. Elimination of sugar-sweetened beverages, such as sodas and sweetened teas; avoidance of calorie-dense fast foods; and routinely bringing food home when eating at restaurants where portion sizes are enormous should be recommended to all patients. Weight loss programs that focus on portion control and provide regular group sessions may lead to the best long-term results.[86] The value of drastically reducing any one component of a diet, such as a very-low-carbohydrate diet, has not been confirmed in large studies,[86,87] so the best recommendation is a well-balanced diet with overall calorie reduction.[88] Many patients have unrealistic weight loss goals in terms of the rate of weight loss, fed by the grandiose claims of magazines and tabloids. A 500-kcal daily deficit is a very aggressive diet that cannot be sustained by many, yet it achieves a weight loss rate of only 1 lb/wk. For someone needing to lose 200 lb, they are looking at a 4-year project of sustaining this degree of caloric deficit. Although this seems disheartening, the data with respect to liver disease indicate that it is probably the process of losing weight and not reaching the final goal that confers the benefits. Discussing this with patients can provide a needed incentive to maintain a pattern of healthy eating despite relatively modest changes over time.

In counseling patients and discussing their commonly expressed frustrations, one must be mindful that there may be significant genetic underpinnings to the lack of progress in improving fitness with the lifestyle changes discussed previously. Before the fit, lean, and athletic disparagingly dismiss as volitional the failed efforts of some to improve their own fitness, one must be mindful of the many known and yet unknown genetic factors that might fully thwart the efforts of even the most earnest and diligent to improve their health through exercise.

SUMMARY

Lifestyle modification is the primary recommendation for patients with NAFLD and especially for those with NASH. Even if and when efficacious pharmacologic interventions are identified, lifestyle changes will likely remain the initial treatment recommendation because new drugs are inevitably expensive and may have unanticipated adverse effects after prolonged use.

In the absence of major randomized controlled trials of lifestyle changes for NASH, one must rely on small or uncontrolled trials, trials that impact surrogate markers, and an evolving understanding of the pathogenesis of NASH. All of these are fraught with difficulty and can be appropriately criticized for their individual weaknesses, but the sum of the data as it currently exists does make a convincing argument for the benefits of weight loss and exercise for NASH.[89–97]

The best recommendation is that all people should consume reasonable portions of a diet that is low in fat; low in simple carbohydrates; devoid of industrial *trans*-fats; and replete with vitamins, minerals, and natural antioxidants, while engaging in aerobic activities at least three times weekly. Unfortunately, these simple goals are surprisingly hard to achieve in an environment of copious amounts of delicious food and busy daily routines that seem to preclude time for exercise. Many of these difficulties can only be overcome by a culture change that values wholesome foods and regular exercise over the convenience of prepared foods and the comfort of minimizing physical activity.

REFERENCES

1. Lee Y, Hirose H, Ohneda M, et al. Beta-cell lipotoxicity in the pathogenesis of non-insulin-dependent diabetes mellitus of obese rats: impairment in adipocyte-beta-cell relationships. Proc Natl Acad Sci U S A 1994;91(23):10878–82.
2. Cusi K. Nonalcoholic fatty liver disease in type 2 diabetes mellitus. Curr Opin Endocrinol Diabetes Obes 2009;16(2):141–9.
3. Han MS, Park SY, Shinzawa K, et al. Lysophosphatidylcholine as a death effector in the lipoapoptosis of hepatocytes. J Lipid Res 2008;49(1):84–97.
4. Day CP, James OF. Steatohepatitis: a tale of two "hits". Gastroenterology 1998; 114(4):842–5.
5. Bradbury MW, Berk PD. Lipid metabolism in hepatic steatosis. Clin Liver Dis 2004;8(3):639–71.
6. Yamaguchi K, Yang L, McCall S, et al. Inhibiting triglyceride synthesis improves hepatic steatosis but exacerbates liver damage and fibrosis in obese mice with nonalcoholic steatohepatitis. Hepatology 2007;45(6):1366–74.
7. Day CP. From fat to inflammation. Gastroenterology 2006;130(1):207–10.
8. Malhi H, Gores GJ. Molecular mechanisms of lipotoxicity in nonalcoholic fatty liver disease. Semin Liver Dis 2008;28(4):360–9.
9. Anderson N, Borlak J. Molecular mechanisms and therapeutic targets in steatosis and steatohepatitis. Pharmacol Rev 2008;60(3):311–57.
10. Schenk S, Saberi M, Olefsky JM. Insulin sensitivity: modulation by nutrients and inflammation. J Clin Invest 2008;118(9):2992–3002.
11. Day CP, James OF. Hepatic steatosis: innocent bystander or guilty party? Hepatology 1998;27(6):1463–6.
12. Sanyal AJ, Campbell-Sargent C, Mirshahi F, et al. Nonalcoholic steatohepatitis: association of insulin resistance and mitochondrial abnormalities. Gastroenterology 2001;120(5):1183–92.
13. Berk PD. Regulatable fatty acid transport mechanisms are central to the pathophysiology of obesity, fatty liver, and metabolic syndrome. Hepatology 2008; 48(5):1362–76.
14. Díaz-Delfín J, Morales M, Caelles C. Hypoglycemic action of thiazolidinediones/peroxisome proliferator-activated receptor γ by inhibition of the c-Jun NH_2-terminal kinase pathway. Diabetes 2007;56(7):1865–71.
15. Perseghin G, Lattuada G, De Cobelli F, et al. Habitual physical activity is associated with intrahepatic fat content in humans. Diabetes Care 2007;30(3):683–8.
16. Belcher G, Schernthaner G. Changes in liver tests during 1-year treatment of patients with type 2 diabetes with pioglitazone, metformin or gliclazide. Diabet Med 2005;22(8):973–9.
17. Loomba R, Lutchman G, Kleiner DE, et al. Clinical trial: pilot study of metformin for the treatment of nonalcoholic steatohepatitis. Aliment Pharmacol Ther 2008;29: 172–82.
18. Teranishi T, Ohara T, Maeda K, et al. Effects of pioglitazone and metformin on intracellular lipid content in liver and skeletal muscle of individuals with type 2 diabetes mellitus. Metabolism 2007;56(10):1418–24.
19. Nair S, Diehl AM, Wiseman M, et al. Metformin in the treatment of nonalcoholic steatohepatitis: a pilot open label trial. Aliment Pharmacol Ther 2004;20(1): 23–8.

20. Schwimmer JB, Middleton MS, Deutsch R, et al. A phase 2 clinical trial of metformin as a treatment for non-diabetic paediatric nonalcoholic steatohepatitis. Aliment Pharmacol Ther 2005;21(7):871–9.
21. Marchesini G, Brizi M, Bianchi G, et al. Metformin in nonalcoholic steatohepatitis (letter). Lancet 2001;358(9285):893–4.
22. Bugianesi E, Gentilcore E, Manini R, et al. A randomized controlled trial of metformin versus vitamin E or prescriptive diet in nonalcoholic fatty liver disease. Am J Gastroenterol 2005;100(5):1082–90.
23. Fukukura Y, Fujiyoshi F, Inoue H, et al. Focal fatty infiltration in the posterior aspect of hepatic segment IV: relationship to pancreaticoduodenal venous drainage. Am J Gastroenterol 2000;95(12):3590–5.
24. Atwell TD, Lloyd RV, Nagorney DM, et al. Peritumoral steatosis associated with insulinomas: appearance at imaging. Abdom Imaging 2008;33(5):571–4.
25. Fregeville A, Couvelard A, Paradis V, et al. Metastatic insulinoma and glucagonoma from the pancreas responsible for specific peritumoral patterns of hepatic steatosis secondary to local effects of insulin and glucagon on hepatocytes. Gastroenterology 2005;129(4):1150, 365.
26. Jolliet P, Leverve X, Pichard C. Acute hepatic steatosis complicating massive insulin overdose and excessive glucose administration. Intensive Care Med 2001;27(1):313–6.
27. Krasnoff JB, Painter PL, Wallace JP, et al. Health-related fitness and physical activity in patients with nonalcoholic fatty liver disease. Hepatology 2008;47(4):1158–66.
28. Tamura Y, Tanaka Y, Sato F, et al. Effects of diet and exercise on muscle and liver intracellular lipid contents and insulin sensitivity in type 2 diabetic patients. J Clin Endocrinol Metab 2005;90(6):3191–6.
29. Black SE, Mitchell E, Freedson PS, et al. Improved insulin action following short-term exercise training: role of energy and carbohydrate balance. J Appl Phys 2005;99(6):2285–93.
30. Gauthier MS, Couturier K, Latour JG, et al. Concurrent exercise prevents high-fat-diet-induced macrovesicular hepatic steatosis. J Appl Phys 2003;94(6):2127–34.
31. Nielsen S, Guo Z, Johnson CM, et al. Splanchnic lipolysis in human obesity. J Clin Invest 2004;113(11):1582–8.
32. Church TS, Kuk JL, Ross R, et al. Association of cardiorespiratory fitness, body mass index, and waist circumference to nonalcoholic fatty liver disease. Gastroenterology 2006;130(7):2023–30.
33. Zelber-Sagi S, Nitzan-Kaluski D, Goldsmith R, et al. Role of leisure-time physical activity in nonalcoholic fatty liver disease: a population-based study. Hepatology 2008;48(6):1791–8.
34. Caldwell SH, Chang CY, Nakamoto RK, et al. Mitochondria in nonalcoholic fatty liver disease. Clin Liver Dis 2004;8(3):595–617.
35. Pessayre D. Role of mitochondria in nonalcoholic fatty liver disease. J Gastroenterol Hepatol 2007;22(Suppl 1):S20–7.
36. Petersen KF, Dufour S, Befroy D, et al. Impaired mitochondrial activity in the insulin-resistant offspring of patients with type 2 diabetes. N Engl J Med 2004;350:664–71.
37. Petersen KF, Dufour S, Shulman GI. Decreased insulin-stimulated ATP synthesis and phosphate transport in muscle of insulin-resistant offspring of type 2 diabetic parents. PLoS Med 2005;2(9):e233.
38. Holloway GP, Bonen A, Spriet LL. Regulation of skeletal muscle mitochondrial fatty acid metabolism in lean and obese individuals. Am J Clin Nutr 2009;89(1):455S–62S.

39. De Filippis E, Alvarez G, Berria R, et al. Insulin-resistant muscle is exercise resistant: evidence for reduced response of nuclear-encoded mitochondrial genes to exercise. Am J Physiol Endocrinol Metab 2008;294(3):E607–14.
40. Stefan N, Thamer C, Staiger H, et al. Genetic variations in *PPARD* and *PPARGC1A* determine mitochondrial function and change in aerobic physical fitness and insulin sensitivity during lifestyle intervention. J Clin Endocrinol Metab 2007;92(5):1827–33.
41. Lowell BB, Shulman GI. Mitochondrial dysfunction and type 2 diabetes. Science 2005;307(5708):384–7.
42. Freeman HC, Hugill A, Dear NT, et al. Deletion of nicotinamide nucleotide transhydrogenase: a new quantitative trait locus accounting for glucose intolerance in C57BL/6J mice. Diabetes 2006;55(7):2153–6.
43. Toye AA, Lippiat JD, Proks P, et al. A genetic and physiological study of impaired glucose homeostasis control in C57BL/6J mice. Diabetologia 2005; 48(4):675–86.
44. Dengel DR, Pratley RE, Hagberg JM, et al. Distinct effects of aerobic exercise training and weight loss on glucose homeostasis in obese sedentary men. J Appl Phys 1996;81(1):318–25.
45. Orchard TJ, Temprosa M, Goldberg R, et al. The effect of metformin and intensive lifestyle intervention on the metabolic syndrome: the Diabetes Prevention Program randomized trial. Ann Intern Med 2005;142(8):611–9.
46. Lindström J, Ilanne-Parikka P, Peltonen M, et al. Sustained reduction in the incidence of type 2 diabetes by lifestyle intervention: follow-up of the Finnish Diabetes Prevention Study. Lancet 2006;368(9548):1673–9.
47. Schenk S, Horowitz JF. Acute exercise increases triglyceride synthesis in skeletal muscle and prevents fatty acid-induced insulin resistance. J Clin Invest 2007; 117(6):1690–8.
48. Tiikkainen M, Bergholm R, Vehkavaara S, et al. Effects of identical weight loss on body composition and features of insulin resistance in obese women with high and low liver fat content. Diabetes 2003;52(3):701–7.
49. Suzuki A, Lindor K, St Saver J, et al. Effect of changes on body weight and lifestyle in nonalcoholic fatty liver disease. J Hepatol 2005;43(6):1060–6.
50. Harrison SA, Fecht W, Brunt EM, et al. Orlistat for overweight subjects with nonalcoholic steatohepatitis: a randomized, prospective trial. Hepatology 2009;49(1):80–6.
51. Marchesini G, Natale S, Manini R, et al. Review article: the treatment of fatty liver disease associated with the metabolic syndrome. Aliment Pharmacol Ther 2005; 22(Suppl 2):37–9.
52. Kashi MR, Torres DM, Harrison SA. Current and emerging therapies in nonalcoholic fatty liver disease. Semin Liver Dis 2008;28(4):396–406.
53. Rafiq N, Younossi ZM. Effects of weight loss on nonalcoholic fatty liver disease. Semin Liver Dis 2008;28(4):427–33.
54. Nobili V, Manco M, Devito R, et al. Lifestyle intervention and antioxidant therapy in children with nonalcoholic fatty liver disease: a randomized, controlled trial. Hepatology 2008;48(1):119–28.
55. Luyckx FH, Desaive C, Thiry A, et al. Liver abnormalities in severely obese subjects: effect of drastic weight loss after gastroplasty. Int J Obes Relat Metab Disord 1998;22(3):222–6.
56. Kral JG, Thung SN, Biron S, et al. Effects of surgical treatment of the metabolic syndrome on liver fibrosis and cirrhosis. Surgery 2004;135(1):48–58.
57. Rozental P, Biava C, Spencer H, et al. Liver morphology and function tests in obesity and during total starvation. Am J Dig Dis 1967;12:198–208.

58. Capron JP, Delamarre J, Dupas JL, et al. Fasting in obesity: another cause of liver injury with alcoholic hyaline? Dig Dis Sci 1982;27:265–8.
59. Verna EC, Berk PD. Role of fatty acids in the pathogenesis of obesity and fatty liver: impact of bariatric surgery. Semin Liver Dis 2008;28(4):407–26.
60. Hu FB, Li TY, Colditz GA, et al. Television watching and other sedentary behaviors in relation to risk of obesity and type 2 diabetes mellitus in women. JAMA 2003; 289(14):1785–91.
61. Schäfer S, Kantartzis K, Machann J, et al. Lifestyle intervention in individuals with normal versus impaired glucose tolerance. Eur J Clin Invest 2007;37(7): 535–43.
62. Elliott SS, Keim NL, Stern JS, et al. Fructose, weight gain, and the insulin resistance syndrome. Am J Clin Nutr 2002;76(5):911–22.
63. Bray GA, Nielsen SJ, Popkin BM. Consumption of high-fructose corn syrup in beverages may play a role in the epidemic of obesity. Am J Clin Nutr 2004; 79(4):537–43.
64. Ouyang X, Cirillo P, Sautin Y, et al. Fructose consumption as a risk factor for nonalcoholic fatty liver disease. J Hepatol 2008;48(6):993–9.
65. Henry RR, Crapo PA, Thorburn AW. Current issues in fructose metabolism. Annu Rev Nutr 1991;11:21–39.
66. Terrier F, Vock P, Cotting J, et al. Effect of intravenous fructose on the P-31 MR spectrum of the liver: dose response in healthy volunteers. Radiology 1989; 171(2):557–63.
67. Teff KL, Elliott SS, Tschop M, et al. Dietary fructose reduces circulating insulin and leptin, attenuates postprandial suppression of ghrelin, and increases triglycerides in women. J Clin Endocrinol Metab 2004;89(6):2963–72.
68. Shapiro A, Mu W, Roncal C, et al. Fructose-induced leptin resistance exacerbates weight gain in response to subsequent high-fat feeding. Am J Physiol Regul Integr Comp Physiol 2008;295(5):R1370–5.
69. Mossoba MM, Kramer JKG, Delmonte P, et al. Official methods for the determination of *Trans* fat. Champaign (IL): AOCS Press; 2003.
70. Ibrahim A, Natrajan S, Ghafoorunissa R. Dietary trans-fatty acids alter adipocyte plasma membrane fatty acid composition and insulin sensitivity in rats. Metabolism 2005;54(2):240–6.
71. Katz AM. Should trans fatty acids be viewed as membrane-active drugs? Atheroscler Suppl 2006;7(2):41–2.
72. Mozaffarian D, Katan MB, Ascherio A, et al. Trans fatty acids and cardiovascular disease. N Engl J Med 2006;354(15):1601–13.
73. Kechagias S, Ernersson Å Dahlqvist O, et al. Fast-food-based hyper-alimentation can induce rapid and profound elevation of serum alanine aminotransferase in healthy subjects. Gut 2008;57(5):649–54.
74. Stender S, Dyerberg J, Astrup A. High levels of industrially produced trans fat in popular fast foods. N Engl J Med 2006;354(15):1650–2.
75. Araya J, Rodrigo R, Videla LA, et al. Increase in long-chain polyunsaturated fatty acid n - 6/n - 3 ratio in relation to hepatic steatosis in patients with nonalcoholic fatty liver disease. Clin Sci (Lond) 2004;106(6):635–43.
76. Tetri LH, Basaranoglu M, Brunt EM, et al. Severe NAFLD with hepatic necroinflammatory changes in mice fed trans fats and a high-fructose corn syrup equivalent. Am J Physiol Gastrointest Liver Physiol 2008;295(5):G987–95.
77. Satchithanandam S, Oles CJ, Spease CJ, et al. Trans, saturated, and unsaturated fat in foods in the United States prior to mandatory trans-fat labeling. Lipids 2004; 39(1):11–8.

78. Eckel RH, Borra S, Lichtenstein AH, et al. Understanding the complexity of trans fatty acid reduction in the American diet: American Heart Association Trans Fat Conference 2006: report of the Trans Fat Conference Planning Group. Circulation 2007;115(16):2231–46.
79. Albers MJ, Harnack LJ, Steffen LM, et al. 2006 marketplace survey of trans-fatty acid content of margarines and butters, cookies and snack cakes, and savory snacks. J Am Diet Assoc 2008;108(2):367–70.
80. Willett WC, Mozaffarian D. Trans fats in cardiac and diabetes risk: an overview. Curr Cardiovasc Risk Rep 2007;1:16–23.
81. Eckel RH, Kris-Etherton P, Lichtenstein AH, et al. Americans' awareness, knowledge, and behaviors regarding fats: 2006–2007. J Am Diet Assoc 2009;109(2):288–96.
82. Borra S, Kris-Etherton PM, Dausch JG, et al. An update of trans-fat reduction in the American diet. J Am Diet Assoc 2007;107(12):2048–50.
83. Jones NL, Killian KJ. Exercise limitation in health and disease. N Engl J Med 2000;343(9):632–41.
84. Bouneva I, Kirby DF. Management of nonalcoholic fatty liver disease: weight control. Clin Liver Dis 2004;8(3):693–713.
85. Eden KB, Orleans CT, Mulrow CD, et al. Does counseling by clinicians improve physical activity? A summary of the evidence for the U.S. Preventive Services Task Force. Ann Intern Med 2002;137(3):208–15.
86. Sacks FM, Bray GA, Carey VJ, et al. Comparison of weight-loss diets with different compositions of fat, protein, and carbohydrates. N Engl J Med 2009; 360(9):859–73.
87. Kirk E, Reeds DN, Finck BN, et al. Dietary fat and carbohydrates differentially alter insulin sensitivity during caloric restriction. Gastroenterology 2009;136(5): 1552–60.
88. Bonow RO, Eckel RH. Diet, obesity, and cardiovascular risk. N Engl J Med 2003; 348:2057–8.
89. Harrison SA, Day CP. Benefits of lifestyle modification in NAFLD. Gut 2007;56(12): 1760–9.
90. Palmer M, Schaffner F. Effect of weight reduction on hepatic abnormalities in overweight patients. Gastroenterology 1990;99(5):1408–13.
91. Ueno T, Sugawara H, Sujaku K, et al. Therapeutic effects of restricted diet and exercise in obese patients with fatty liver. J Hepatol 1997;27(1):103–7.
92. Kugelmas M, Hill DB, Vivian B, et al. Cytokines and NASH: a pilot study of the effects of lifestyle modification and vitamin E. Hepatology 2003;38:413–9.
93. Hickman IJ, Jonsson JR, Prins JB, et al. Modest weight loss and physical activity in overweight patients with chronic liver disease results in sustained improvements in alanine aminotransferase, fasting insulin, and quality of life. Gut 2004; 53(3):413–9.
94. Vajro P, Mandato C, Franzese A, et al. Vitamin E treatment in pediatric obesity-related liver disease: a randomized study. J Pediatr Gastroenterol Nutr 2004;38(1):48–55.
95. Huang MA, Greenson JK, Chao C, et al. One-year intense nutritional counseling results in histological improvement in patients with nonalcoholic steatohepatitis: a pilot study. Am J Gastroenterol 2005;100(5):1072–81.
96. Wang C-L, Liang L, Fu J-F, et al. Effect of lifestyle intervention on nonalcoholic fatty liver disease in Chinese obese children. World J Gastroenterol 2008; 14(10):1598–602.
97. Nobili V, Manco M, Devito R, et al. Effect of vitamin E on aminotransferase levels and insulin resistance in children with nonalcoholic fatty liver disease. Aliment Pharmacol Ther 2006;24(11–12):1553–61.

Pharmacologic Therapy of Non-Alcoholic Steatohepatitis

Vlad Ratziu, MD, PhD[a,*], Shira Zelber-Sagi, RD, PhD[b,c]

KEYWORDS

- Non-alcoholic steatohepatitis • Steatosis • Fibrosis
- Glitazones • Ursodesoxycholic acid • Sartans
- Orlistat • Hepatoprotectants

Specific therapy for non-alcoholic steatohepatitis (NASH) is needed because of the potential severity of this liver disease.[1] Many studies have shown that patients with NASH have an increased overall mortality compared with an age- and sex-matched control population.[2–4] Specifically, liver-related mortality is increased nine- to tenfold,[2,4] and different reports have confirmed that cirrhosis is an independent cause of death,[2,3] third only to neoplastic and cardiovascular causes. NASH is a recognized cause of cryptogenic cirrhosis[5] and, increasingly, of hepatocellular carcinoma.[6,7] Therefore, there is a clear unmet medical need for NASH therapy.

IS THERE A NEED FOR PHARMACOLOGIC THERAPY IN NASH?

Although diet and lifestyle changes are a rational first-line therapy in NASH, many patients fail to comply with these measures or to implement them on a long-term basis. Weight- loss trials typically demonstrate reduced compliance with the diet after the first few months,[8–11] and weight loss among participants will at best average 3 to 4 kg after 2 to 4 years.[11,12] The lack of a strong and sustainable effect of diet and lifestyle changes in NASH has been demonstrated,[11] and it appears less and less probable that diet alone will be able to control the epidemics of obesity at a population level.[12] Low compliance is also the rule for increased physical activity,[13] on average 20% after 2 years follow up.[14] Moreover, many patients cannot exercise because of fatigue, arthrosis and cardiovascular comorbidities.[15] Although diet and lifestyle

[a] Université Pierre et Marie Curie, Assistance Publique Hôpitaux de Paris, Hôpital Pitié Salpêtrière, 47-83 Bd de l'Hôpital, Paris 75013, France
[b] The Liver Unit, Department of Gastroenterology, Tel Aviv Sourasky Medical Center, 6 Weizmann Street, Tel Aviv 64239, Israel
[c] School of Public Health, Haifa University, Haifa, Israel
* Corresponding author.
E-mail address: vratziu@teaser.fr (V. Ratziu).

Clin Liver Dis 13 (2009) 667–688
doi:10.1016/j.cld.2009.07.001
liver.theclinics.com
1089-3261/09/$ – see front matter

changes should be tried first, pharmacologic therapy for NASH will be needed when these measures fail to significantly improve the liver condition.

INDICATIONS FOR TREATMENT

The indications for treatment have not been established. The spectrum of non-alcoholic fatty liver disease (NAFLD) covers bland steatosis and steatohepatitis. Currently it is believed that only steatohepatitis carries a significant risk of liver disease progression, while the risk associated with bland steatosis is largely extrahepatic—worsening of the insulin resistance phenotypic complications. Therefore first-line diet and lifestyle changes should be enforced in any patient with NAFLD, but pharmacologic therapy specifically aimed at improving the liver condition is most certainly necessary only in patients with steatohepatitis.

Which patients with steatohepatitis are eligible for specific pharmacologic therapy is also an open question. Obviously the aim of such therapy would be to improve liver injury to halt or slow down progression of the liver disease. Just like in any other chronic liver disease, and, in particular, chronic viral hepatitis, patients with bridging fibrosis (Brunt stage 3) are at high risk of progression and therefore in need of specific liver-directed therapy. Arguably, patients at earlier stages but with cumulating risk factors of liver fibrosis (age older than 50, diabetes, arterial hypertension, or severe insulin resistance) also could be candidates for such therapy. Lastly, it is important that an integrative approach combining nonpharmacologic measures and pharmacologic therapy be defined in carefully planned, future trials. It will be important to assess, not only the additional effect of any pharmacologic agent over diet and lifestyle interventions, but also the best timing for its initiation.

PHARMACOLOGIC THERAPY IN NASH: TWO BROAD AVENUES OF RESEARCH

Insulin resistance is an almost universal finding in primary NASH.[16] It is believed to be the main driving force behind excessive fat accumulation in the liver,[17] but it may also play a role in the initiation and perpetuation of steatohepatitis and progression of fibrogenesis.[18] Therefore, improvement of insulin sensitivity is an obvious target for a candidate pharmacologic agent in NASH (**Fig. 1**). This approach assumes that correcting insulin resistance will improve liver injury indirectly through a reduction in necroinflammation and subsequently an inhibition or a halt to the progression of fibrosis. At best, this is a lengthy process, but it carries the advantage of temporarily correcting the main and supposedly causal underlying disorder. Unfortunately, some of the available trials with insulin-sensitizing molecules such as the glitazones, have shown that in some patients, the mere correction of insulin resistance is not sufficient to improve liver injury.[19] An alternative approach therefore would be to develop drugs that are targeted specifically at improving liver inflammation and blocking liver fibrosis irrespective of any effect on insulin resistance (see **Fig. 1**). Such anti-inflammatory or antifibrotic agents fall in the category of hepatoprotectants (some of which are listed in **Table 1**); they do not necessarily target pathways of liver cell-injury specific for NASH, but NASH would be one of their main clinical applications given the impressive epidemiologic burden of this disease.

This article reviews the salient findings of the main clinical trials in adult human NASH and their limitations. It does not discuss trials designed for obese or diabetic populations irrespective of the liver injury and which subsequently analyzed the impact of those drugs on liver transaminases or on the noninvasive assessment of liver fat.

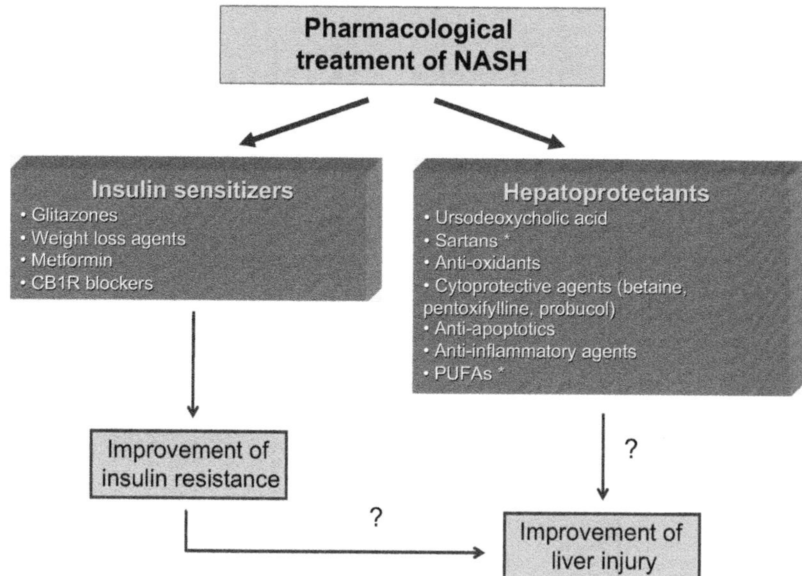

Fig. 1. Candidate pharmacologic agents for treatment of NASH. *Also have insulin sensitizing properties.

INSULIN-SENSITIZING AGENTS

Glitazones

Mode of action

Glitazones are agonists of PPAR-gamma (peroxisome proliferator-activated receptor) nuclear receptors, and they have been in use for treating type 2 diabetes for almost a decade. These insulin-sensitizing agents promote the differentiation of large, insulin-resistant adipocytes into small, metabolically active, insulin-sensitive adipocytes. This results in a modification of fat-derived metabolic and hormonal signals, mainly a reduction in the release of free fatty acids, a reduction of tumor necrosis factor α (TNF-α) and resistin expression, and an increase in adiponectin production. The net result is an increase in the storage of fatty acids in adipose tissue, a reduction of hepatic glucose production, and a higher uptake of glucose by the muscles. This redistribution of fat from ectopic tissues (liver, muscle) to the adipose tissue is probably the main determinant of the insulin-sensitizing action of this class of drugs.

Human trials in NASH

Table 2 summarizes the available studies on glitazones in human NASH that reported on end-of-treatment histology. Four randomized and two open-label studies have been published so far. These studies are very heterogeneous as far as

- Molecules in use (rosiglitazone or pioglitazone), the dose under study (two different doses for each molecule)
- Length of exposure (6 or 12 months)
- Inclusion or not of patients with diabetes, or with normal transaminases, simple guidance, or protocol-defined requirements of dietary restrictions
- Existence of a run-in phase

Table 1
Main clinical trials of different drug treatments in patients with NAFLD/NASH

Medication/ Author & Year of Publication	Number of Participants Completing Follow-up	Design	Dosage mg/d*	Duration Month	Cointerventions	Significant Concomitant Weight Loss	Outcomes Significant Improvement: Biochemical (Liver Enzymes)	Radiological	Histologic
Orlistat									
Harrison 2004[54]	10	SA	120×3	6	Diet1400 kcal /d	Yes	Yes	NA	NS
Zelber-Sagi 2006[57]	44	RCT, DB, PC	120×3	6	Diet 25 kcal/kg ideal body weight/d	Yes, equal in both arms	No difference between arms	No difference between arms	No difference between arms
Hussein 2007[55]	14	SA	120×3	6	Diet 25 kcal/kg body weight/d	Yes	Yes	NA	Yes for steatosis
Harrison 2009[56]	41	RCT, OL	120×3 & vitamin E (800 IU)	9	Diet1400 kcal/d & vitamin E (800 IU)	Yes, equal in both arms	No difference between arms	NA	No difference between arms
Omega-3 fatty acids									
Capanni 2006[124]	56	CT	1000	12	No	No	Yes	Yes	NA
Tanaka 2008[125]	23	SA	2700	12	Dietary advice	No	Yes	Yes	NS

Vitamin E									
Hasegawa 2001[70]	9 (with repeated biopsies)	SA	300 mg	12	Diet 30 kcal/kg body weight/d	Yes	Yes	NA	NS
Kugelmas 2003[71]	16	RCT, SB	800 IU	3	Diet plus aerobic exercise	Yes	No difference between arms	NA	NA
Harrison 2003[72]	45	RCT, DB, PC	Vitamins E 1000 IU & C 1000 mg	6	Diet 1600 kcal/d plus exercise program	No	No	NA	No difference between arms
Betaine									
Abdelmalek 2001[89]	7	SA	20,000 IU	12	No	No	Yes	NA	Yes for fibrosis
Pentoxifylline									
Adams 2004[105]	11	SA	1600	12	Dietary advice	Yes, slightly	Yes	NA	NA
Satapathy 2007[107]	9	SA	1200	12	No	Yes, slightly	Yes	NA	Yes for overall grading
Probucol									
Merat 2003[109]	17	SA	500	6	No	No	Yes	NA	NA
Merat 2003[110]	27	RCT, DB, PC	500	6	No	No	Yes	NA	NA
Merat 2008[111]	8	SA	500	12	No	No	Yes	Yes	Yes for steatosis and necroinflammation

Abbreviations: CT, controlled trial; DB, double blind; NA, not available; NS, not significant; OL, open label; PC, placebo controlled; RCT, randomized controlled trial; SA, single arm; SB, single blind.
* unless otherwise noted.

Table 2
Glitazone trials with available end-of-treatment histology

	Drug (Dose/d), n	Comparator, n	Treatment Duration	End of Treatment Histology, n (Drug/PLB)	% with Diabetes	Change Versus Placebo (*P*)		
						Steatosis	Ballooning/Lobular Inflammation	Fibrosis
Randomized controlled trials								
Sanyal, 2004[24]	Pioglitazone (30 mg) + vitamin E, N=10	Vitamin E, N=10	6 months	18 (9/9)	0%	I (NA)	NC/NA	NC
Belfort, 2006[20]	Pioglitazone (45 mg) N= 26	Placebo N= 21	6 months	47(26/21)	48%	I (< 0.001)	I (< 0.02)/I (< 0.01)	NC
Ratziu, 2008[19]	Rosiglitazone (8 mg), N=32	Placebo, N=32	1 year	63 (32/31)	33%	I (< 0.02)	NC/NC	NC
Aithal, 2008[21]	Pioglitazone (30 mg), N=37	Placebo, N=37	1 year	61(31/30)	0%	NC	I (< 0.01)/NC	I (0.05)
Open-label trials								
Tetri, 2003[22]	Rosiglitazone (8 mg), N=25	None	1 year	22	NA	—	—	—
Promrat, 2004[23]	Pioglitazone (30 mg), N=18	None	1 year	18	0%	—	—	—

Abbreviations: I, improved; NA, not available; NC, no change.

Moreover, these studies are small in sample size, and it is therefore difficult to have a clear understanding on their effect on liver injury in human NASH.

Efficacy of glitazones in human adult NASH

The most reproducible effect of glitazones in human NASH is a significant reduction in transaminase levels and a reduction in steatosis. The reduction in transaminases occurs early on therapy (starting month 4 of treatment) and is sustained throughout the treatment period. The magnitude of reduction ranges between 30% and 60%, while normalization of alanine aminotransferase (ALT) ranges widely between 38% and 100%. Reductions in transaminase levels correlated significantly with improvement in insulin sensitivity and loss of liver fat.[19,20] Steatosis is the histologic feature most reliably improved by glitazones. With one exception,[21] all trials analyzed here have shown that glitazones reduce steatosis significantly more often than placebo. In the one negative trial, 25% of the patients had a very low level of baseline steatosis, from 5% to 25%,[21] which might make differences between groups harder to detect. Despite an overall efficacy, there seems to be a considerable heterogeneity in the individual response to glitazones. In the few studies that have reported this information, only 47% to 65% of treated patients experienced an improvement in steatosis.[19,20,22]

Although the biochemical response and the antisteatogenic effect have been documented, the efficacy on the other histologic lesions is rather uncertain. For instance, four studies documented a significant improvement in ballooning in patients treated with both glitazones.[20,22–24] The proportion of patients with improved hepatocyte ballooning ranged between 32% and 54% of treated patients.[20,22–24] Only one of the two controlled studies, however, has shown that this improvement was significant versus placebo.

Intralobular inflammation was improved in most[20,21,23] but not all[19] studies that reported on it, although not always with a high level of significance.[21] In the latter study using lower doses of pioglitazone, the improvement versus placebo was not significant despite a 1-year therapy. Portal inflammation was either unchanged[19,21,23] or worsened in one study with rosiglitazone.[22]

Very few studies have reported on the changes in the non-alcoholic steatohepatitis activity score (NAS) owing to its more recent publication, and the results are contrasting. In a 6-month study, the score improved in 46% of pioglitazone-treated patients by 2 points or more, versus only 14% in the placebo group (P = .02).[20] It is not reported, however, if this reduction is caused mainly by the reduction in steatosis that is part of the score. Another study with rosiglitazone for a longer period did not demonstrate significant changes in NAS score with rosiglitazone or placebo.[19]

Only three studies,[20,21] including an uncontrolled one,[23] showed improvement of fibrosis on glitazone therapy. In these three trials, in which all patients used pioglitazone, improvement occurred in 29% to 61% of treated patients. When changes in the active arm were compared with changes in the placebo arm for controlled trials, however, improvement of fibrosis was still significant in only one study with a marginal level of statistical significance (see **Table 2**). Only two studies specifically assessed changes in perisinusoidal fibrosis, one clearly documenting no change[19] and the other reporting a qualitative improvement.[22]

Unfortunately, any beneficial effects induced by glitazones seem to be short-lived if the drug is discontinued. Two studies included a follow-up after stopping pioglitazone[25] or rosiglitazone.[19] Both showed within 3 months a swift return to baseline levels of transaminases[19] and a worsening of insulin sensitivity with return to baseline levels of both the homeostasis model assessment (HOMA) index and adiponectin 1 year later. Histologic follow-up data off-therapy, which are available for only a small uncontrolled series of nine patients treated with pioglitazone in an open-label trial,[25] showed that steatosis, lobular inflammation, and the composite histologic activity score significantly worsened 1 year after stopping pioglitazone. A similar trend was observed for ballooning. Histologic criteria for the diagnosis of steatohepatitis, which disappeared in all but one patient after 1 year of pioglitazone therapy, were again present in most patients.[25] Although the authors report no worsening of hepatic fibrosis, this most probably reflects the short delay off-therapy.

The main drawback of using glitazones is their safety profile. Weight gain is a frequent adverse effect, mainly because of the expansion of the peripheral adipose tissue[26] and therefore usually not reversible after cessation of therapy. Although aesthetically and psychologically this can be considered undesirable by patients already overweight or obese, it is not associated with an increased cardiometabolic risk. An increased risk of fractures in the upper and lower distal limbs also has been documented with both glitazones in women but not in men.[27] A more serious adverse effect of both glitazones is the potential for worsening heart failure. There is a considerable debate over a potentially increased risk of myocardial infarction with rosiglitazone, which is labeled with a black box warning for this adverse effect. A large randomized study with a 5.5-year follow-up confirmed a twofold increase in the risk of heart failure with rosiglitazone but not that of myocardial infarction or overall cardiovascular morbidity or mortality compared with standard glucose-lowering drugs.[28]

In conclusion, the available trials of glitazones in NASH show that overall, the reduction in transaminases and loss of steatosis are the two most robust and reproducible hepatic effects of glitazones. It is important to note, however, that the beneficial effect of the reduction in liver fat has been debated, as some animal studies have challenged the concept that all liver fat is bad. Blocking esterification of fatty acids in triglycerides resulted in a higher level of hepatic oxidative stress, more inflammation and hepatic cell injury, and more fibrosis in animals fed a methionine choline-deficient (MCD) diet.[29] This, however, might not be relevant to human NASH, a disease causally associated with insulin resistance, where reduction of liver fat is probably simply a marker of improvement in insulin sensitivity. Beyond the antisteatogenic effect, about half of the studies have shown an improvement in all aspects of necroinflammation, but the improvement in fibrosis appears to be at best marginal. Future studies will need to better characterize nonresponders, to determine whether longer treatment duration results in additional histologic improvement, and if at least some of the hepatic effects are independent from the insulin-sensitizing effects, as some animal models suggest.[30,31] Pioglitazone and rosiglitazone have similar insulin-sensitizing potency and result in similar glycemic control in diabetes. The only notable differences consist in the lipid profile (an increase in serum triglycerides with rosiglitazone but not with pioglitazone), although to what extent this is detrimental in human NASH has not been established. Therefore, different study designs most probably account for the discrepant results obtained in trials published so far. The use of both glitazones is safe in patients with well-preserved liver function and there is no significant concern about hepatotoxicity. There is no reason to believe so far that more advanced fibrosis will result in a higher rate of adverse events.

Metformin

Earlier experimental data provided initial enthusiasm for the use of metformin for treating fatty liver. In the insulin-resistant ob/ob mouse model, metformin was able to reduce steatosis, serum transaminases and hepatic TNF-α expression, concomitantly with an improvement in insulin sensitivity and associated metabolic disturbances.[32] Shortly thereafter, an open-label trial of small sample size showed an improvement in serum transaminases in people with NAFLD.[33] This was confirmed in two other randomized studies.[34,35] Interestingly, an open-label study showed a breakthrough of ALT levels starting month 6 of therapy (initial decline followed by an increase),[36] pointing to the absence of a sustained effect on therapy, while a more recent open-label study showed no overall significant reduction in ALT values after 1 year of metformin therapy.[37] Metformin therapy can induce weight loss,[38] and it is possible that changes in weight during treatment might account for some of these discordant findings. For instance, in one study, 19% of treated patients lost more than 10 kg in weight, and ALT reduction was significant in these patients.[37] Data on histology are conflicting and overall point to a lack of histologic benefit, although most of the available studies are of small sample size. Two randomized trials showed no effect,[35,39] and one open-label trial showed only an improvement in hepatic cell injury (ballooning).[37] Only one study has shown a significant improvement in all histologic lesions in the metformin arm[34]; however the comparator arm did not undergo end-of-treatment liver biopsy, thus precluding any relevant conclusion to be drawn. In a study comparing metformin with rosiglitazone in patients with type 2 diabetes, Tiikainen and colleagues[40] suggested that the absence of effect of metformin could be caused by its very weak antisteatogenic effect (measured by proton spectroscopy) and the absence of induction of circulating adiponectin. The latter point, together with the absence of reduction of histologic steatosis, since has been confirmed.[37] Results from a much larger US NASH clinical research network (CRN) study comparing metformin with pioglitazone should be available in early 2010. Until then, there are no convincing data on the efficacy of metformin in human NASH.

Weight-Loss Agents: Orlistat

Orlistat is a reversible inhibitor of gastric and pancreatic lipases, blocking the absorption of around 30% of dietary triglycerides. This results in a modest reduction in weight (3 kg less than placebo[41]) sufficient to improve glycemic control[41–46] and reduce the incidence of type 2 diabetes in obese subjects.[42,43,46] There is some speculation related to possible weight-loss independent effects,[42,44,47] which could be related to the reduction in plasma free fatty acid (FFA) levels,[47] a significant modulator of insulin sensitivity.[48–52]

In a small case series, weight loss induced by diet plus orlistat resulted in clinical and histopathological improvement of NASH patients.[53] Two small uncontrolled trials demonstrated a beneficial effect of diet combined with orlistat on liver enzymes and histologic features including fibrosis following 6 months treatment.[54,55] In a study by Harrison and colleagues,[54] out of 10 obese NASH patients, fibrosis improved by 1 point in three, and one patient had a one-stage worsening. Steatosis improved in six patients, ranging from a 10% to 30% improvement. Hussein and colleagues[55] treated 14 obese NASH patients for 6 months with diet combined with orlistat. The treatment led to an average weight reduction of 5.3% of initial weight, resulting in significant reduction in liver enzymes and steatosis and a nonsignificant reduction in inflammation and fibrosis. Because both studies lacked control groups, the changes observed do not necessarily reflect any unique property of orlistat beyond weight loss.

Only two small randomized trials are available.[56,57] One of them[57] included 44 NAFLD patients, but only 22 underwent end-of-treatment liver biopsy. Additionally, treatment was of short duration (6 months). Both groups improved to the same extent in terms of weight loss, ALT reduction (although more pronounced in the orlistat group), and reduction in histologic steatosis (by 50%), which might reflect the strict behavioral weight-loss program enforced throughout the study period in both arms.[57] The assessment of fatty liver by ultrasound suggested an even greater improvement in the orlistat arm, although this was not confirmed by histology. The small number of patients with control liver biopsy and the short treatment exposure precludes any interpretation of the histologic data provided.

Another randomized, open-label trial compared diet plus vitamin E (800 IU) daily with or without orlistat for 9 months in 41 NASH patients.[56] Again, orlistat did not enhance weight loss or improve liver enzymes, measures of insulin resistance, and histopathology to a higher degree than placebo. The patients who improved liver histology also lost weight, whether on placebo or on orlistat. This allowed the authors to calculate that in this small series, a weight reduction of at least 9% is necessary to start observing improvement in the inflammatory activity and fibrosis.[56] The rather disappointing results of these two trials could be because of the strict dietary counseling. Although this was aimed at reducing gastrointestinal adverse effects of orlistat, it also might have induced weight loss in both groups, therefore obscuring the effect of orlistat and exposing a type 2 error.

HEPATOPROTECTIVE AGENTS

Ursodeoxycholic Acid

Ursodeoxycholic acid (UDCA) is a naturally occurring bile acid with distinct hepatoprotective activities.[58,59] An early nonrandomized study demonstrated an efficacy on ALT but also on steatosis reduction.[60] A subsequent, larger, multicentric, randomized, North American trial, however, failed to demonstrate any effect of UDCA on ALT or histology. The reasons for this lack of efficacy are not clear, especially because other studies have documented an improvement in ALT levels in NASH[61] or in hepatitis C, with a clear dose–effect relationship in the latter case.[62] Another randomized study showed a biochemical improvement with UDCA but no histologic improvement. Only the patients receiving both UDCA and vitamin E showed an improvement in steatosis as compared with the placebo or UDCA-only arms.[63] Recently a French multicentric trial tested high-dose UDCA (HD-UDCA, 28 to 35 mg/kg) in 126 patients randomized to receive placebo or HD-UDCA for 1 year. The results confirmed a significant reduction in ALT and gamma glutamyl transferase (GGT) values in the HD-UDCA arm, and a reduction in FibroTest (Biopredictive, Paris, France), a serum fibrosis marker.[64,65] Surprisingly there was an improvement in serum glucose, HBA1c, and surrogate markers of insulin resistance (serum insulin, HOMA levels) that were independent of weight variation. Although overall a reduction in ALT levels correlates with improvement in necroinflammation,[66] larger studies with histologic endpoints are needed to confirm that beyond biochemical improvement HD-UDCA induces a histologic remission.

Vitamin E

Vitamin E (alpha-tocopherol) is an inexpensive and well-tolerated molecule with antioxidant properties. In vitro and animal studies showed that vitamin E decreased the levels of transforming growth factor-β, a profibrogenic cytokine, ameliorated liver necrosis and fibrosis,[67,68] and prevented hepatic stellate cell activation.[69]

In an uncontrolled trial, a 1-year alpha-tocopherol treatment (300 IU/d) resulted in reduced steatosis in six out of nine NASH patients and reduced inflammation and fibrosis in five, although this may be attributed to weight loss that occurred with diet during the run-in phase. Interestingly, liver enzymes were reduced significantly after alpha-tocopherol treatment[70] but not with diet alone in the run-in phase.

In a small, short-term, pilot trial, 16 NASH patients were randomized to lifestyle modification (diet and exercise) with or without vitamin E at a dose of 800 IU for a period of 12 weeks. Vitamin E supplementation provided no statistically significant improvement in serum aminotransferase levels.[71]

It has been suggested that vitamin C enhances regeneration of oxidized vitamin E[72,73] and therefore that the association of both vitamins might improve the overall antioxidant potency. A double-blind, randomized, placebo-controlled trial of 45 NASH patients tested the association of vitamin C and vitamin E (at a daily dose of 1000 mg and 1000 IU, respectively).[72] After 6 months of treatment, there was no improvement in ALT or aspartate aminiotransferase (AST), or any histologic benefit for necroinflammation and fibrosis when comparing with the placebo group.[72]

In recent years, randomized controlled trials (RCTs) tested vitamin E treatment in combination with another drug[63] or as an additional treatment arm versus drug treatment.[34] As mentioned previously, the combination of UDCA with vitamin E had beneficial effects over the UDCA monotherapy arm in a Swiss trial that included 16 patients per arm treated for 2 years.[63] The combination therapy significantly reduced serum transaminases, sometimes to normal values. It also reduced necroinflammatory activity and steatosis, while there was no histologic benefit with standard-dose UDCA alone.[63] In an open-label, randomized trial, nondiabetic NAFLD patients were given metformin or vitamin E (800 IU/d) or diet for 12 months. Vitamin E was significantly less potent in reducing transaminases and achieving normal ALT than metformin.[34] Thus far, there are insufficient data to support the use of vitamin E supplements for patients with NAFLD.

Sartans

Three different lines of arguments make sartans or angiotensin receptor blockers (ARBs) attractive candidates for treating NASH. First, the renin–angiotensin system seems to be involved NAFLD development. Transgenic mice overexpressing renin develop steatosis, which subsequently progresses to steatohepatitis and fibrosis.[74] The livers of these animals exhibit a proinflammatory gene induction profile (in particular TNF-α), an increased production of reactive oxygen species, and apoptosis,[74] all very reminiscent of human NASH. Valsartan, which is an ARB, is able to significantly improve steatosis accumulation.[74]

Second, some of the ARBs are also partial PPARγ agonists. They induce beneficial effects on glucose and lipid metabolism without some of the adverse effects of full agonists (such as glitazones), particularly fluid retention and edema.[75] Telmisartan seems to have the strongest PPARγ activity, followed by irbesartan and to a lesser degree by losartan and one of its metabolites, EXP 3174.[76] Animal studies have shown that telmisartan increases caloric expenditure, protects against diet-induced weight gain, reduces accumulation of visceral and subcutaneous fat, promotes adipocyte differentiation into smaller insulin sensitive adipocytes, and reduces liver fat.[77] Similar data in people are yet to follow, but a large study has shown that losartan reduces the incidence of new-onset diabetes,[78] while a meta-analysis confirmed a significant reduction of incident type 2 diabetes with both angiotensin-converting enzyme (ACE) inhibitors and ARBs.[79]

Third, the renin–angiotensin system is activated in liver fibrogenesis.[80] Angiotensin 2 activates stellate cells (a process mediated through the induction of oxidative stress by nicotinamide adenine dinucleotide phosphate [NADPH] oxidase)[81] and exacerbates liver fibrosis in vivo.[82] Conversely, angiotensin 2 antagonists[83] and ACE inhibitors[84] attenuate fibrosis progression in vivo. Taken together, these data suggest that some of the ARBs have both insulin-sensitizing and hepatoprotective, particularly antifibrotic, effects that could be beneficial in NASH. As a proof of principle, it has been shown that olmesartan has mild antisteatogenic and strong antifibrotic and anti-inflammatory properties in the MCD model, an experimental NASH model in rats.[85]

Despite this wealth of experimental evidence in favor of this class of molecules, very few studies have been performed in people. In an open-label study of seven patients with NASH and arterial hypertension (half of whom were diabetics) treated for 1 year with losartan, a Japanese team showed reduction in transaminase levels and improvement in hepatic necroinflammation in five patients, although, as predicted, there was no insulin-sensitizing effect (measured by HOMA scores) and no loss of liver fat by histology.[86] There was a potentially interesting antifibrotic effect as evidenced by a reduction in fibrotic stage in four patients and a reduction of plasma TGF-β1 concentration and of hepatic stellate cell activation[87] (measured by α-smooth muscle actin immunostaining). These histologic data, however, are not yet convincing given the small sample size, the open-label design, and the reality of sampling error.

Betaine

An attractive hypothesis in the pathogenesis of NAFLD is that a decrease in S-adenosylmethionine (SAM), a substance that protects the liver against fatty infiltration, may lead to steatosis.[88,89] Betaine acts as a methyl donor in an alternative pathway for the remethylation of homocysteine to methionine. SAM, which is the activated form of methionine, converts phosphatidyl–ethanolamine to phosphatidylcholine. Phosphatidylcholine is an important constituent of lipoproteins involved in the transport of fat from the liver and hence prevents hepatic fat accumulation.[89–91] Betaine and methionine itself have been shown to increase SAM levels and to protect against steatosis in animal models of alcoholic liver disease.[92] Furthermore, betaine is essential for cellular membrane integrity and hepatoprotection.[89,93–95] Betaine and phosphatidylcholine supplements are safe, inexpensive, and widely available. There are almost no studies testing their efficacy in human NASH, however. One small pilot trial tested the effects of treatment with betaine in 10 patients, 7 of whom completed 1 year of treatment. Betaine significantly improved serum ALT, AST, hepatic steatosis, inflammation, and fibrosis. These results are very preliminary, but further trials with these compounds should be encouraged.

Pentoxifylline

Extensive evidence supports a central role of TNF-α and other proinflammatory cytokines in the development of obesity-associated insulin resistance, fatty liver, and the progression from fatty liver to NASH.[96] TNF-α triggers the production of additional cytokines that collectively recruit inflammatory cells, which destroy hepatocytes and induce fibrogenesis.[97] Circulating TNF-α levels have been demonstrated to be significantly higher in patients with NASH as compared with controls.[98,99] Pentoxifylline (PTX) is a methylxanthine compound known to inhibit the production of TNF-α.[100,101] Some studies demonstrated that PTX decreases serum transaminases and hepatic inflammation in experimental models of NASH in rodents such as the high-fat diet[102] or the MCD diet.[103] Others reported negative results.[104]

Two pilot uncontrolled trials have evaluated the possible role of PTX for treating biopsy-proven NASH in people.[105,106] Both demonstrated a reduction in serum transaminases after 1 year[105] or even 6 months of treatment.[106] Insulin sensitivity also improved in one of the studies.[106] Encouraging histologic results have been presented after 1 year of therapy in nine patients (reduction of necroinflammation in 5 patients, reduction of fibrosis in four out of six), although in an uncontrolled trial.[107] Tolerance, however, was an issue, with study withdrawals because of nausea.[105] Adams and colleagues[105] demonstrated a significant reduction in transaminase levels after 1 year of treatment with PTX in 20 patients. Almost half of the patients withdrew from the study, however, primarily because of nausea, and others reported an increase in gastrointestinal side effects.[106]

In the largest RCT trial of PTX so far, 30 patients were randomized (2:1) to PTX 1200 mg daily versus placebo for 12 months.[108] Twenty-six patients completed the entire duration of therapy. A significant improvement in serum transaminases, steatosis, and ballooning was documented in the completers of the PTX group. The most common adverse effects were mild headache and abdominal cramps, but without difference between the two groups and no withdrawals for adverse effects.[108] Although results are encouraging, larger RCTs are warranted, and a way to minimize adverse effects should be considered.

Probucol

Probucol is a lipid-lowering agent that is also a phenolic antioxidant that promotes endogenous antioxidants and can act as a free radical scavenger. Three trials have tested probucol in NASH, all by the same investigators. In an uncontrolled trial, probucol significantly reduced liver enzymes in 17 NASH patients.[109] These results were confirmed in a double-blind RCT in 27 NASH patients treated with either 500 mg/d probucol daily for 6 months or placebo. The AST and ALT mean levels decreased in the probucol arm significantly more than in the control arm.[110] In both trials, there was no weight loss that could have confounded the biochemical response. A recent single-arm trial (500 mg/d, eight patients) of a longer duration (1 year) suggested a histologic improvement in hepatic steatosis and necroinflammation but not in fibrosis.[111]

Probucol also was tested in combination with pantetheine (an agent that promotes fatty acid oxidation and reduces serum triglycerides) in an uncontrolled trial. Sixteen NASH patients were treated with pantetheine (600 mg/d) and probucol (500 mg/d) for 1 year. The mean AST and ALT significantly decreased, and inflammation was improved in four out of eight patients with repeated biopsy.[112]

Omega-3 Polyunsaturated Fatty Acids

Fish oil is composed primarily of omega-3 fatty acids, which, along with omega-6 fatty acids, constitute the essential fatty acids. Fish, marine animals, and nuts are particularly rich in omega-3 fatty acids, whereas omega-6 fatty acids are concentrated in animal products, vegetable oils, and transfatty acids typical of the modern Western diet. The current Western diets have an omega-6/omega-3 fatty acid ratio of around 16:1, in sharp contrast with primitive diets that were closer to 1:1. Because downstream products of omega-6 are proinflammatory, and those of omega-3 are anti-inflammatory, it is possible that this unbalanced fatty acids ratio has an effect on hepatic pathology.[113]

Insulin resistance is accompanied by a change in the composition of fatty acids in serum and tissues, with a deficiency of omega-3 polyunsaturated fatty acids (PUFA).[114,115] Dietary fatty acid composition modifies hepatic lipid metabolism.[116] For instance, long-chain fatty acids present in fish oil are natural ligands of peroxisome proliferator-activated receptor α (PPARα), a group of nuclear receptors that modulate lipid metabolism in hepatocytes.[117] Low levels of circulating n-3 PUFA, with a consequent increase of the n-6/n-3 fatty acid ratio, impair PPARα activity in the liver. This phenomenon is associated with a higher hepatic uptake of circulating free fatty acids, a decrease of hepatocyte fatty acid oxidation, a reduced synthesis of fatty acid transport proteins (ie, VLDL), and an up-regulation of lipogenic transcription factors such as sterol regulatory element binding protein-1c (SREBP-1c).[118–120] The net effect is in favor of an excessive fat accumulation in the liver. Previous experimental studies have shown that diets enriched with n-3 PUFA increase insulin sensitivity,[121] reduce intrahepatic triglyceride content, and ameliorate steatohepatitis in rodents.[122] In ob/ob mice, dietary PUFA markedly decreased the mature form of SREBP-1c and thereby reduced the hepatic expression of lipogenic genes such as fatty acid synthase and stearoyl-CoA desaturase 1. Consequently, the liver triglyceride content and plasma ALT levels decreased.[122] Levy and colleagues compared rats that were fed carbohydrate-enriched diets (controls), fish oil, or lard for 4 weeks. In fish oil-fed animals, the liver triglyceride concentration was lower than in control and lard-fed animals, respectively. The fish oil feeding blunted the normal postprandial decline in fatty acid degradation genes (PPARα, CPT1, and ACO) and blunted the normal postprandial rise in triglyceride synthesis genes (SREBP1-c, FAS, SCD-1). Therefore, fish oil ingestion decreased the propensity for hepatic triglyceride storage.[116] Moreover, it has been shown that an increased omega-3 hepatic concentration protects the liver in the acute D-galactosamine/lipopolysaccaride hepatitis model. This effect results from a reduction in the inflammatory response.[123] This provides good rationale for a beneficial effect of omega 3 polyunsaturated fatty acids not only for the first steatogenic hit, but also for subsequent proinflammatory hits.

Support for the protective role of omega-3 PUFA in people comes from two pilot clinical trials. The first is a nonrandomized open-label controlled trial that assessed the effect of a 1-year n-3 PUFA supplementation at a dose of 1000 mg/d in 42 NAFLD patients versus 14 patients who refused the treatment and were analyzed as controls. PUFA supplementation significantly decreased serum liver enzymes (ALT, AST, GGT) and reduced liver fat (as measured by ultrasonography) compared with controls.[124]

The second is a noncontrolled trial in 23 NASH patients who were supplemented with 2700 mg/d of eicosapentaenoic acid (EPA) (one of the major components of n-3 polyunsaturated fatty acids) for 12 months. Serum ALT levels were improved significantly. Seven of the 23 patients underwent post-treatment liver biopsy, which showed improvement of hepatic steatosis and fibrosis, hepatocyte ballooning, and lobular inflammation in six patients.[125] In both trials, body weight remained unchanged.

Two observational studies also provide further evidence of a protective association. A case–control study intended to evaluate whether patients with NASH (N = 45) had a specific dietary pattern as compared with a sample of 856 controls, matched for sex and age.[126] Diet history was assessed using a semiquantitative food frequency questionnaire. A significantly higher intake of n-6 fatty acids ($P = .003$) and n-6/n-3 ratio ($P < .001$) was found in NASH patients. These results suggest that the quality and combination of fat intake may be more relevant than its isolated amount; an excessive amount of n-6 fatty acids could be implicated in promoting necroinflammation.[126]

A recent cross-sectional study was performed in a subsample (N = 349) of the Israeli National Health and Nutrition Survey. Researchers screened for NAFLD by abdominal ultrasound and assessed diet history using a semiquantitative food frequency questionnaire. Consistent with the findings of Cortez-Pinto and colleagues, this study demonstrated a higher meat intake ($P < .001$) and a tendency ($P = .056$) towards a lower intake of fish rich in omega-3 in NAFLD patients. Because n-6 fatty acids are abundant in meat, these data suggest a higher intake of n-6/n-3 ratio in NAFLD patients.[127] Taken together, these findings suggest that omega-3 fatty acid supplementation could be an attractive adjunctive therapy in NASH patients.

CHALLENGES IN DEMONSTRATING THERAPEUTIC EFFICACY IN NASH CLINICAL TRIALS

The negative results of some of the agents discussed previously highlight some of the methodological challenges for therapeutic research in NASH. First, in some trials, there is a significant rate of spontaneous improvement, which may be caused by inherent changes in lifestyle and diet once patients are included in a trial. Controlled trials are therefore mandatory. This, however, raises an additional question regarding the optimal way to implement the accompanying dietary treatment and lifestyle changes during the trial. When professional dietary advice is provided in a protocol-based manner together with behavioral therapy sessions or any other mandatory, structured interventions, participants in the trial can lose weight to a point that the effects of the drug itself will be obscured, especially in small sample size trials. This was proven in trials with a run-in period, where both groups experienced a significant decline in transaminases.[20] In some circumstances, a strict adherence to dietary instructions is almost mandatory to avoid adverse effects of the active drug (as it is the case with orlistat). It is therefore important to design the trial in such a way that any real additional benefit of a drug over successful lifestyle intervention is not missed. The need for randomization is also crucial, as patients might differ considerably in their lifestyle, implementation of lifestyle changes, dietary patterns, and attitudes toward diet. Blinding can be a challenging issue in case of drugs with almost signature adverse effects (such as diarrhea with orlistat or weight gain with glitazones). Furthermore, dietary composition itself, regardless of weight loss, can affect NAFLD. Thus, the ideal comparison between treatment groups would best include dietary intake assessment (sugar and saturated fat intake), and compliance to dietary treatment beyond weight loss, which is a challenge because its self-reported nature.

A second important aspect is that the results should be expressed by comparing the magnitude of improvement between groups. A trial should be considered positive, not if there is an intragroup improvement, but rather if the magnitude of improvement is higher in the active arm versus the control arm.

A third aspect is the rather limited sample size of currently available trials. Probably the main explanation for this is that liver biopsy, which is necessary for diagnosing and evaluating therapeutic effects, is an invasive procedure. Future efforts should be directed toward identifying and validating noninvasive diagnostic procedures, not only for fibrosis, but also for steatosis and inflammation (steatohepatitis).

SUMMARY

Owing to its recognition as a frequent disease with a potential for a significantly increased liver-related mortality, NASH became in recent years an unmet medical need of major importance in hepatology. Diet and lifestyle changes always should be a first-line therapy. In many patients, however, implementation is difficult, and compliance is poor. Therefore, drug therapy is often the only therapeutic possibility. Hopefully, a new era of specifically targeted therapies for this condition is beginning. Given the complexity of the mechanisms involved in insulin resistance, necroinflammatory damage, and hepatic fibrogenesis, simply correcting insulin resistance will not be enough in many candidates for treatment. Tailoring therapy with hepatoprotective and insulin-sensitizing agents in non- or partial responders is a very attractive option for future therapeutic strategies.

REFERENCES

1. Ratziu V, Poynard T. Assessing the outcome of nonalcoholic steatohepatitis? It's time to get serious. Hepatology 2006;44:802–5.
2. Ong JP, Pitts A, Younossi ZM. Increased overall mortality and liver-related mortality in nonalcoholic fatty liver disease. J Hepatol 2008;49:608–12.

3. Adams LA, Lymp JF, St Sauver J, et al. The natural history of nonalcoholic fatty liver disease: a population-based cohort study. Gastroenterology 2005;129: 113–21.
4. Ekstedt M, Franzen LE, Mathiesen UL, et al. Long-term follow-up of patients with NAFLD and elevated liver enzymes. Hepatology 2006;44:865–73.
5. Caldwell SH, Crespo DM. The spectrum expanded: cryptogenic cirrhosis and the natural history of nonalcoholic fatty liver disease. J Hepatol 2004;40:578–84.
6. Ratziu V, Poynard T. Hepatocellular carcinoma in NAFLD. In: Farrell G, George J, De la Hall P, editors. Fatty liver disease. NASH and related disorders. West Sussex (UK): Blackwell Publishing; 2005. p. 263–75.
7. El-Serag HB, Hampel H, Javadi F. The association between diabetes and hepatocellular carcinoma: a systematic review of epidemiologic evidence. Clin Gastroenterol Hepatol 2006;4:369–80.
8. Brehm BJ, Seeley RJ, Daniels SR, et al. A randomized trial comparing a very low carbohydrate diet and a calorie-restricted low fat diet on body weight and cardiovascular risk factors in healthy women. J Clin Endocrinol Metab 2003; 88:1617–23.
9. Foster GD, Wyatt HR, Hill JO, et al. A randomized trial of a low-carbohydrate diet for obesity. N Engl J Med 2003;348:2082–90.
10. Yancy WS Jr, Olsen MK, Guyton JR, et al. A low-carbohydrate, ketogenic diet versus a low-fat diet to treat obesity and hyperlipidemia: a randomized, controlled trial. Ann Intern Med 2004;140:769–77.
11. Sacks FM, Bray GA, Carey VJ, et al. Comparison of weight-loss diets with different compositions of fat, protein, and carbohydrates. N Engl J Med 2009; 360:859–73.
12. Katan MB. Weight-loss diets for the prevention and treatment of obesity. N Engl J Med 2009;360:923–5.
13. Erlichman J, Kerbey AL, James WP. Physical activity and its impact on health outcomes. Paper 2. Prevention of unhealthy weight gain and obesity by physical activity: an analysis of the evidence. Obes Rev 2002;3:273–87.
14. Dunn AL, Marcus BH, Kampert JB, et al. Comparison of lifestyle and structured interventions to increase physical activity and cardiorespiratory fitness: a randomized trial. JAMA 1999;281:327–34.
15. Skarfors ET, Wegener TA, Lithell H, et al. Physical training as treatment for type 2 (noninsulin-dependent) diabetes in elderly men. A feasibility study over 2 years. Diabetologia 1987;30:930–3.
16. Marchesini G, Brizi M, Morselli-Labate AM, et al. Association of nonalcoholic fatty liver disease with insulin resistance. Am J Med 1999;107:450–5.
17. Browning JD, Horton JD. Molecular mediators of hepatic steatosis and liver injury. J Clin Invest 2004;114:147–52.
18. Bugianesi E, McCullough AJ, Marchesini G. Insulin resistance: a metabolic pathway to chronic liver disease. Hepatology 2005;42:987–1000.
19. Ratziu V, Giral P, Jacqueminet S, et al. Rosiglitazone for nonalcoholic steatohepatitis: one-year results of the randomized placebo-controlled Fatty Liver Improvement with Rosiglitazone Therapy (FLIRT) Trial. Gastroenterology 2008; 135:100–10.
20. Belfort R, Harrison SA, Brown K, et al. A placebo-controlled trial of pioglitazone in subjects with nonalcoholic steatohepatitis. N Engl J Med 2006;355:2297–307.
21. Aithal GP, Thomas JA, Kaye PV, et al. Randomized, placebo-controlled trial of pioglitazone in nondiabetic subjects with nonalcoholic steatohepatitis. Gastroenterology 2008;135:1176–84.

22. Neuschwander-Tetri BA, Brunt EM, Wehmeier KR, et al. Improved nonalcoholic steatohepatitis after 48 weeks of treatment with the PPAR-gamma ligand rosiglitazone. Hepatology 2003;38:1008–17.
23. Promrat K, Lutchman G, Uwaifo GI, et al. A pilot study of pioglitazone treatment for nonalcoholic steatohepatitis. Hepatology 2004;39:188–96.
24. Sanyal AJ, Mofrad PS, Contos MJ, et al. A pilot study of vitamin E versus vitamin E and pioglitazone for the treatment of nonalcoholic steatohepatitis. Clin Gastroenterol Hepatol 2004;2:1107–15.
25. Lutchman G, Modi A, Kleiner DE, et al. The effects of discontinuing pioglitazone in patients with nonalcoholic steatohepatitis. Hepatology 2007;46:424–9.
26. Balas B, Belfort R, Harrison SA, et al. Pioglitazone treatment increases whole body fat but not total body water in patients with nonalcoholic steatohepatitis. J Hepatol 2007;47:565–70.
27. Loke YK, Singh S, Furberg CD. Long-term use of thiazolidinediones and fractures in type 2 diabetes: a meta-analysis. CMAJ 2009;180:32–9.
28. Home PD, Pocock SJ, Beck-Nielsen H, et al. Rosiglitazone evaluated for cardiovascular outcomes in oral agent combination therapy for type 2 diabetes (RECORD): a multicentre, randomised, open-label trial. Lancet 2009;(373): 2125–35.
29. Yamaguchi K, Yang L, McCall S, et al. Inhibiting triglyceride synthesis improves hepatic steatosis but exacerbates liver damage and fibrosis in obese mice with nonalcoholic steatohepatitis. Hepatology 2007;45:1366–74.
30. Galli A, Crabb DW, Ceni E, et al. Antidiabetic thiazolidinediones inhibit collagen synthesis and hepatic stellate cell activation in vivo and in vitro. Gastroenterology 2002;122:1924–40.
31. Marra F, Efsen E, Romanelli RG, et al. Ligands of peroxisome proliferator-activated receptor gamma modulate profibrogenic and proinflammatory actions in hepatic stellate cells. Gastroenterology 2000;119:466–78.
32. Lin HZ, Yang SQ, Chuckaree C, et al. Metformin reverses fatty liver disease in obese, leptin-deficient mice. Nat Med 2000;6:998–1003.
33. Marchesini G, Brizi M, Bianchi G, et al. Metformin in nonalcoholic steatohepatitis. Lancet 2001;358:893–4.
34. Bugianesi E, Gentilcore E, Manini R, et al. A randomized controlled trial of metformin versus vitamin E or prescriptive diet in nonalcoholic fatty liver disease. Am J Gastroenterol 2005;100:1082–90.
35. Uygun A, Kadayifci A, Isik AT, et al. Metformin in the treatment of patients with nonalcoholic steatohepatitis. Aliment Pharmacol Ther 2004;19:537–44.
36. Nair S, Diehl AM, Wiseman M, et al. Metformin in the treatment of nonalcoholic steatohepatitis: a pilot open-label trial. Aliment Pharmacol Ther 2004; 20:23–8.
37. Loomba R, Lutchman G, Kleiner DE, et al. Clinical trial: pilot study of metformin for the treatment of nonalcoholic steatohepatitis. Aliment Pharmacol Ther 2008; Oct 9. [Epub ahead of print].
38. Knowler WC, Barrett-Connor E, Fowler SE, et al. Reduction in the incidence of type 2 diabetes with lifestyle intervention or metformin. N Engl J Med 2002; 346:393–403.
39. Haukeland JW, Konopski Z, Loberg EM, et al. A randomized placebo-controlled trial with metformin in patients with NAFLD [abstract]. Hepatology 2008;48:62A.
40. Tiikkainen M, Hakkinen AM, Korsheninnikova E, et al. Effects of rosiglitazone and metformin on liver fat content, hepatic insulin resistance, insulin clearance, and

gene expression in adipose tissue in patients with type 2 diabetes. Diabetes 2004;53:2169–76.

41. Rucker D, Padwal R, Li SK, et al. Long-term pharmacotherapy for obesity and overweight: updated meta-analysis. BMJ 2007;335:1194–9.
42. Heymsfield SB, Segal KR, Hauptman J, et al. Effects of weight loss with orlistat on glucose tolerance and progression to type 2 diabetes in obese adults. Arch Intern Med 2000;160:1321–6.
43. Hollander PA, Elbein SC, Hirsch IB, et al. Role of orlistat in the treatment of obese patients with type 2 diabetes. A 1-year randomized double-blind study. Diabetes Care 1998;21:1288–94.
44. Kelley DE, Bray GA, Pi-Sunyer FX, et al. Clinical efficacy of orlistat therapy in overweight and obese patients with insulin-treated type 2 diabetes: a 1-year randomized controlled trial. Diabetes Care 2002;25:1033–41.
45. Miles JM, Leiter L, Hollander P, et al. Effect of orlistat in overweight and obese patients with type 2 diabetes treated with metformin. Diabetes Care 2002;25: 1123–8.
46. Torgerson JS, Hauptman J, Boldrin MN, et al. XENical in the prevention of diabetes in obese subjects (XENDOS) study: a randomized study of orlistat as an adjunct to lifestyle changes for the prevention of type 2 diabetes in obese patients. Diabetes Care 2004;27:155–61.
47. Kelley DE, Kuller LH, McKolanis TM, et al. Effects of moderate weight loss and orlistat on insulin resistance, regional adiposity, and fatty acids in type 2 diabetes. Diabetes Care 2004;27:33–40.
48. Kelley DE, Williams KV, Price JC, et al. Plasma fatty acids, adiposity, and variance of skeletal muscle insulin resistance in type 2 diabetes mellitus. J Clin Endocrinol Metab 2001;86:5412–9.
49. Griffin ME, Marcucci MJ, Cline GW, et al. Free fatty acid-induced insulin resistance is associated with activation of protein kinase C theta and alterations in the insulin-signaling cascade. Diabetes 1999;48:1270–4.
50. Kim JK, Fillmore JJ, Chen Y, et al. Tissue-specific overexpression of lipoprotein lipase causes tissue-specific insulin resistance. Proc Natl Acad Sci U S A 2001; 98:7522–7.
51. Santomauro AT, Boden G, Silva ME, et al. Overnight lowering of free fatty acids with Acipimox improves insulin resistance and glucose tolerance in obese diabetic and nondiabetic subjects. Diabetes 1999;48:1836–41.
52. Ryysy L, Hakkinen AM, Goto T, et al. Hepatic fat content and insulin action on free fatty acids and glucose metabolism, rather than insulin absorption are associated with insulin requirements during insulin therapy in type 2 diabetic patients. Diabetes 2000;49:749–58.
53. Harrison SA, Ramrakhiani S, Brunt EM, et al. Orlistat in the treatment of NASH: a case series. Am J Gastroenterol 2003;98:926–30.
54. Harrison SA, Fincke C, Helinski D, et al. A pilot study of orlistat treatment in obese, nonalcoholic steatohepatitis patients. Aliment Pharmacol Ther 2004;20:623–8.
55. Hussein O, Grosovski M, Schlesinger S, et al. Orlistat reverse fatty infiltration and improves hepatic fibrosis in obese patients with nonalcoholic steatohepatitis (NASH). Dig Dis Sci 2007;52:2512–9.
56. Harrison SA, Fecht W, Brunt EM, et al. Orlistat for overweight subjects with nonalcoholic steatohepatitis: A randomized, prospective trial. Hepatology 2009;49:80–6.
57. Zelber-Sagi S, Kessler A, Brazowsky E, et al. A double-blind randomized placebo-controlled trial of orlistat for the treatment of nonalcoholic fatty liver disease. Clin Gastroenterol Hepatol 2006;4:639–44.

58. Beuers U. Drug insight: mechanisms and sites of action of ursodeoxycholic acid in cholestasis. Nat Clin Pract Gastroenterol Hepatol 2006;3:318–28.
59. Bellentani S. Immunomodulating and antiapoptotic action of ursodeoxycholic acid: where are we and where should we go? Eur J Gastroenterol Hepatol 2005;17:137–40.
60. Laurin J, Lindor KD, Crippin JS, et al. Ursodeoxycholic acid or clofibrate in the treatment of nonalcohol-induced steatohepatitis: a pilot study. Hepatology 1996; 23:1464–7.
61. Kiyici M, Gulten M, Gurel S, et al. Ursodeoxycholic acid and atorvastatin in the treatment of nonalcoholic steatohepatitis. Can J Gastroenterol 2003;17:713–8.
62. Omata M, Yoshida H, Toyota J, et al. A large-scale, multicentre, double-blind trial of ursodeoxycholic acid in patients with chronic hepatitis C. Gut 2007;56: 1747–53.
63. Dufour JF, Oneta CM, Gonvers JJ, et al. Randomized placebo-controlled trial of ursodeoxycholic acid with vitamin E in nonalcoholic steatohepatitis. Clin Gastroenterol Hepatol 2006;4:1537–43.
64. Poynard T, Morra R, Halfon P, et al. Meta-analyses of FibroTest diagnostic value in chronic liver disease. BMC Gastroenterol 2007;7:40.
65. Ratziu V, Massard J, Charlotte F, et al. Diagnostic value of biochemical markers (FibroTest-FibroSURE) for the prediction of liver fibrosis in patients with nonalcoholic fatty liver disease. BMC Gastroenterol 2006;6:6.
66. Suzuki A, Lymp J, Sauver JS, et al. Values and limitations of serum aminotransferases in clinical trials of nonalcoholic steatohepatitis. Liver Int 2006;26: 1209–16.
67. Parola M, Leonarduzzi G, Biasi F, et al. Vitamin E dietary supplementation protects against carbon tetrachloride-induced chronic liver damage and cirrhosis. Hepatology 1992;16:1014–21.
68. Parola M, Muraca R, Dianzani I, et al. Vitamin E dietary supplementation inhibits transforming growth factor beta 1 gene expression in the rat liver. FEBS Lett 1992;308:267–70.
69. Houglum K, Venkataramani A, Lyche K, et al. A pilot study of the effects of d-alpha-tocopherol on hepatic stellate cell activation in chronic hepatitis C. Gastroenterology 1997;113:1069–73.
70. Hasegawa T, Yoneda M, Nakamura K, et al. Plasma transforming growth factor beta-1 level and efficacy of alpha-tocopherol in patients with nonalcoholic steatohepatitis: a pilot study. Aliment Pharmacol Ther 2001;15: 1667–72.
71. Kugelmas M, Hill DB, Vivian B, et al. Cytokines and NASH: a pilot study of the effects of lifestyle modification and vitamin E. Hepatology 2003;38: 413–9.
72. Harrison SA, Torgerson S, Hayashi P, et al. Vitamin E and vitamin C treatment improves fibrosis in patients with nonalcoholic steatohepatitis. Am J Gastroenterol 2003;98:2485–90.
73. Chan AC. Partners in defense, vitamin E and vitamin C. Can J Physiol Pharmacol 1993;71:725–31.
74. Wei Y, Clark SE, Morris EM, et al. Angiotensin II-induced non-alcoholic fatty liver disease is mediated by oxidative stress in transgenic TG(mRen2)27(Ren2) rats. J Hepatol 2008;49:417–28.
75. Sharma AM. Telmisartan: the ACE of ARBs? Hypertension 2006;47:822–3.
76. Kurtz TW. New treatment strategies for patients with hypertension and insulin resistance. Am J Med 2006;119:S24–30.

77. Sugimoto K, Qi NR, Kazdova L, et al. Telmisartan but not valsartan increases caloric expenditure and protects against weight gain and hepatic steatosis. Hypertension 2006;47:1003–9.
78. Dahlof B, Devereux RB, Kjeldsen SE, et al. Cardiovascular morbidity and mortality in the Losartan Intervention For Endpoint reduction in hypertension study (LIFE): a randomised trial against atenolol. Lancet 2002;359:995–1003.
79. Scheen AJ. Renin–angiotensin system inhibition prevents type 2 diabetes mellitus. Part 1. A meta-analysis of randomised clinical trials. Diabetes Metab 2004; 30:487–96.
80. Paizis G, Cooper ME, Schembri JM, et al. Up-regulation of components of the renin–angiotensin system in the bile duct-ligated rat liver. Gastroenterology 2002;123:1667–76.
81. Bataller R, Schwabe RF, Choi YH, et al. NADPH oxidase signal transduces angiotensin II in hepatic stellate cells and is critical in hepatic fibrosis. J Clin Invest 2003;112:1383–94.
82. Bataller R, Gabele E, Parsons CJ, et al. Systemic infusion of angiotensin II exacerbates liver fibrosis in bile duct-ligated rats. Hepatology 2005;41:1046–55.
83. Ramalho LN, Ramalho FS, Zucoloto S, et al. Effect of losartan, an angiotensin II antagonist, on secondary biliary cirrhosis. Hepatogastroenterology 2002;49: 1499–502.
84. Jonsson JR, Clouston AD, Ando Y, et al. Angiotensin-converting enzyme inhibition attenuates the progression of rat hepatic fibrosis. Gastroenterology 2001; 121:148–55.
85. Hirose A, Ono M, Saibara T, et al. Angiotensin II type 1 receptor blocker inhibits fibrosis in rat nonalcoholic steatohepatitis. Hepatology 2007;45:1375–81.
86. Yokohama S, Yoneda M, Haneda M, et al. Therapeutic efficacy of an angiotensin II receptor antagonist in patients with nonalcoholic steatohepatitis. Hepatology 2004;40:1222–5.
87. Yokohama S, Tokusashi Y, Nakamura K, et al. Inhibitory effect of angiotensin II receptor antagonist on hepatic stellate cell activation in nonalcoholic steatohepatitis. World J Gastroenterol 2006;12:322–6.
88. Rozental P, Biava C, Spencer H, et al. Liver morphology and function tests in obesity and during total starvation. Am J Dig Dis 1967;12:198–208.
89. Abdelmalek MF, Angulo P, Jorgensen RA, et al. Betaine, a promising new agent for patients with nonalcoholic steatohepatitis: results of a pilot study. Am J Gastroenterol 2001;96:2711–7.
90. Hirata F, Axelrod J. Phospholipid methylation and biological signal transmission. Science 1980;209:1082–90.
91. Hirata F, Viveros OH, Diliberto EJ Jr, et al. Identification and properties of two methyltransferases in conversion of phosphatidylethanolamine to phosphatidylcholine. Proc Natl Acad Sci U S A 1978;75:1718–21.
92. Barak AJ, Beckenhauer HC, Junnila M, et al. Dietary betaine promotes generation of hepatic S-adenosylmethionine and protects the liver from ethanol-induced fatty infiltration. Alcohol Clin Exp Res 1993;17:552–5.
93. Kashi MR, Torres DM, Harrison SA. Current and emerging therapies in nonalcoholic fatty liver disease. Semin Liver Dis 2008;28:396–406.
94. Mato JM, Corrales FJ, Lu SC, et al. S-adenosylmethionine: a control switch that regulates liver function. FASEB J 2002;16:15–26.
95. Patrick L. Nonalcoholic fatty liver disease: relationship to insulin sensitivity and oxidative stress. Treatment approaches using vitamin E, magnesium, and betaine. Altern Med Rev 2002;7:276–91.

96. Carter-Kent C, Zein NN, Feldstein AE. Cytokines in the pathogenesis of fatty liver and disease progression to steatohepatitis: implications for treatment. Am J Gastroenterol 2008;103:1036–42.
97. Tilg H, Diehl AM. Cytokines in alcoholic and nonalcoholic steatohepatitis. N Engl J Med 2000;343:1467–76.
98. Hui JM, Hodge A, Farrell GC, et al. Beyond insulin resistance in NASH: TNF-alpha or adiponectin? Hepatology 2004;40:46–54.
99. Wigg AJ, Roberts-Thomson IC, Dymock RB, et al. The role of small intestinal bacterial overgrowth, intestinal permeability, endotoxaemia, and tumour necrosis factor alpha in the pathogenesis of nonalcoholic steatohepatitis. Gut 2001;48:206–11.
100. Neuner P, Klosner G, Schauer E, et al. Pentoxifylline in vivo down-regulates the release of IL-1 beta, IL-6, IL-8, and tumour necrosis factor-alpha by human peripheral blood mononuclear cells. Immunology 1994;83:262–7.
101. Duman DG, Ozdemir F, Birben E, et al. Effects of pentoxifylline on TNF-alpha production by peripheral blood mononuclear cells in patients with nonalcoholic steatohepatitis. Dig Dis Sci 2007;52:2520–4.
102. Yalniz M, Bahcecioglu IH, Kuzu N, et al. Amelioration of steatohepatitis with pentoxifylline in a novel nonalcoholic steatohepatitis model induced by high-fat diet. Dig Dis Sci 2007;52:2380–6.
103. Koppe SW, Sahai A, Malladi P, et al. Pentoxifylline attenuates steatohepatitis induced by the methionine choline-deficient diet. J Hepatol 2004;41:592–8.
104. Vial P, Riquelme A, Pizarro M, et al. Pentoxifylline does not prevent either liver damage or early profibrogenic events in a rat model of nonalcoholic steatohepatitis. Ann Hepatol 2006;5:25–9.
105. Adams LA, Zein CO, Angulo P, et al. A pilot trial of pentoxifylline in nonalcoholic steatohepatitis. Am J Gastroenterol 2004;99:2365–8.
106. Satapathy SK, Garg S, Chauhan R, et al. Beneficial effects of tumor necrosis factor-alpha inhibition by pentoxifylline on clinical, biochemical, and metabolic parameters of patients with nonalcoholic steatohepatitis. Am J Gastroenterol 2004;99:1946–52.
107. Satapathy SK, Sakhuja P, Malhotra V, et al. Beneficial effects of pentoxifylline on hepatic steatosis, fibrosis, and necroinflammation in patients with nonalcoholic steatohepatitis. J Gastroenterol Hepatol 2007;22:634–8.
108. Rinella M, Koppe S, Brunt EM, et al. Pentoxifillin improves ALT and histology in patients with NASH: a double-blind, placebo-controlled trial. In: Digestive disease week. Chicago. 2009.
109. Merat S, Malekzadeh R, Sohrabi MR, et al. Probucol in the treatment of nonalcoholic steatohepatitis: an open-labeled study. J Clin Gastroenterol 2003;36:266–8.
110. Merat S, Malekzadeh R, Sohrabi MR, et al. Probucol in the treatment of nonalcoholic steatohepatitis: a double-blind randomized controlled study. J Hepatol 2003;38:414–8.
111. Merat S, Aduli M, Kazemi R, et al. Liver histology changes in nonalcoholic steatohepatitis after one year of treatment with probucol. Dig Dis Sci 2008;53:2246–50.
112. Tokushige K, Hashimoto E, Yatsuji S, et al. Combined pantethine and probucol therapy for Japanese patients with nonalcoholic steatohepatitis. Hepatol Res 2007;37:872–7.
113. Lee S, Gura KM, Puder M. Omega-3 fatty acids and liver disease. Hepatology 2007;45:841–5.

114. Borkman M, Storlien LH, Pan DA, et al. The relation between insulin sensitivity and the fatty-acid composition of skeletal muscle phospholipids. N Engl J Med 1993;328:238–44.
115. Storlien LH, Baur LA, Kriketos AD, et al. Dietary fats and insulin action. Diabetologia 1996;39:621–31.
116. Levy JR, Clore JN, Stevens W. Dietary n-3 polyunsaturated fatty acids decrease hepatic triglycerides in Fischer 344 rats. Hepatology 2004;39:608–16.
117. Reddy JK. Nonalcoholic steatosis and steatohepatitis. III. Peroxisomal beta-oxidation, PPAR alpha, and steatohepatitis. Am J Physiol Gastrointest Liver Physiol 2001;281:G1333–9.
118. Araya J, Rodrigo R, Videla LA, et al. Increase in long-chain polyunsaturated fatty acid n - 6/n - 3 ratio in relation to hepatic steatosis in patients with nonalcoholic fatty liver disease. Clin Sci (Lond) 2004;106:635–43.
119. Ip E, Farrell G, Hall P, et al. Administration of the potent PPARalpha agonist, Wy-14,643, reverses nutritional fibrosis and steatohepatitis in mice. Hepatology 2004;39:1286–96.
120. Clarke SD. Nonalcoholic steatosis and steatohepatitis. I. Molecular mechanism for polyunsaturated fatty acid regulation of gene transcription. Am J Physiol Gastrointest Liver Physiol 2001;281:G865–9.
121. Storlien LH, Kraegen EW, Chisholm DJ, et al. Fish oil prevents insulin resistance induced by high-fat feeding in rats. Science 1987;237:885–8.
122. Sekiya M, Yahagi N, Matsuzaka T, et al. Polyunsaturated fatty acids ameliorate hepatic steatosis in obese mice by SREBP-1 suppression. Hepatology 2003;38:1529–39.
123. Schmocker C, Weylandt KH, Kahlke L, et al. Omega-3 fatty acids alleviate chemically induced acute hepatitis by suppression of cytokines. Hepatology 2007;45:864–9.
124. Capanni M, Calella F, Biagini MR, et al. Prolonged n-3 polyunsaturated fatty acid supplementation ameliorates hepatic steatosis in patients with nonalcoholic fatty liver disease: a pilot study. Aliment Pharmacol Ther 2006;23:1143–51.
125. Tanaka N, Sano K, Horiuchi A, et al. Highly purified eicosapentaenoic acid treatment improves nonalcoholic steatohepatitis. J Clin Gastroenterol 2008;42:413–8.
126. Cortez-Pinto H, Jesus L, Barros H, et al. How different is the dietary pattern in nonalcoholic steatohepatitis patients? Clin Nutr 2006;25:816–23.
127. Zelber-Sagi S, Nitzan-Kaluski D, Goldsmith R, et al. Long-term nutritional intake and the risk for nonalcoholic fatty liver disease (NAFLD): a population-based study. J Hepatol 2007;47:711–7.

Non-Alcoholic Fatty Liver Disease: Is Bariatric Surgery the Answer?

Anjana A. Pillai, MD[a], Mary E. Rinella, MD[b,*]

KEYWORDS

- Non-alcoholic fatty liver disease
- Non-alcoholic steatohepatitis • Bariatric surgery
- Roux-en-Y gastric bypass • Gastric banding

Non-alcoholic fatty liver disease (NAFLD) encompasses a spectrum of disease states ranging from simple steatosis to non-alcoholic steatohepatitis (NASH) to end-stage liver disease (ESLD). Fatty liver is the most common cause of liver disease in the United States, affecting approximately one-third of the general population and more than three-fourths of obese patients.[1–3] NASH is distinguished from simple steatosis by the presence of inflammation and ballooning degeneration on the background of hepatic steatosis.

The World Health Organization estimates that 1 billion people worldwide are overweight and 300 million are obese.[4] In the United States alone, greater than one-third of adults older than 20 years of age are reported as being obese (defined by a body mass index [BMI; calculated as the weight in kilograms divided by height in meters squared] $\geq$30 kg/m^2) and by 2025 this number is expected to increase to 45% to 50%.[5,6] In an analysis of mid-life mortality, overweight patients had a 20% to 40% increase and obese individuals had an overwhelming 200% to 300% increase in mortality compared with nonsmoking people of the same age.[7]

NAFLD/NASH represents the hepatic manifestation of the metabolic syndrome that also includes dyslipidemia, central obesity, hypertension (HTN), and insulin resistance (NCEP/ATP III criteria, 2004) (**Table 1**). Most patients with NAFLD are overweight or obese. This excess adipose tissue is typically in a truncal distribution, representing predominantly visceral adipose tissue. Insulin resistance is the hallmark of NAFLD and likely contributes to disease progression.[8–11] The presence of diabetes mellitus

[a] Department of Transplant Surgery, Northwestern University, Feinberg School of Medicine, 675 N. St. Clair Avenue, Galter 17-200, Chicago, IL 60611, USA
[b] Division of Hepatology, Northwestern University, Feinberg School of Medicine, 303 E. Chicago Avenue, Searle 10-541, Chicago, IL 60611, USA
* Corresponding author.
E-mail address: mrinella@nmff.org (M.E. Rinella).

Clin Liver Dis 13 (2009) 689–710
doi:10.1016/j.cld.2009.07.012
1089-3261/09/$ – see front matter

Table 1
Diagnostic criteria for the metabolic syndrome[a]

Criteria	NCEP ATP III
Central obesity (waist circumference)	>102 cm (men) >88 cm (women)
Fasting plasma glucose concentration (mmol/L)	>5.6 (>110 mg/dL)
Blood pressure (mm Hg)	>130/85
Fasting triglycerides (mmol/L)	>1.7 (150 mg/dL)
High-density cholesterol (mmol/L)	<1.0 (<45 mg/dL) (men) <1.3 (<50 mg/dL) (women)

[a] Requires the presence of 3 or more of the 5 features from NCEP ATP III: National Cholesterol Education Program, Third Adult Treatment Panel (2004).

(DM) and obesity are 2 key clinical risk factors for development of cirrhosis in a patient with NAFLD.[12,13] Approximately three-fourths of patients with diabetes or obesity are estimated to have NAFLD. Given the increase in the incidence of both these conditions, a staggering number of Americans have or will develop fatty liver disease.[13] Several studies have shown that the severity of fibrosis progression is closely related to the degree of central obesity and insulin resistance or overt diabetes, with estimated rates of ESLD ranging from 5% to 20% in 10 years.[14–18]

From a physiologic perspective, obesity itself represents a chronic, inflammatory condition resulting from the failure of the normal homeostatic regulation of energy intake, storage, and use.[19,20] Visceral adipose tissue secretes an abundance of proinflammatory cytokines that cause alterations in intrahepatic insulin signaling, leading to insulin resistance, which then exacerbates obesity-associated hepatic steatosis, and contributes to inflammation and progressive fibrogenesis.[19,20] The subcutaneous and visceral fat depots are metabolically distinct. Visceral adipose tissue contains more immature adipocytes and inflammatory cells, resulting in more metabolic activity than subcutaneous adipose tissue. To illustrate this, Klein and colleagues[21] examined the effect of liposuction on metabolic parameters in obese subjects. Despite a large amount of weight loss from subcutaneous fat removal, no changes were observed in obesity-related metabolic derangements or proinflammatory cytokines. In the setting of obesity, visceral adipose tissue undergoes hypertrophy and infiltration with macrophages. These changes result in the release of a plethora of adipocytokines that exacerbate insulin resistance, perpetuate a proinflammatory state, and culminate in worsening hepatic steatosis and injury (**Fig. 1**). Hepatic insulin resistance results, leading to an inability of insulin to stimulate glycogen synthesis and suppress gluconeogenesis, thus failing to downregulate hepatic glucose production in times of caloric excess.[22] The chronic inflammatory state induced by obesity has been implicated in the pathogenesis of several other diseases common to the metabolic syndrome including atherosclerosis, obstructive sleep apnea (OSA), and hypercoagulability. An increased risk for malignancy in obese patients is in part a result of chronic inflammation in this setting.[23]

The distinction between simple hepatic steatosis and NASH is important because their natural history is distinct. Only 3% of patients with simple steatosis developing cirrhosis compared with up to 20% in patients with NASH. Rafiq and colleagues[24] recently demonstrated that subjects with biopsy-proven NASH had increased liver-related mortality compared with their non-NASH counterparts. In addition, diabetic patients with NAFLD had an increase in both liver-related and overall mortality.[24]

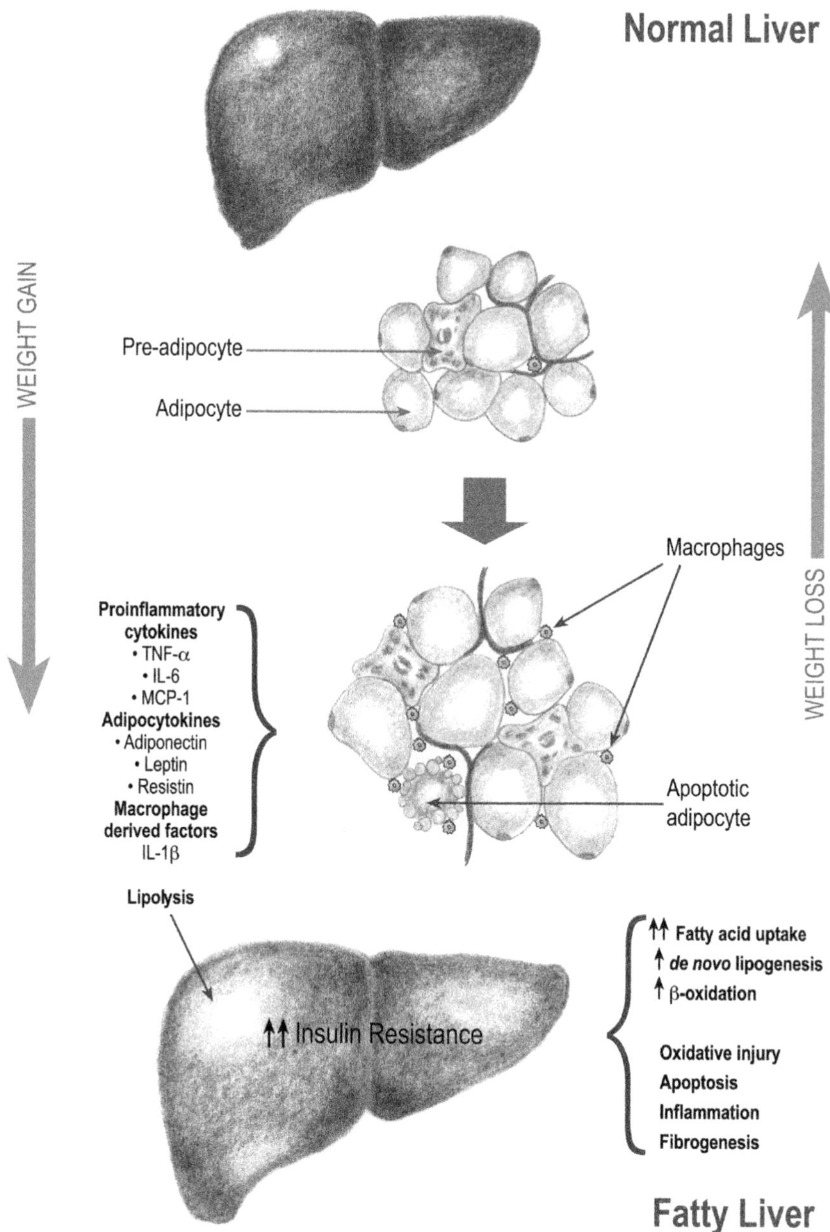

Fig. 1. Alterations in adipose and hepatic tissue related to weight change.

Even in the absence of steatohepatitis (NASH), emerging data continue to confirm that hepatic steatosis is an independent risk factor for cardiovascular disease and mortality.[25–29] Several studies have demonstrated that coronary artery disease surpasses liver-related complications as the most common cause of death in patients with NAFLD.[18,24,30] This result is likely due to the interplay between NAFLD and risk factors for the metabolic syndrome, which can lead to increased atheroma formation and abnormalities in endothelial function.[25,31–34] Targher and colleagues[28] demonstrated NAFLD was an independent predictor for cardiovascular mortality in a cohort of type 2 diabetic patients. In addition, Adams and colleagues[26] confirmed that cardiovascular complications caused 25% of deaths compared with only 13% of liver-related deaths in patients with NAFLD.

In summary, NAFLD not only contributes to the development of liver-related morbidity and mortality, it is a predisposing factor for cardiovascular disease and malignancy. Thus, any intervention must ameliorate comorbid risk factors, specifically central obesity and insulin resistance that contribute to the progression of liver disease. Sustained weight loss can be beneficial in preventing and even reversing NAFLD; however, it is often difficult to achieve in this patient population with diet and exercise alone.

DIET AND EXERCISE

Although lifestyle modifications (nutritional counseling and regular exercise) are the first line of treatment, with the goal of increasing energy consumption while decreasing caloric intake, there is significant concern in the literature as to whether these practices alone are sufficient in this population. Several studies examined the efficacy of weight loss on diet and exercise in obese patients with NASH/NAFLD.[35–37] A pilot study performed by Huang and colleagues enrolled 23 patients with biopsy-proven NASH to receive standard nutritional counseling for 1 year aimed at reducing insulin resistance and weight. At the end of the year, repeat liver biopsies demonstrated that 9 of the 15 patients had histologic improvement of NASH, although this was not statistically significant.[35] Ueno and colleagues similarly examined the effects of a restricted diet and exercise regimen (walking or jogging) in obese Japanese subjects. After 3 months, the treated group had significant improvements in aminotransferases, total cholesterol, fasting glucose, BMI, and steatosis compared with the controls.[37] As encouraging as these reports may be, meaningful and sustained weight loss is hard to achieve by diet and exercise alone, and even harder to maintain in this population. In fact, in the select group of patients who achieve their weight loss goals, the majority often rebound in weight to levels at or above their preintervention weight.

ANTIOBESITY MEDICATIONS

Other alternatives to lifestyle modifications include antiobesity medications such as orlistat and sibutramine. Orlistat inhibits gastric and pancreatic lipase, blocking the absorption of long-chain fatty acids and cholesterol, leading to a 30% decrease in fat absorption.[38] Sibutramine enhances satiety by inhibiting serotonin and norepinephrine reuptake.[38] Several small studies examined the role of these medications on patients with NASH/NAFLD[39–41] and showed improvements in BMI, aminotransaminases, steatosis, and to a smaller degree, fibrosis. Harrison et al, prospectively studied the combination of Orlistat with caloric restriction in overweight patients with NASH to determine its effects on weight loss and liver histology.[42] The authors concluded that subjects who lost $\geq$ 5% of their body weight improved insulin resistance and steatosis while those who lost $\geq$ 9% achieved changes in liver histology including improvement in ballooning, inflammation and NAFLD activity score. Ongoing large, randomized controlled studies are needed to fully determine the long-term benefits of these drugs on NAFLD/NASH patients. Another promising medication is rimonabant, a selective cannabinoid type 1 receptor (CB1) antagonist, which was approved as a weight loss agent in several countries outside the United States. In

2 large, randomized controlled multicenter trials, rimonabant proved to be effective in improving metabolic parameters by attaining sustained weight loss, and improving lipid profiles and insulin sensitivity.[43,44] Independent of weight loss, CB1 antagonists seem to decrease de novo lipogenesis, among other lipid metabolic effects, making them attractive agents for the treatment of NAFLD. However, preliminary studies examining the efficacy of this drug in patients with NASH were terminated due to reports of adverse psychiatric outcomes including suicide.[45] Nevertheless, the mechanism of action of these medications are quite promising and newer peripherally acting cannabinoid receptor antagonists are in development which should eliminate the centrally acting side effects leading to the unfavorable psychiatric problems.

BARIATRIC SURGERY

Given the limitations rendered by behavioral modifications and pharmacologic agents in maintaining sustained weight loss, bariatric surgery is as an attractive option in reversing many of the risk factors associated with NASH/NAFLD. Over the last decade, the short- and long-term benefits of bariatric surgery in morbidly obese patients have been well established and may provide a promising treatment modality for patients with NAFLD/NASH. Bariatric surgery was first introduced as a treatment modality for achieving weight loss in obese subjects in the 1950s. According to the National Institutes of Health (NIH) guidelines, bariatric surgery can be considered in individuals whose BMI is greater than 40 kg/m^2 or in persons with a BMI 35 kg/m^2 or over who have high-risk comorbidities such as heart disease, DM, hyperlipidemia, and OSA.[46] Although obesity-related liver disease is a major complication of obesity, leading to liver failure in many and the need for liver transplantation in some, it is not yet considered per se a comorbidity of obesity with respect to bariatric surgery.

Since its inception, marked improvements in surgical technique and experience have allowed for several different surgical options with the ability to tailor each procedure to the need of the individual patient. The number of bariatric surgeries has steadily increased in recent years due to the worldwide increase in the incidence of obesity and its recognized associated mortality, improved reimbursement from insurance carriers, and the lack of long-term effectiveness of nonsurgical treatments.[7,47,48] Technological advances in the field have improved safety, decreased duration of hospital stay and, most notably, reduced in-hospital mortality from 0.89% in 1998 to 0.19% in 2004.[47,49]

Bariatric surgeries are categorized by the mechanism by which they induce weight loss: purely restrictive procedures, purely malabsorptive procedures, or those that combine both. The type of surgery performed is influenced by patient comorbidities as well as by patient and institutional/surgeon preference.

RESTRICTIVE PROCEDURES

Restrictive procedures achieve weight loss by creating a limited gastric reservoir. Limiting gastric space leads to early satiety and diminishes caloric intake. Options include vertical banded gastroplasty (VBG), adjustable gastric banding (AGB), and sleeve gastrectomy. These procedures are less invasive and less complex than malabsorptive procedures, but achieve a lesser degree of weight loss than surgeries with a malabsorptive component. Because of this, restrictive procedures are often preferred for high-risk surgical patients.

VBG consists of partitioning the stomach with 4 parallel rows of staples, then applying a vertical band to the external gastric surface at the opening between the upper gastric pouch and the body of the stomach (the “stoma”). The band is placed

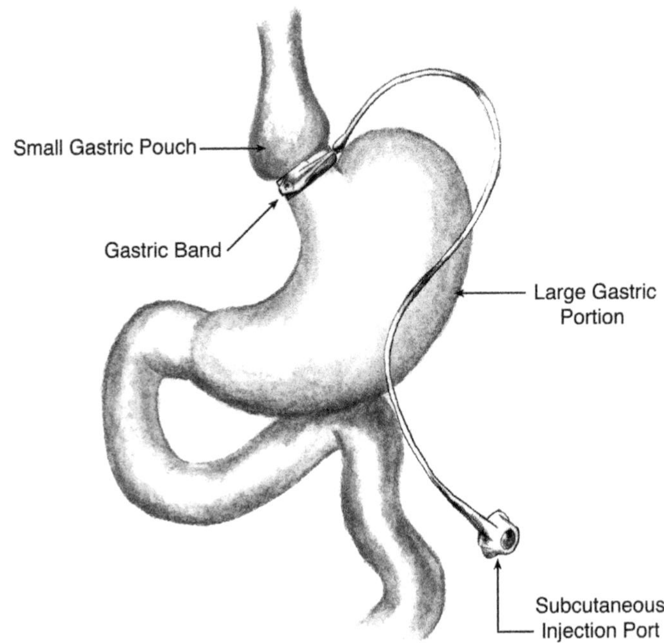

Fig. 2. Adjustable gastric banding.

to prevent dilatation of the stoma. Although this procedure gained popularity in the 1980s, it has since been abandoned due to a failure to produce sustained weight-loss results as well as complications of persistent vomiting, reflux disease, and band erosion.[47]

Failure of VBG led to AGB (**Fig. 2**), which can be performed via an open or laparoscopic approach. In this procedure, a band or collar is placed around the upper stomach 1 to 2 cm below the gastroesophageal junction, creating a 30-mL gastric pouch. Stomach constriction is variable and is adjusted by modifying the amount of saline injected into a subcutaneous port, which is linked to a balloon within the confines of the band.[47] This procedure is appealing in that it is a quick and less invasive approach that can be adjusted postoperatively to achieve the desired amount of gastric restriction.

MALABSORPTIVE PROCEDURES

Malabsorptive procedures involve bypassing variable lengths of the small intestine to minimize available intestinal absorptive surface, resulting in a "short gut syndrome." The most notorious of the malabsorptive procedures is the jejunoileal (JI) bypass, which is no longer performed. The JI bypass was first introduced in the 1950s, and gained popularity in the 1960s and early 1970s due to its ability to achieve remarkable weight loss in obese individuals. The procedure involved bypassing approximately 90% to 95% of the length of the small intestine to create a surgical short gut and a long blind loop. Unfortunately, it was plagued with significant morbidity and mortality due to severe weight loss and electrolyte disturbances. There were reports of hepatic failure, nephrolithiasis, and autoimmune problems that persisted years after surgery.[47,50] Some patients presented with cirrhosis whereas others developed overt hepatic failure soon after undergoing JI bypass. Prior studies assessing the effects of weight loss using a very low calorie formula in morbidly obese patients demonstrated that patients who lost more than 1.6 kg per week were at a higher risk for developing portal fibrosis and inflammation.[51] Proposed mechanisms of liver failure with JI bypass similarly include rapid weight loss causing massive mobilization of visceral fatty acids to the liver via the portal circulation, and bacterial overgrowth in the blind loop leading to endotoxin release and altered intestinal permeability. Thus a combination of increased lipolysis and excess exposure to endotoxin or other proinflammatory factors may stress pathways that manage lipid excess, perpetuate oxidative injury, and promote further recruitment of proinflammatory and profibrogenic cytokines. Due to these multiple complications, the JI bypass has now been abandoned.

COMBINATION RESTRICTIVE AND MALABSORPTIVE PROCEDURES

Both the Roux-en-Y gastric bypass (RYGB) (**Fig. 3**) and the biliopancreatic diversion (BPD) (**Fig. 4**A, B) have malabsorptive as well as restrictive elements. The gastric bypass was first developed in the 1970s, and has dramatically evolved in the last 30 years to become the most commonly performed bariatric procedure in the United States. More than 90% of gastric bypass procedures are performed laparoscopically, leading to less postoperative pain, shorter hospital stay, and a quicker overall recovery.[43] The procedure consists of dividing the upper portion of the stomach to create a 20- to 30-mL gastric pouch followed by a reestablishment of gastrointestinal continuity with a gastrojejunostomy. The Roux-en-Y limb is created using variable lengths of small intestine, allowing the surgeon to alter the degree of surgically induced malabsorption. The biliopancreatic limb is approximately 30 to 60 cm in length, and is the limb of jejunum extending from the ligament of Treitz to the

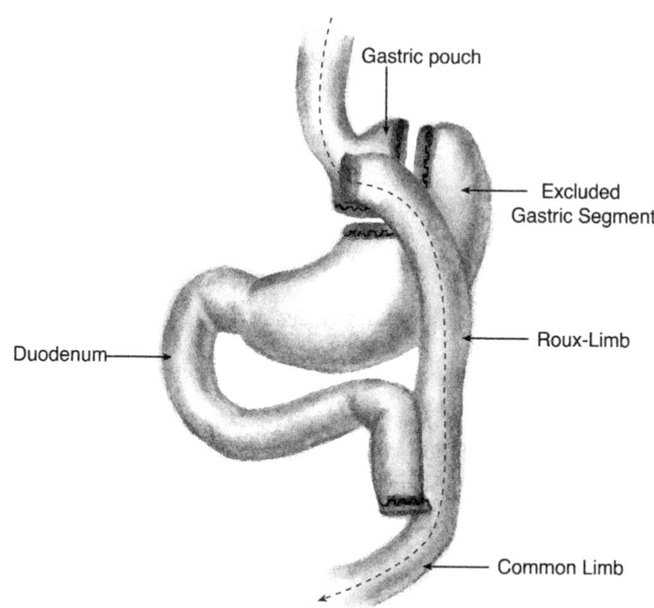

Fig. 3. Roux-en-Y gastric bypass.

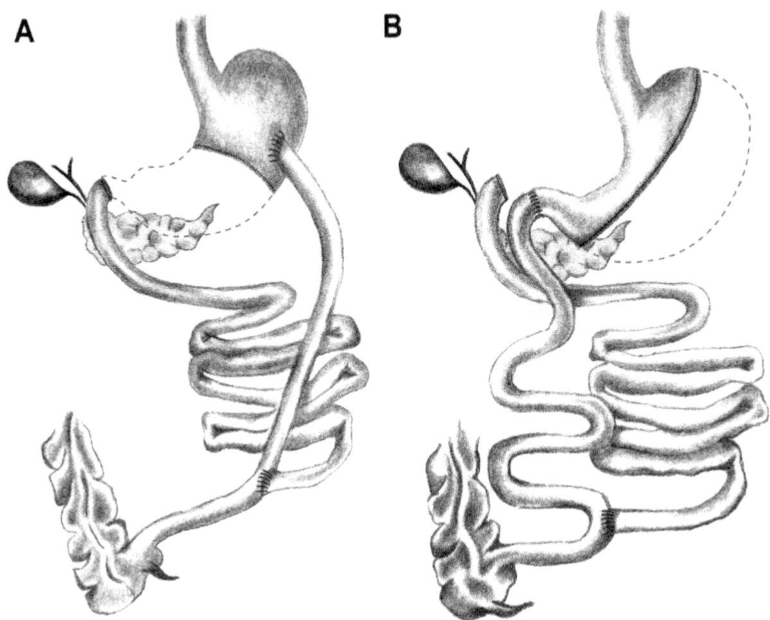

Fig. 4. (*A*) Biliopancreatic diversion. (*B*) Biliopancreatic diversion with duodenal switch.

jejunojejunostomy. This juncture is where the nutrient stream, bile, and pancreatic secretions come together.[47] The alimentary limb is the Roux limb from the gastrojejunostomy to the jejunojejunostomy, and is approximately 75 to 150 cm in length. Ingested nutrients in the absence of bile and pancreatic juice are transmitted via this limb. The common channel is the portion of the small intestine from the jejunojejunostomy extending distally to the ileocecal valve, and is highly variable in length.[47]

The biliopancreatic diversion (BPD) was initially developed in 1979 to avoid the stasis associated with intestinal bypass by maintaining a flow of bile and pancreatic juice through the biliopancreatic limb.[52] The BPD involves a subtotal gastrectomy (50%–80%) and differs from the RYGB in that the jejunojejunostomy is very distal, creating a common channel ranging from 50 to 100 cm in length (see **Fig. 4**A). The BPD with duodenal switch consists of a sleeve gastrectomy whereby the greater curvature of the stomach is resected vertically, creating a long tubular stomach along the lesser curvature (see **Fig. 4**B). The pylorus is preserved to avoid dumping seen in the BPD without duodenal switch, and an ileoduodenostomy is constructed distal to the pylorus.[53] In this procedure, the alimentary and biliopancreatic limbs are usually equal in length.

THE IMPACT OF BARIATRIC SURGERY ON MORBIDITY AND MORTALITY

Morbid obesity is associated with increased mortality and morbidity due to its association with many disease states. The life expectancy of severely obese persons is estimated to be reduced by 5 to 20 years.[54] Two recent landmark studies confirmed the benefits of bariatric surgery in not only achieving substantial weight loss and improving the comorbidities of obesity but also in reducing mortality.

In 2004, Buchwald and colleagues[55] performed a meta-analysis of 136 studies examining over 22,000 patients to review the impact of bariatric surgery on weight loss and obesity-related comorbidities. According to the study, the mean percentage of excess weight loss 2 years following surgery was 61.2% for all bariatric surgery procedures, and ranged from 47.5% for gastric banding (GB), to 61.6% for RYGB, to 70.1% for with or without duodenal switch. Regarding type 2 diabetes, more than 75% of patients had complete resolution of their disease after surgery and in the remaining patients, more than 50% had significant improvement. The more pronounced effect on comorbid conditions seen in RYGB and BPD may in part be related to changes in gut peptides that occur after these procedures.

In a retrospective cohort study, Adams and colleagues[56] compared 7925 surgical patients to 7925 matched severely obese controls, followed for a mean of 7.1 years. The study concluded that adjusted long-term mortality from all causes decreased by 40% in the surgery group compared with controls. Specifically, compared with controls the surgically treated group had a 56% decrease in mortality from cardiovascular disease, a 92% decrease in mortality from diabetes, and a 60% decrease in mortality from cancer.

In a similar study in 2004, Sjöström and colleagues[57] summarized the findings of a large, prospectively controlled study of Swedish obese subjects that matched obese subjects who underwent gastric surgery by VBG, RYGB, and AGB to conventionally treated obese patients. After 10 years, there was a 1.6% increase over the inclusion weight in controls whereas the surgical group maintained a weight loss of 16.1% ($P<.001$). Of note, 2- and 10-year rates of recovery from diabetes, dyslipidemia, and HTN were vastly greater in the surgical group. Mean changes in weight loss and amelioration of risk factors were significantly higher in subjects treated by RYGB than in those who underwent VBG or AGB. More recently, the same group addressed the importance of weight loss on overall mortality in a prospectively controlled study that examined more than 4000 obese Swedish subjects over a 16-year period.[58] Cumulative overall mortality was drastically reduced in the bariatric surgery group compared with subjects who received conventional treatment. The unadjusted overall hazard ratio was 0.76 in the surgery group ($P=.04$); however, the study was not powered to determine whether this favorable survival effect of surgery is based on merely weight loss or amelioration of risk factors.

EFFECTS OF BARIATRIC SURGERY ON NON-ALCOHOLIC FATTY LIVER DISEASE HISTOLOGY

The bariatric population is an interesting one in which to study NAFLD because it encompasses the entire spectrum of disease. Most patients undergoing bariatric surgery have some degree of hepatic steatosis: approximately 25% have NASH and 1% to 3% will have cirrhosis incidentally found in the operating room. In the absence of large, randomized controlled trials, the available literature evaluating the effects of obesity surgery on NAFLD/NASH is limited to case series involving small numbers of patients from a single institution, retrospective studies, and prospective observational reports. There is also a great degree of variability between studies regarding patient selection or the type of surgery performed. Furthermore, many do not specifically comment on improvement or resolution of NASH or have defined histologic criteria to assess the full spectrum of the disease. **Table 2** summarizes selected studies that specifically reported changes in liver histology after bariatric surgery.

The initial experience with the effects of bariatric surgery on liver disease was not favorable, given the complications associated with JI bypass. Scattered reports of hepatic decompensation after other bariatric procedures have since surfaced. The first reported case of fatal hepatic decompensation after biliopancreatic diversion was in 1992. A patient died of liver failure from acute steatohepatitis with cholestasis after an 83% excess weight loss over 10 months.[71] More recently, in a case series of 3 severely obese patients (BMI 49–86 kg/m^2) undergoing RYGB with an extended Roux

Table 2
The effects of bariatric surgery on liver histology in NAFLD patients

Study	Surgery	Total/NASH, N	Cirrhosis, N	Mean Initial BMI	Mean Interval to Second Biopsy (months)	Mean Excess Weight Loss	Histology				
							Steatosis	Ballooning	Inflammation	Fibrosis	NASH Resolution
Dixon, 2004[73]	AGB	36/23	1	47 (±10.6)	25.6	52%	↓	↓	↓	↓	82%
Dixon et al, 2006[65]	AGB	60/30		45.9 (±7.4)	29.5	32%	↓	Not reported	↓	↓	80%
Mattar et al, 2005[61]	RYGB (41) SG (23) AGB (6)	70	2	56 (±11)	15	59%	↓	Not reported	↓	↓	Not reported
Mathurin et al, 2006[62]	BIB (71) AGB (100)	121/24		49 (±8)	12	19%	↓	Not reported	Not reported	↑	75%
Kral et al, 2004[74]	BPD	104	11	31 (±8)	41	34%	↓	Not reported	↓	↓/↑	Not reported
Mottin et al, 2005[59]	RYGB	90		46.7 (±0.88)	12	81.4%	↓	Not reported	Not reported	Not reported	Not reported
Clark et al, 2005[60]	RYGB	16		51.1 (±6.1)	10	35.4%	↓	↓	↓	↓	Not reported
Csendes et al, 2006[63]	RYGB	16/4	1	44.3	17.5	72%	↓	↓	↓	↑	100%
de Almeida et al, 2006[64]	RYGB	16		53.4 (±8.8)	23.5	42%	↓	↓	↓	↓/↑	Not reported
Barker et al, 2006[66]	RYGB	19/19	1	47 (±4.4)	21.4	52.4%	↓	↓	↓	↓/↑	89%
Liu et al, 2007[67]	RYGB	39/23		47.7 (±6.2)	18	Not reported	↓	↓	↓	↓/↑	100%
Furuya et al, 2007[68]	RYGB	18/12	1	51.7 (±7.4)	24	60%	↓	↓	Not reported	↓	Not reported

Abbreviations: AGB, adjustable gastric banding; BIB, biliointestinal bypass; BPD, biliopancreatic diversion; RYGB, Roux-en-Y gastric bypass; SG, sleeve gastrectomy.

limb (225 cm), all were found to have severe hepatic dysfunction 7 to 17 months following weight loss surgery.[72] None of the patients were reported to be grossly cirrhotic at the time of surgery or had known liver disease before surgery; however, preoperative liver biopsies were not obtained. All biopsies at the time of hepatic decompensation showed severe steatosis, steatohepatitis, or gross cirrhosis. One could extrapolate from the JI bypass literature that decompensation in these patients could have been attributed to the profound malabsorption and stasis caused by the extended Roux limb. This study underscores the importance of balancing maximal weight loss with safety, particularly in patients with underlying hepatic disease. Patients with significant liver disease are less likely to tolerate surgery with a large malabsorptive component.

Many studies attempted to address whether bariatric surgery is effective in improving or even eliminating NAFLD (see **Table 2**). These studies were not uniform in the surgery performed, length of follow-up, or reporting of histologic changes. However, there are general trends suggested by the available data. Various surgical approaches can have distinct effects on weight loss and comorbidities depending on the degree of malabsorption induced and differential effects on gut peptides, most notably glucagonlike peptide-1 (GLP-1) and peptide YY (PYY).

In the 1990s, several retrospective studies showed that most patients had significant improvement in hepatic steatosis or fibrosis after bariatric surgery (RYGB, VBG, or GB) with a subset of patients developing increased fibrosis, steatosis, and steatohepatitis after surgery.[69,70,75] Unfortunately, data were not reported regarding the timing of follow-up biopsies or patient characteristics in those subjects that progressed.

Several studies reported changes in liver histology after purely restrictive procedures such as the adjustable gastric band. Dixon and colleagues[73] performed laparoscopic AGB on 36 morbidly obese patients with NAFLD, and compared liver biopsies performed intraoperatively with those after weight loss, with a mean follow-up period of 25.6 months. As expected, improvements were seen in diabetes, HTN, and the rest of the metabolic syndromes. Mean excess weight loss in this cohort was 51% and follow-up liver biopsies showed significant improvements in steatosis, pericellular fibrosis, and necroinflammatory scores. Complete resolution of NASH was seen in 82% of subjects. In this study there were no reports of worsening liver histology after bariatric surgery.

Mixed restrictive and malabsorptive studies showed similar promise in lowering NASH-related comorbidities. RYGB was the most commonly performed bariatric operation in most studies. Mean excess weight loss ranged from 35% to 80% in approximately 250 patients.[59–61,62,64,66–68] The largest of these series from Mottin and colleagues[59] examined 90 patients who had a mean excess weight loss of 81.4%. In those studies that reported amelioration of comorbidities, most patients had marked improvement or resolution of metabolic risk factors including diabetes, HTN, and dyslipidemia.[60,64,68] Although histologic end points on paired liver biopsies varied greatly between studies, nearly all showed striking improvement in steatosis, resolution or reduction of hepatocellular ballooning, and a decrease in the fibrosis score.[59,60,63,66–68] Complete resolution or improvement in the degree of NASH/NAFLD was well described in several of the studies as well.[63,64,66–68] A small number of patients developed an increase in their fibrosis score after surgery.[63,66,67]

Kral and colleagues[74] examined the effects of BPD in 689 severely obese patients, of whom 104 had the paired liver biopsies necessary for pre- and postoperative comparisons. In this cohort, 2% of the patients were found to have incidental cirrhosis, 8 of whom were included in this analysis. Inflammation resolved in 60% of patients and a significant improvement in steatosis was noted that correlated with weight loss.

Severe fibrosis also improved in 27% of patients, including 5 of 8 patients with cirrhosis. In contrast, 40% of patients developed fibrosis, 3 of whom developed cirrhosis on repeat biopsy (2 had stage III fibrosis and 1 had no fibrosis on index biopsy). Many of those who progressed had lower serum albumin levels, suggesting they may have had significant underlying liver disease. Mattar and colleagues[61] examined paired liver biopsies in 70 NAFLD patients who underwent RYGB (41), laparoscopic sleeve gastrectomy (23), or LAGB (6). Sleeve gastrectomy was performed in "high-risk" patients as part of a 2-step procedure to RYGB. Although the degree of excess weight lost after restrictive procedures was less pronounced than after RGB, 39% versus 68% (P<.001), respectively, differences in histologic end points between the groups were not statistically significant. Of the variables examined, lower preoperative BMI, younger age, and female sex were significantly associated with improvements in the NASH score.

In an interesting study by Mathurin and colleagues,[62] insulin sensitivity and histology were compared with preoperative values in 171 severely obese patients after biliointestinal bypass (71) or GB (100) 1 year after surgery. The biliointestinal bypass consisted of jejunoileostomy coupled with colecystojejunal ansastamosis.[76] Severe steatosis significantly improved in 77% of patients and NASH disappeared in 75%. The mean fibrosis score increased significantly in all patients 1 year after surgery (from 0.14 to 0.38, P<.0001); however, it is unclear whether the magnitude of increase (0.24) and the mean fibrosis on the second biopsy are clinically meaningful. Patients with persistent severe steatosis after surgery were found to have more insulin resistance compared with those subjects with minimal or moderate steatosis, irrespective of the type of weight loss surgery performed. These data reconfirm insulin resistance as the hallmark of NAFLD and ultimately, if insulin resistance is still present postoperatively despite significant weight loss, it is likely that liver disease will persist as well.

Klein and colleagues[77] carefully studied the role of gastric bypass surgery on the metabolic and hepatic abnormalities of 7 extremely obese NAFLD patients (BMI >50 kg/m^2) before and after surgery, and examined histology and gene expression in paired biopsy samples. Steatosis was significantly reduced, although inflammation and fibrosis did not change significantly. However, despite an apparent lack of improvement in fibrosis, hepatic gene expression of several profibrogenic cytokines clearly demonstrated a reduction as a result of surgery, suggesting that bariatric surgery does favorably impact fibrogenesis.

All studies using standard RYGB, BPD, or AGB have consistently demonstrated improvement in steatosis on follow-up liver biopsy. Most studies demonstrated a reduction in inflammation and ballooning if reported, although the effect of bariatric surgery on fibrosis has been more inconsistent. Liver biopsy sampling may play a role; however, other factors such as the extent and rapidity of weight loss likely regulate the expression of proinflammatory and profibrogenic cytokines. Overall, based on the available information, procedures with a malabsorptive component are more likely to be associated with mild worsening of liver disease, although they seem to be well tolerated and beneficial in most patients. Laparoscopic AGB has become the procedure of choice in many centers, and may in general terms be a better choice for patients with more significant liver disease.

CONSEQUENCES OF BARIATRIC SURGERY INDEPENDENT OF WEIGHT LOSS: THE ROLE OF GUT PEPTIDES

Recent data suggest that the improvements in metabolic syndrome comorbidities seen after bariatric surgery may not be solely due to weight loss. Complex changes in gut hormones likely contribute to improved appetite and glucose control. Improvements in insulin sensitivity are a result of weight loss, but can be seen after surgery before any significant weight loss has occurred. Specifically, postprandial increases in GLP-1, a peptide associated with satiety and insulin sensitivity, have been consistently demonstrated.[78,79] Such increases in GLP-1 occur early and persist, in contrast to diet-induced weight loss or purely restrictive procedures such as LAGB.[80–83] Peptide YY (PYY), which is cosecreted with GLP-1, has significant effects on food intake and gastric motility. PYY also increases after RYGB to a greater extent than after AGB, and likely contributes to the decrease in appetite seen after gastric bypass surgery.[83] In animal models, increased levels of GLP-1 have been shown to decrease hepatic steatosis and hepatic gluconeogenesis. Case reports suggest there may be a benefit in humans as well, although prospective clinical trials are needed to confirm this.[84–86]

The effects of RYGB on leptin levels are less clear. The effects of RYGB may not entirely be due to weight loss, offering another mechanism by which bypass surgery improves glucose homeostasis.[82,83] It is well known that a decrease in leptin action, due either to a deficiency of or resistance to the hormone, plays a role in the development of steatosis and insulin resistance. The role of leptin in human NASH remains controversial. Whereas Chitturi and colleagues[87] compared 47 NASH patients with 47 controls and concluded that leptin levels were significantly higher in their NASH cohort, a study by Chalasani and colleagues[88] found no significant difference in leptin levels between 26 patients with NAFLD and 20 matched controls. Although animal data have shown a correlation of leptin levels with hepatic fibrosis, this has not been clearly demonstrated in human studies.[89,90]

Ghrelin, an orexigenic hormone involved in the regulation of hunger, gut motility, and energy expenditure, is primarily secreted by the oxyntic glands of the gastric fundus. Ghrelin increases hunger when infused into humans and decreases after caloric restriction.[91] Some investigators have demonstrated an attenuation of the ghrelin response to fasting after bypass surgery, although this remains controversial.[91,92] Not surprisingly, ghrelin does not seem to decrease after purely restrictive procedures such as AGB.[93] There are virtually no data on the direct hepatic effects of these gut peptide changes that occur after bariatric surgery, although a recent study demonstrated expedited suppression of glucose-stimulated hepatic glucose production in patients several years after AGB.[77,94] Small studies have attempted to address the role of ghrelin in human NASH, although no decisive information has emerged. As a deeper understanding of the role of gut hormones in surgically induced weight loss evolves, more detailed hypotheses will be developed to explore the potential effects of gut hormones on NAFLD.

PATIENT SELECTION: IS BARIATRIC SURGERY SAFE IN PATIENTS WITH ADVANCED DISEASE?

Morbidly obese patients are at an increased risk of unexpected cirrhosis due to the nearly uniform presence of fatty liver disease. Cirrhosis is discovered during bariatric surgery in 1% to 3% of patients without a history or suspicion of liver disease.[95,96] It is from this retrospective experience that investigators have extrapolated on the safety of bariatric surgery in patients with cirrhosis. In an international questionnaire study, of 91 patients discovered to be cirrhotic at the time of bariatric surgery, 4 deaths were reported in the perioperative period (4%), 6 late deaths were attributed to liver failure (7%), and 11 patients were reported to have progressive hepatic dysfunction (12%).[95] Despite these findings, 60% of respondents recommended proceeding with bariatric surgery after the intraoperative diagnosis of cirrhosis. The limitations of this study make it difficult to stratify the true risks of bariatric surgery in cirrhotic patients. More recently, Dallal and colleagues[96] analyzed 2000 morbidly obese patients who underwent laparoscopic RYGB and again identified cirrhosis in 1.4% of the overall cohort. When compared with the entire cohort, cirrhotics were significantly more prone to be heavier (BMI 53 vs 48), older (age 50 vs 45 years), more likely to be male (relative risk=1.3), and have a higher incidence of diabetes (70% vs 21%) and HTN (67% vs 21%). However, in contrast to the previous study, the 30-day mortality was low (zero) and adverse outcomes were generally minor and limited. This stark contrast in mortality is likely due to the fact that all patients in the current study were compensated cirrhotics (as evidenced by normal synthetic function, lack of ascites, or obvious portal hypertension) and exclusively underwent laparoscopic surgery. In the former study, the degree of hepatic compensation was not included, and multiple types of procedures were performed. Based on the limitations of both studies, prospective, well-controlled studies addressing the safety of bariatric surgery in patients with advanced liver disease are needed to stratify the risk for patients with NASH cirrhosis, and to better understand those that might benefit from such an intervention.

Extrapolating from retrospective data of cirrhotics meeting bariatric surgical criteria (see **Table 2**), it seems that well-compensated patients may not only tolerate, but actually benefit from bariatric surgery.[74] Surgery may offer them the potential to either reverse or stabilize ongoing liver injury. Based on these potential benefits, it is the authors' practice to consider bariatric surgery in patients with mild decompensation (mild ascites or other manifestations of portal hypertension). However, as an added safety measure, the authors perform pretransplant evaluations in case further hepatic decompensation might be precipitated by the bariatric intervention. In such cases, it is crucial that the potential risks involved with this approach be clearly discussed with the patient. Given the potential for complications in these patients, the approach should be cautious and involve a collaborative effort between the bariatric surgeon, the hepatologist and, potentially, a transplant surgeon. As of now, only those patients that meet the criteria of BMI 35 or more with comorbidities (not including NAFLD), or a BMI greater than 40 are eligible for surgery. Many, but not all patients with NASH will fulfill these criteria. Thus, patients with advanced NASH who have not yet developed cirrhosis and who meet the criteria for surgery should be considered for the procedure, as it may offer an opportunity to decrease or attenuate ongoing liver injury. Until more decisive prospective data emerge, the potential benefit to the modestly overweight patient with advanced NASH will not be known.

NON-ALCOHOLIC FATTY LIVER DISEASE AFTER LIVER TRANSPLANTATION

NASH typically takes decades to progress to cirrhosis; however, recent work has demonstrated that disease recurrence after liver transplantation for NASH or cryptogenic cirrhosis may occur at an accelerated rate. Ong and colleagues[97] demonstrated that the incidence of NAFLD after transplant was 24.4% (15.7% with histologic confirmation of NASH) in a group of patients transplanted for cryptogenic cirrhosis over a mean follow-up of 26 months. Contos and colleagues[98] showed that recurrent hepatic steatosis approached 100% by 5 years after liver transplant in a series of 30 patients with NASH-related or cryptogenic cirrhosis compared with 25% in a cohort of age- and weight-matched controls with alcohol-related disease. Weight gain is common after liver transplantation, as are obesity-associated comorbidities. These factors are compounded by immunosuppressive regimens that often lead to or exacerbate preexisting diabetes, and HTN. Reports of de novo development of NAFLD after liver transplantation have also been documented in a few case reports.[99,100]

Several groups demonstrated good outcomes in patients undergoing bariatric surgery during or after liver transplantation, although literature is limited to individual case reports.[101–103] Campsen and colleagues[104] recently published a case report of AGB performed in a young morbidly obese woman (BMI 42) with DM, HTN, and OSA who underwent adjustable GB during liver transplantation. Six months after surgery, the patient experienced a 45% excess weight loss with resolution of her HTN, DM, and OSA. This novel approach requires careful patient selection, as well as close collaboration and expertise between the transplant team and bariatric surgeons. The first reported case series of an open RYGB performed on 2 morbidly obese post liver transplant recipients was documented in 2001 by Duchini and colleagues.[102] Both patients had recurrent NASH after liver transplantation and were successfully treated with gastric bypass surgery with resultant weight loss, normalization of liver enzymes, and improvement in histologic and metabolic parameters. In 2005, the first successful laparoscopic RYGB was reported on a morbidly obese (BMI 54 kg/m^2) hepatitis C virus patient 2 years after orthotopic liver transplant.[103] These patients were well compensated with normal hepatic synthetic function. Furthermore, due to the challenging nature of an abdominal operation in post transplant recipients, it is crucial that the bariatric surgeons have significant operative experience and, ideally, access to a liver transplant surgeon.

CHALLENGES IN THE INTERPRETATION AND DESIGN OF FUTURE STUDIES

Many studies confirmed the high prevalence of fatty liver in the bariatric surgery population and suggested that weight loss surgery can attenuate or even reverse liver injury related to NASH. The major limitation of this current body of literature is its heterogeneity regarding type of surgery performed, preoperative use of very low calorie diets (VLCD), and study design. Many centers are routinely initiating a VLCD, defined as a total daily energy intake of between 400 and 800 kcal, for a specified duration of time before surgery. This type of intervention successfully decreases liver size and fat content, as reported in a study by Lewis and colleagues[105] in which patients were given a 6-week course of VLCD before undergoing AGB. Others have shown that with rapid weight loss induced by a VLCD preoperatively, a reduction in liver volume, particularly of the left lobe, improves visualization of the stomach and simplifies the operation.[106] The use of an intragastric balloon for preoperative weight reduction before gastric bypass surgery in superobese patients has also been reported by a few groups. Alfalah and colleagues used this method in 10 superobese patients (mean BMI 64$\pm$7 kg/m^2) who were identified as potential candidates for laparoscopic RYGB.[107,108]

As prospective studies are designed, preoperative techniques for the reduction of liver size will need to be clearly defined and preferably standardized. Rapid weight loss could have obvious effects on baseline histology obtained on the day of surgery, including a reduction, or even possibly an increase in hepatic steatosis as a result of massive lipolysis. Furthermore, as has been demonstrated in recent studies, rapid weight loss can result in an increase in necroinflammation that may not accurately represent the patient's baseline. The timing of the biopsy intraoperatively is also very important and should be documented. All biopsies ideally should be performed at the beginning of the case to minimize the presence of "surgical hepatitis," which could be confused with lobular inflammation related to NASH. The etiology of such histologic changes has not been clearly defined, although manipulation of the liver and the systemic effects of anesthesia likely play a role.

FUTURE DIRECTIONS

There is a clear trend favoring less invasive techniques in virtually all areas of medicine. This approach has already begun to promote the development of endoscopic techniques to achieve sustained weight loss. A handful of small studies has evaluated the efficacy of endoscopically placed gastric balloons. Although such options have promise, several limitations of these procedures will need to be overcome before they can be safely recommended to patients. Bariatric surgical options continue to evolve, and the eventual introduction of endoscopic techniques may broaden the spectrum of eligible patients to include higher-risk surgical patients as well as those not meeting weight and comorbidity criteria for bariatric surgery.[109–112]

Current estimates suggest that the obesity epidemic will be a pervasive problem for years to come, and this is reflected in the significant increase in obesity-related publications and focused research funding. Bariatric surgery significantly impacts many obesity-related comorbidities and likely will play a role in the prevention or treatment of advanced liver disease secondary to NASH. However, well-designed prospective trials will be essential to confirm this and to more accurately identify NASH patients who are most likely to benefit from bariatric surgery.

ACKNOWLEDGMENT

Thanks to Christine de Sayve for the original drawings provided for the figures in this article.

REFERENCES

1. Browning JD, Szczepaniak LS, Dobbins R, et al. Prevalence of hepatic steatosis in an urban population in the United States: impact of ethnicity. Hepatology 2004;40:1387–95.
2. Lazo M, Clark JM. The epidemiology of no-nalcoholic fatty liver disease: a global perspective. Semin Liver Dis 2008;28:339–50.
3. Wanless IR, Lentz JS. Fatty liver hepatitis (steatohepatitis) and obesity: an autopsy study with analysis of risk factors. Hepatology 1990;12:1106–10.
4. World Health Organization, obesity and overweight, 2009. Available at: http://www.who.int/dietphysicalactivity/media/en/gsfs_obesity.pdf. Accessed July, 2009.
5. CDC/NCHS, National Health and Nutrition Examination Survey, 2005–2006. Available at: http://www.cdc.gov/nchs/products/pubs/pubd/hestats/overweight/overweight_adult.pdf. Accessed July, 2009.
6. Burke A, Lucey MR. Non-alcoholic fatty liver disease, non-alcoholic steatohepatitis and orthotopic liver transplantation. Am J Transplant 2004;4:686–93.
7. Adams KF, Schatzkin A, Harris TB, et al. Overweight, obesity, and mortality in a large prospective cohort of persons 50 to 71 years old. N Engl J Med 2006;355:763–78.
8. Vuppalanchi R, Chalasani N. Nonalcoholic fatty liver disease and nonalcoholic steatohepatitis: selected practical issues in their evaluation and management. Hepatology 2009;49:306–17.
9. Chitturi S, Abeygunasekera S, Farrell GC, et al. NASH and insulin resistance: insulin hypersecretion and specific association with the insulin resistance syndrome. Hepatology 2002;35:373–9.

10. Marchesini G, Bugianesi E, Forlani G, et al. Nonalcoholic fatty liver, steatohepatitis, and the metabolic syndrome. Hepatology 2003;37:917–23.
11. Pagano G, Pacini G, Musso G, et al. Nonalcoholic steatohepatitis, insulin resistance, and metabolic syndrome: further evidence for an etiologic association. Hepatology 2002;35:367–72.
12. Ratziu V, Giral P, Charlotte F, et al. Liver fibrosis in overweight patients. Gastroenterology 2000;118:1117–23.
13. Angulo P, Keach JC, Batts KP, et al. Independent predictors of liver fibrosis in patients with nonalcoholic steatohepatitis. Hepatology 1999;30:1356–62.
14. Powell EE, Cooksley WG, Hanson R, et al. The natural history of nonalcoholic steatohepatitis: a follow-up study of forty-two patients for up to 21 years. Hepatology 1990;11:74–80.
15. Hui JM, Kench JG, Chitturi S, et al. Long-term outcomes of cirrhosis in nonalcoholic steatohepatitis compared with hepatitis C. Hepatology 2003;38:420–7.
16. Harrison SA, Di Bisceglie AM. Advances in the understanding and treatment of nonalcoholic fatty liver disease. Drugs 2003;63:2379–94.
17. Fassio E, Alvarez E, Dominguez N, et al. Natural history of nonalcoholic steatohepatitis: a longitudinal study of repeat liver biopsies. Hepatology 2004;40:820–6.
18. Adams LA, Angulo P. Recent concepts in non-alcoholic fatty liver disease. Diabet Med 2005;22:1129–33.
19. Dandona P, Aljada A, Bandyopadhyay A. Inflammation: the link between insulin resistance, obesity and diabetes. Trends Immunol 2004;25:4–7.
20. Kaplan LM. Leptin, obesity, and liver disease. Gastroenterology 1998;115:997–1001.
21. Klein S, Fontana L, Young VL, et al. Absence of an effect of liposuction on insulin action and risk factors for coronary heart disease. N Engl J Med 2004;350:2549–57.
22. Samuel VT, Liu ZX, Qu X, et al. Mechanism of hepatic insulin resistance in nonalcoholic fatty liver disease. J Biol Chem 2004;279:32345–53.
23. Calle EE, Rodriguez C, Walker-Thurmond K, Thun MJ, et al. Overweight, obesity, and mortality from cancer in a prospectively studied cohort of U.S. adults. N Engl J Med 2003;348:1625–38.
24. Rafiq N, Bai C, Fang Y, et al. Long-term follow-up of patients with nonalcoholic fatty liver. Clin Gastroenterol Hepatol 2009;7:234–8.
25. Bugianesi E. Nonalcoholic fatty liver disease (NAFLD) and cardiac lipotoxicity: another piece of the puzzle. Hepatology 2008;47:2–4.
26. Adams LA, Lymp JF, St Sauver J, et al. The natural history of nonalcoholic fatty liver disease: a population-based cohort study. Gastroenterology 2005;129:113–21.
27. Loria P, Lonardo A, Bellentani S, et al. Non-alcoholic fatty liver disease (NAFLD) and cardiovascular disease: an open question. Nutr Metab Cardiovasc Dis 2007;17:684–98.
28. Targher G, Bertolini L, Padovani R, et al. Increased prevalence of cardiovascular disease in type 2 diabetic patients with non-alcoholic fatty liver disease. Diabet Med 2006;23:403–9.
29. Kadayifci A, Tan V, Ursell PC, et al. Clinical and pathologic risk factors for atherosclerosis in cirrhosis: a comparison between NASH-related cirrhosis and cirrhosis due to other aetiologies. J Hepatol 2008;49:595–9.
30. Ong JP, Pitts A, Younossi ZM. Increased overall mortality and liver-related mortality in non-alcoholic fatty liver disease. J Hepatol 2008;49:608–12.

31. Brea A, Mosquera D, Martin E, et al. Nonalcoholic fatty liver disease is associated with carotid atherosclerosis: a case-control study. Arterioscler Thromb Vasc Biol 2005;25:1045–50.
32. Targher G. Associations between liver histology and early carotid atherosclerosis in subjects with nonalcoholic fatty liver disease. Hepatology 2005;42: 974–5 [discussion: 975].
33. Targher G, Bertolini L, Padovani R, et al. Associations between liver histology and carotid intima-media thickness in patients with nonalcoholic fatty liver disease. Arterioscler Thromb Vasc Biol 2005;25:2687–8.
34. Villanova N, Moscatiello S, Ramilli S, et al. Endothelial dysfunction and cardiovascular risk profile in nonalcoholic fatty liver disease. Hepatology 2005;42:473–80.
35. Huang MA, Greenson JK, Chao C, et al. One-year intense nutritional counseling results in histological improvement in patients with non-alcoholic steatohepatitis: a pilot study. Am J Gastroenterol 2005;100:1072–81.
36. Palmer M, Schaffner F. Effect of weight reduction on hepatic abnormalities in overweight patients. Gastroenterology 1990;99:1408–13.
37. Ueno T, Sugawara H, Sujaku K, et al. Therapeutic effects of restricted diet and exercise in obese patients with fatty liver. J Hepatol 1997;27:103–7.
38. Clark JM. Weight loss as a treatment for nonalcoholic fatty liver disease. J Clin Gastroenterol 2006;40(Suppl 1):S39–43.
39. Harrison SA, Fincke C, Helinski D, et al. A pilot study of orlistat treatment in obese, non-alcoholic steatohepatitis patients. Aliment Pharmacol Ther 2004; 20:623–8.
40. Hatzitolios A, Savopoulos C, Lazaraki G, et al. Efficacy of omega-3 fatty acids, atorvastatin and orlistat in non-alcoholic fatty liver disease with dyslipidemia. Indian J Gastroenterol 2004;23:131–4.
41. Sabuncu T, Nazligul Y, Karaoglanoglu M, et al. The effects of sibutramine and orlistat on the ultrasonographic findings, insulin resistance and liver enzyme levels in obese patients with non-alcoholic steatohepatitis. Rom J Gastroenterol 2003;12:189–92.
42. Harrison SA, Fecht W, Brunt EM, et al. Orlistat for overweight subjects with nonalcoholic steatohepatitis: A randomized, prospective trial. Hepatology 2009;49:80–6.
43. Pi-Sunyer FX, Aronne LJ, Heshmati HM, et al, RIO-North America Study Group. Effect of rimonabant, a cannabinoid-1 receptor blocker, on weight and cardiometabolic risk factors in overweight or obese patients: RIO-North America: a randomized controlled trial. JAMA 2006;295:761–75.
44. Van Gaal LF, Rissanen AM, Scheen AJ, et al, RIO-Europe Study Group. Effects of the cannabinoid-1 receptor blocker rimonabant on weight reduction and cardiovascular risk factors in overweight patients: 1-year experience from the RIO-Europe study. Lancet 2005;365:1389–97.
45. Kashi MR, Torres DM, Harrison SA. Current and emerging therapies in nonalcoholic fatty liver disease. Semin Liver Dis 2008;28:396–406.
46. NIH conference. Gastrointestinal surgery for severe obesity. Consensus Development Conference Panel. Ann Intern Med 1991.
47. Elder KA, Wolfe BM. Bariatric surgery: a review of procedures and outcomes. Gastroenterology 2007;132:2253–71.
48. Tsai AG, Asch DA, Wadden TA. Insurance coverage for obesity treatment. J Am Diet Assoc 2006;106:1651–5.
49. Zhao Y, Encinosa W. CT bariatric surgery utilization and outcomes in 1998 and 2004. Statistical brief #23. Rockville (MD): Agency for Healthcare Research and Quality; January 2007.

50. Verna EC, Berk PD. Role of fatty acids in the pathogenesis of obesity and fatty liver: impact of bariatric surgery. Semin Liver Dis 2008;28:407–26.
51. Andersen T, Gluud C, Franzmann MB, et al. Hepatic effects of dietary weight loss in morbidly obese subjects. J Hepatol 1991;12:224–9.
52. Scopinaro N, Gianetta E, Civalleri D, et al. Bilio-pancreatic bypass for obesity: II. Initial experience in man. Br J Surg 1979;66:618–20.
53. Marceau P, Biron S, Bourque RA, et al. Biliopancreatic diversion with a new type of gastrectomy. Obes Surg 1993;3:29–35.
54. Fontaine KR, Redden DT, Wang C, et al. Years of life lost due to obesity. JAMA 2003;289:187–93.
55. Buchwald H, Avidor Y, Braunwald E, et al. Bariatric surgery: a systematic review and meta-analysis. JAMA 2004;292:1724–37.
56. Adams TD, Gress RE, Smith SC, et al. Long-term mortality after gastric bypass surgery. N Engl J Med 2007;357:753–61.
57. Sjostrom L, Lindroos AK, Peltonen M, et al. Lifestyle, diabetes, and cardiovascular risk factors 10 years after bariatric surgery. N Engl J Med 2004;351: 2683–93.
58. Sjostrom L, Narbro K, Sjostrom CD, et al. Effects of bariatric surgery on mortality in Swedish obese subjects. N Engl J Med 2007;357:741–52.
59. Mottin CC, Moretto M, Padoin AV, et al. Histological behavior of hepatic steatosis in morbidly obese patients after weight loss induced by bariatric surgery. Obes Surg 2005;15:788–93.
60. Clark JM, Alkhuraishi AR, Solga SF, et al. Roux-en-Y gastric bypass improves liver histology in patients with non-alcoholic fatty liver disease. Obes Res 2005;13:1180–6.
61. Mattar SG, Velcu LM, Rabinovitz M, et al. Surgically-induced weight loss significantly improves nonalcoholic fatty liver disease and the metabolic syndrome. Ann Surg 2005;242:610–7 [discussion: 618–20].
62. Mathurin P, Gonzalez F, Kerdraon O, et al. The evolution of severe steatosis after bariatric surgery is related to insulin resistance. Gastroenterology 2006;130: 1617–24.
63. Csendes A, Smok G, Burgos AM. Histological findings in the liver before and after gastric bypass. Obes Surg 2006;16:607–11.
64. de Almeida SR, Rocha PR, Sanches MD, et al. Roux-en-Y gastric bypass improves the nonalcoholic steatohepatitis (NASH) of morbid obesity. Obes Surg 2006;16:270–8.
65. Dixon JB, Bhathal PS, O'Brien PE. Weight loss and non-alcoholic fatty liver disease: falls in gamma-glutamyl transferase concentrations are associated with histologic improvement. Obes Surg 2006;16:1278–86.
66. Barker KB, Palekar NA, Bowers SP, et al. Non-alcoholic steatohepatitis: effect of Roux-en-Y gastric bypass surgery. Am J Gastroenterol 2006;101:368–73.
67. Liu X, Lazenby AJ, Clements RH, et al. Resolution of nonalcoholic steatohepatitis after gastric bypass surgery. Obes Surg 2007;17:486–92.
68. Furuya CK Jr, de Oliveira CP, de Mello ES, et al. Effects of bariatric surgery on nonalcoholic fatty liver disease: preliminary findings after 2 years. J Gastroenterol Hepatol 2007;22:510–4.
69. Luyckx FH, Desaive C, Thiry A, et al. Liver abnormalities in severely obese subjects: effect of drastic weight loss after gastroplasty. Int J Obes Relat Metab Disord 1998;22:222–6.
70. Ranlov I, Hardt F. Regression of liver steatosis following gastroplasty or gastric bypass for morbid obesity. Digestion 1990;47:208–14.

71. Grimm IS, Schindler W, Haluszka O. Steatohepatitis and fatal hepatic failure after biliopancreatic diversion. Am J Gastroenterol 1992;87:775–9.
72. Cotler SJ, Vitello JM, Guzman G, et al. Hepatic decompensation after gastric bypass surgery for severe obesity. Dig Dis Sci 2004;49:1563–8.
73. Dixon JB, Bhathal PS, Hughes NR, et al. Nonalcoholic fatty liver disease: improvement in liver histological analysis with weight loss. Hepatology 2004; 39:1647–54.
74. Kral JG, Thung SN, Biron S, et al. Effects of surgical treatment of the metabolic syndrome on liver fibrosis and cirrhosis. Surgery 2004;135:48–58.
75. Silverman EM, Sapala JA, Appelman HD. Regression of hepatic steatosis in morbidly obese persons after gastric bypass. Am J Clin Pathol 1995;104:23–31.
76. Eriksson F. Biliointestinal bypass. Int J Obes 1981;5:437–47.
77. Klein S, Mittendorfer B, Eagon JC, et al. Gastric bypass surgery improves metabolic and hepatic abnormalities associated with nonalcoholic fatty liver disease. Gastroenterology 2006;130:1564–72.
78. Laferrere B, Heshka S, Wang K, et al. Incretin levels and effect are markedly enhanced 1 month after Roux-en-Y gastric bypass surgery in obese patients with type 2 diabetes. Diabetes Care 2007;30:1709–16.
79. le Roux CW, Welbourn R, Werling M, et al. Gut hormones as mediators of appetite and weight loss after Roux-en-Y gastric bypass. Ann Surg 2007;246:780–5.
80. Bose M, Olivan B, Teixeira J, et al. Do incretins play a role in the remission of type 2 diabetes after gastric bypass surgery: what are the evidence? Obes Surg 2009;19:217–29.
81. Korner J, Bessler M, Cirilo LJ, et al. Effects of Roux-en-Y gastric bypass surgery on fasting and postprandial concentrations of plasma ghrelin, peptide YY, and insulin. J Clin Endocrinol Metab 2005;90:359–65.
82. Korner J, Bessler M, Inabnet W, et al. Exaggerated glucagon-like peptide-1 and blunted glucose-dependent insulinotropic peptide secretion are associated with Roux-en-Y gastric bypass but not adjustable gastric banding. Surg Obes Relat Dis 2007;3:597–601.
83. Korner J, Inabnet W, Conwell IM, et al. Differential effects of gastric bypass and banding on circulating gut hormone and leptin levels. Obesity (Silver Spring) 2006;14:1553–61.
84. Ding X, Saxena NK, Lin S, et al. Exendin-4, a glucagon-like protein-1 (GLP-1) receptor agonist, reverses hepatic steatosis in ob/ob mice. Hepatology 2006; 43:173–81.
85. Lee YS, Shin S, Shigihara T, et al. Glucagon-like peptide-1 gene therapy in obese diabetic mice results in long-term cure of diabetes by improving insulin sensitivity and reducing hepatic gluconeogenesis. Diabetes 2007;56:1671–9.
86. Tushuizen ME, Bunck MC, Pouwels PJ, et al. Incretin mimetics as a novel therapeutic option for hepatic steatosis. Liver Int 2006;26:1015–7.
87. Chitturi S, Farrell G, Frost L, et al. Serum leptin in NASH correlates with hepatic steatosis but not fibrosis: A manifestation of lipotoxicity? Hepatology 2002;36: 403–9.
88. Chalasani N, Crabb DW, Cummings OW, et al. Does leptin play a role in the pathogenesis of human nonalcoholic steatohepatitis? Am J Gastroenterol 2003;98:2771–6.
89. Angulo P, Alba LM, Petrovic LM, et al. Leptin, insulin resistance, and liver fibrosis in human nonalcoholic fatty liver disease. J Hepatol 2004;41:943–9.
90. Javor ED, Ghany MG, Cochran EK, et al. Leptin reverses nonalcoholic steatohepatitis in patients with severe lipodystrophy. Hepatology 2005;41:753–60.

91. Cummings DE, Weigle DS, Frayo RS, et al. Plasma ghrelin levels after diet-induced weight loss or gastric bypass surgery. N Engl J Med 2002;346:1623–30.
92. Faraj M, Havel PJ, Phelis S, et al. Plasma acylation-stimulating protein, adiponectin, leptin, and ghrelin before and after weight loss induced by gastric bypass surgery in morbidly obese subjects. J Clin Endocrinol Metab 2003;88: 1594–602.
93. Foschi D, Corsi F, Colombo F, et al. Different effects of vertical banded gastroplasty and Roux-en-Y gastric bypass on meal inhibition of ghrelin secretion in morbidly obese patients. J Invest Surg 2008;21:77–81.
94. Goldfine AB, Mun EC, Devine E, et al. Patients with neuroglycopenia after gastric bypass surgery have exaggerated incretin and insulin secretory responses to a mixed meal. J Clin Endocrinol Metab 2007;92:4678–85.
95. Brolin RE, Bradley LJ, Taliwal RV. Unsuspected cirrhosis discovered during elective obesity operations. Arch Surg 1998;133:84–8.
96. Dallal RM, Mattar SG, Lord JL, et al. Results of laparoscopic gastric bypass in patients with cirrhosis. Obes Surg 2004;14:47–53.
97. Ong J, Younossi ZM, Reddy V, et al. Cryptogenic cirrhosis and posttransplantation nonalcoholic fatty liver disease. Liver Transpl 2001;7:797–801.
98. Contos MJ, Cales W, Sterling RK, et al. Development of nonalcoholic fatty liver disease after orthotopic liver transplantation for cryptogenic cirrhosis. Liver Transpl 2001;7:363–73.
99. Garcia RF, Morales E, Garcia CE, et al. Recurrent and de novo nonalcoholic steatohepatitis following orthotopic liver transplantation. Arq Gastroenterol 2001;38:247–53.
100. Poordad F, Gish R, Wakil A, et al. De novo non-alcoholic fatty liver disease following orthotopic liver transplantation. Am J Transplant 2003;3:1413–7.
101. Butte JM, Devaud N, Jarufe NP, et al. Sleeve gastrectomy as treatment for severe obesity after orthotopic liver transplantation. Obes Surg 2007;17:1517–9.
102. Duchini A, Brunson ME. Roux-en-Y gastric bypass for recurrent nonalcoholic steatohepatitis in liver transplant recipients with morbid obesity. Transplantation 2001;72:156–9.
103. Tichansky DS, Madan AK. Laparoscopic Roux-en-Y gastric bypass is safe and feasible after orthotopic liver transplantation. Obes Surg 2005;15:1481–6.
104. Campsen J, Zimmerman M, Shoen J, et al. Adjustable gastric banding in a morbidly obese patient during liver transplantation. Obes Surg 2008;18: 1625–7.
105. Lewis MC, Phillips ML, Slavotinek JP, et al. Change in liver size and fat content after treatment with Optifast very low calorie diet. Obes Surg 2006; 16:697–701.
106. Benjaminov O, Beglaibter N, Gindy L, et al. The effect of a low-carbohydrate diet on the nonalcoholic fatty liver in morbidly obese patients before bariatric surgery. Surg Endosc 2007;21:1423–7.
107. Alfalah H, Philippe B, Ghazal F, et al. Intragastric balloon for preoperative weight reduction in candidates for laparoscopic gastric bypass with massive obesity. Obes Surg 2006;16:147–50.
108. Frutos MD, Morales MD, Lujan J, et al. Intragastric balloon reduces liver volume in super-obese patients, facilitating subsequent laparoscopic gastric bypass. Obes Surg 2007;17:150–4.
109. Lopasso FP, Sakai P, Gazi BM, et al. A pilot study to evaluate the safety, tolerance, and efficacy of a novel stationary antral balloon (SAB) for obesity. J Clin Gastroenterol 2008;42:48–53.

110. Ricci G, Bersani G, Rossi A, et al. Bariatric therapy with intragastric balloon improves liver dysfunction and insulin resistance in obese patients. Obes Surg 2008;18:1438–42.
111. Trande P, Mussetto A, Mirante VG, et al. Efficacy, tolerance and safety of new intragastric air-filled balloon (heliosphere BAG) for obesity: the experience of 17 cases. Obes Surg 2008. DOI: 10.1007/s11695-008-9786-2.
112. Dumonceau JM. Evidence-based review of the bioenterics intragastric balloon for weight loss. Obes Surg 2008;18:1611–7.

Index

Note: Page numbers of article titles are in **boldface** type.

Clin Liver Dis 13 (2009) 711–719
doi:10.1016/S1089-3261(09)00073-7
1089-3261/09/$ – see front matter

Moving?

Make sure your subscription moves with you!

To notify us of your new address, find your **Clinics Account Number** (located on your mailing label above your name), and contact customer service at:

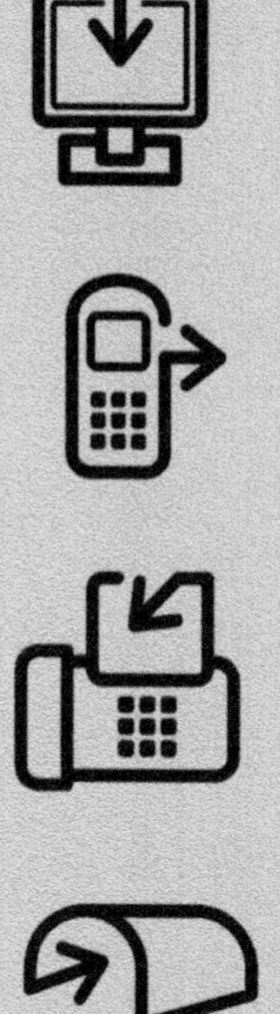

Email: journalscustomerservice-usa@elsevier.com

800-654-2452 **(subscribers in the U.S. & Canada)**
314-447-8871 **(subscribers outside of the U.S. & Canada)**

Fax number: 314-447-8029

Elsevier Health Sciences Division
Subscription Customer Service
3251 Riverport Lane
Maryland Heights, MO 63043

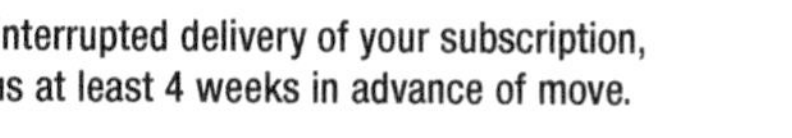
*To ensure uninterrupted delivery of your subscription, please notify us at least 4 weeks in advance of move.

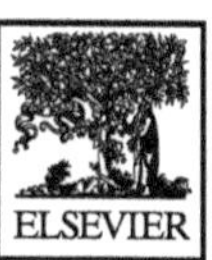

United States Postal Service

Statement of Ownership, Management, and Circulation
(All Periodicals Publications Except Requestor Publications)

1. Publication Title	2. Publication Number	3. Filing Date
Clinics in Liver Disease	0 1 6 - 7 5 4	9/15/09
4. Issue Frequency: Feb, May, Aug, Nov	5. Number of Issues Published Annually: 4	6. Annual Subscription Price: $218.00

7. Complete Mailing Address of Known Office of Publication (*Not printer*) (*Street, city, county, state, and ZIP+4®*)

Elsevier Inc.
360 Park Avenue South
New York, NY 10010-1710

Contact Person: Stephen Bushing
Telephone (Include area code): 215-239-3688

8. Complete Mailing Address of Headquarters or General Business Office of Publisher (*Not printer*)

Elsevier Inc., 360 Park Avenue South, New York, NY 10010-1710

9. Full Names and Complete Mailing Addresses of Publisher, Editor, and Managing Editor (*Do not leave blank*)

Publisher (*Name and complete mailing address*)

John Schrefer , Elsevier, Inc., 1600 John F. Kennedy Blvd. Suite 1800, Philadelphia, PA 19103-2899

Editor (*Name and complete mailing address*)

Kerry Holland, Elsevier, Inc., 1600 John F. Kennedy Blvd. Suite 1800, Philadelphia, PA 19103-2899

Managing Editor (*Name and complete mailing address*)

Catherine Bewick, Elsevier, Inc., 1600 John F. Kennedy Blvd. Suite 1800, Philadelphia, PA 19103-2899

10. Owner (*Do not leave blank. If the publication is owned by a corporation, give the name and address of the corporation immediately followed by the names and addresses of all stockholders owning or holding 1 percent or more of the total amount of stock. If not owned by a corporation, give the names and addresses of the individual owners. If owned by a partnership or other unincorporated firm, give its name and address as well as those of each individual owner. If the publication is published by a nonprofit organization, give its name and address.*)

Full Name	Complete Mailing Address
Wholly owned subsidiary of	4520 East-West Highway
Reed/Elsevier, US holdings	Bethesda, MD 20814

11. Known Bondholders, Mortgagees, and Other Security Holders Owning or Holding 1 Percent or More of Total Amount of Bonds, Mortgages, or Other Securities. If none, check box → None

Full Name	Complete Mailing Address
N/A	

12. Tax Status (*For completion by nonprofit organizations authorized to mail at nonprofit rates*) (*Check one*)
The purpose, function, and nonprofit status of this organization and the exempt status for federal income tax purposes:
Has Not Changed During Preceding 12 Months
Has Changed During Preceding 12 Months (*Publisher must submit explanation of change with this statement*)

PS Form 3526, September 2007 (Page 1 of 3 (Instructions Page 3)) PSN 7530-01-000-9931 **PRIVACY NOTICE**: See our Privacy policy in www.usps.com

13. Publication Title: Clinics in Liver Disease
14. Issue Date for Circulation Data Below: August 2009

15. Extent and Nature of Circulation			Average No. Copies Each Issue During Preceding 12 Months	No. Copies of Single Issue Published Nearest to Filing Date
a. Total Number of Copies (*Net press run*)			950	900
b. Paid Circulation (By Mail and Outside the Mail)	(1)	Mailed Outside-County Paid Subscriptions Stated on PS Form 3541. (*Include paid distribution above nominal rate, advertiser's proof copies, and exchange copies*)	306	286
	(2)	Mailed In-County Paid Subscriptions Stated on PS Form 3541 (*Include paid distribution above nominal rate, advertiser's proof copies, and exchange copies*)		
	(3)	Paid Distribution Outside the Mails Including Sales Through Dealers and Carriers, Street Vendors, Counter Sales, and Other Paid Distribution Outside USPS®	177	185
	(4)	Paid Distribution by Other Classes Mailed Through the USPS (e.g. First-Class Mail®)		
c. Total Paid Distribution (*Sum of 15b (1), (2), (3), and (4)*) ►			483	471
d. Free or Nominal Rate Distribution (By Mail and Outside the Mail)	(1)	Free or Nominal Rate Outside-County Copies Included on PS Form 3541	75	77
	(2)	Free or Nominal Rate In-County Copies Included on PS Form 3541		
	(3)	Free or Nominal Rate Copies Mailed at Other Classes Through the USPS (e.g. First-Class Mail)		
	(4)	Free or Nominal Rate Distribution Outside the Mail (Carriers or other means)		
e. Total Free or Nominal Rate Distribution (Sum of 15d (1), (2), (3) and (4)			75	77
f. Total Distribution (Sum of 15c and 15e) ►			558	548
g. Copies not Distributed (See instructions to publishers #4 (page #3)) ►			392	352
h. Total (Sum of 15f and g)			950	900
i. Percent Paid (15c divided by 15f times 100) ►			86.56%	85.95%

16. Publication of Statement of Ownership

If the publication is a general publication, publication of this statement is required. Will be printed in the **November 2009** issue of this publication. Publication not required

17. Signature and Title of Editor, Publisher, Business Manager, or Owner

Stephen R. Bushing – Subscription Services Coordinator — Date: September 15, 2009

I certify that all information furnished on this form is true and complete. I understand that anyone who furnishes false or misleading information on this form or who omits material or information requested on the form may be subject to criminal sanctions (including fines and imprisonment) and/or civil sanctions (including civil penalties).

PS Form **3526**, September 2007 (Page 2 of 3)

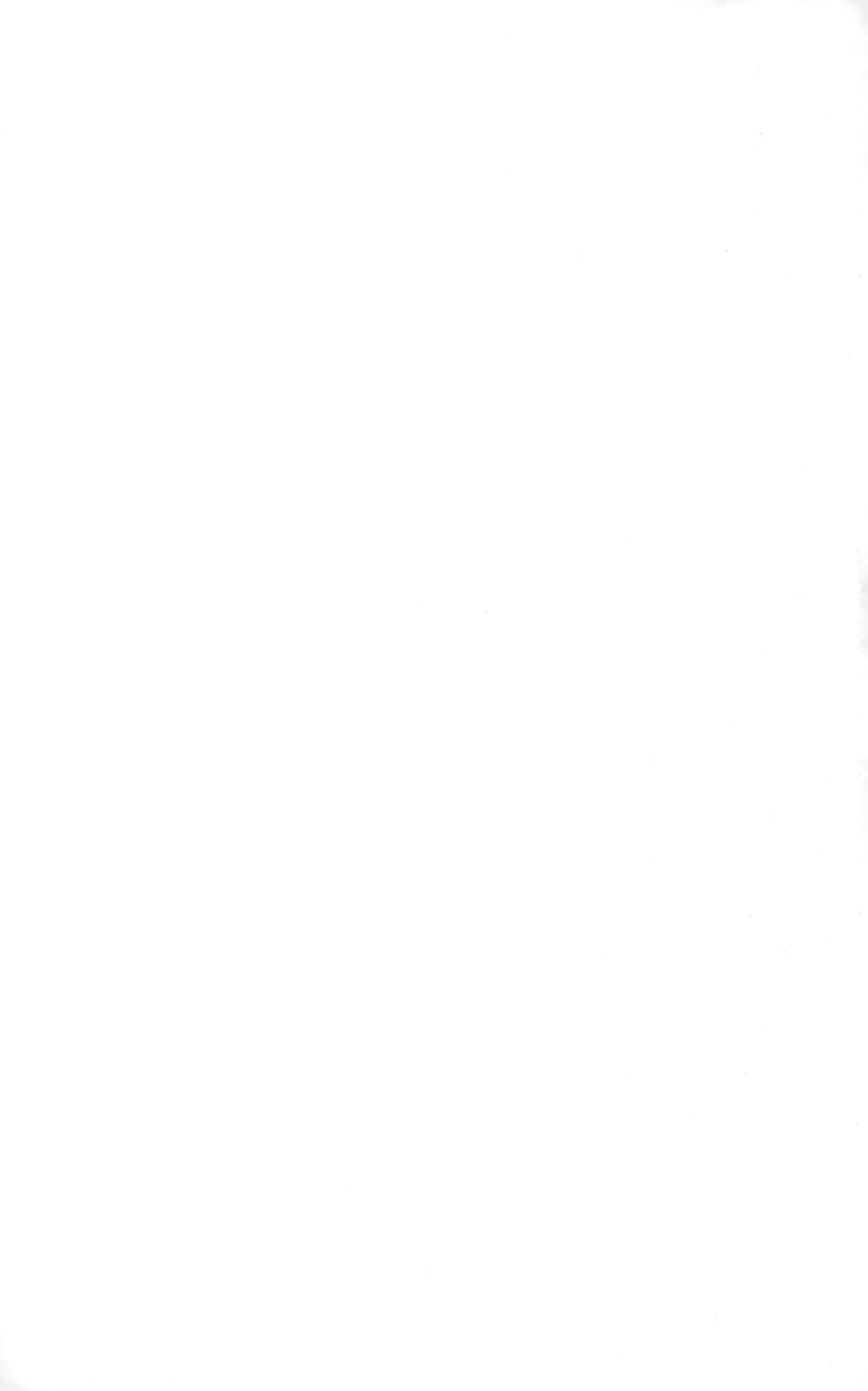

Printed and bound by CPI Group (UK) Ltd, Croydon, CR0 4YY
03/10/2024
01040450-0002